Benchmark Papers in Human Physiology

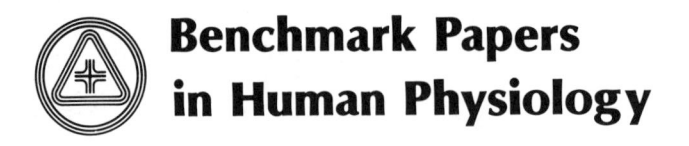

Series Editor: L. L. Langley
School of Medicine
University of Missouri, Kansas City

VOLUME

1. HOMEOSTASIS: Origins of the Concept/*L. L. Langley*
2. CONTRACEPTION/*L. L. Langley*
3. MICROCIRCULATION/*Mary P. Wiedeman*
4. CARDIOVASCULAR PHYSIOLOGY/*James V. Warren*
5. PULMONARY AND RESPIRATORY PHYSIOLOGY, Part I/*Julius H. Comroe, Jr.*
6. PULMONARY AND RESPIRATORY PHYSIOLOGY, PART II/*Julius H. Comroe, Jr.*
7. INFANT NUTRITION/*Doris H. Merritt*
8. THE HEART AND CIRCULATION/*Peter A. Chevalier*
9. TEMPERATURE, PART I: Arts and Concepts/*Theodor H. Benzinger*
10. TEMPERATURE, PART II: Thermal Homeostasis/*Theodor H. Benzinger*
11. AGING/*Geraldine M. Emerson*
12. CELL MEMBRANE PERMEABILITY AND TRANSPORT/*G. R. Kepner*
13. HYPERTENSION: The Renal Basis/*David B. Gordon*
14. HYPOTHALAMIC HORMONES/*James R. Sowers*
15. HIGH ALTITUDE PHYSIOLOGY/*John B. West*

RELATED TITLES IN BENCHMARK PAPERS IN BEHAVIOR

VOLUME

1. HORMONES AND SEXUAL BEHAVIOR/*Carol Sue Carter*
6. PSYCHOPHYSIOLOGY/*Stephen W. Porges and Michael G. H. Coles*
12. CRITICAL PERIODS/*John Paul Scott*
13. THERMOREGULATION/*Evelyn Satinoff*

**Benchmark Papers
in Human Physiology / 14**

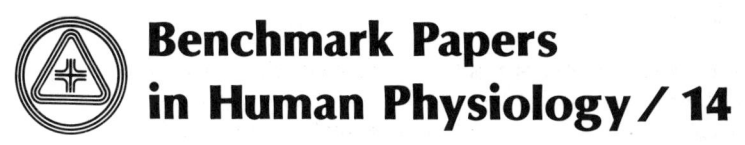

A BENCHMARK® Books Series

HYPOTHALAMIC HORMONES

Edited by

JAMES R. SOWERS

University of Missouri
at Kansas City

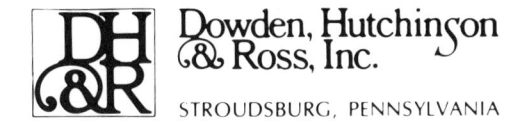

Dowden, Hutchinson & Ross, Inc.

STROUDSBURG, PENNSYLVANIA

Copyright © 1980 by **Dowden, Hutchinson & Ross, Inc.**
Benchmark Papers in Human Physiology, Volume 14
Library of Congress Catalog Card Number: 79-19856
ISBN: 0-87933-358-8

All rights reserved. No part of this book covered by the copyrights hereon may be reproduced or transmitted in any form or by any means—graphic, electronic, or mechanical, including photocopying, recording, taping, or information storage and retrieval systems—without written permission of the publisher.

82 81 80 1 2 3 4 5
Manufactured in the United States of America.

LIBRARY OF CONGRESS CATALOGING IN PUBLICATION DATA
Main entry under title:
Hypothalamic hormones.

  (Benchmark papers in human physiology; 14)
  Includes indexes.
  1. Hypothalamic hormones—Addresses, essays, lectures. 2. Hypothalamo-hypophyseal system—Addresses, essays, lectures. 3. Neuroendocrinology—Addresses, essays, lectures. I. Sowers, James R., 1942-
QP572.H9H92   612.8   79-19856
ISBN 0-87933-358-8

Distributed world wide by Academic Press,
a subsidiary of Harcourt Brace Jovanovich,
Publishers.

SERIES EDITOR'S FOREWORD

James R. Sowers, a young physician trained in endocrinology, is destined to become important in the field of hypothalamic hormones. I had the pleasure, and the good fortune, to recruit Dr. Sowers to join our faculty. He had just finished his fellowship in endocrinology under Jerome Hershman at UCLA. Solidly trained, he has continued his investigations here at the University of Missouri, Kansas City School of Medicine. He knows and loves this subject.

This subject is dear to my heart as well. In 1942 I published a paper about the influence of stress on the adrenal cortex. At that time a plethora of reports was appearing about the influence of various types of stress on the adrenal and about emotional trauma on the thyroid and the gonads. There was thus the strong implication that the nervous system and the endocrine system were linked. But no one, at that time, knew how. I had plans to repeat my procedures after placing lesions in the hypothalamus, but I never got around to it. In retrospect, that series of experiments may well have provided an important clue. The fact of the matter is that Dr. Geoffrey Harris published his perceptive paper in 1947; the rest of the story, a fascinating one that has spawned Nobel prizes, is related in this volume. It is an unfinished story, one that is changing with remarkable speed and acceleration. Certainly additional Nobel Laureates will emerge in this field. A second volume will be needed very soon.

L. L. LANGLEY

PREFACE

This book represents an attempt to choose and elucidate some of the more important articles that have contributed to development of the relatively new but rapidly expanding field of neuroendocrinology. The emphasis in this review has been placed on the earlier studies that laid the foundation for understanding the role of the brain in controlling the integration and selectivity of hypophysial hormone secretion.

I am indebted to two people who played an integral role in the preparation of this book. Mark Funk, an outstanding clinical medical librarian at the University of Missouri-Kansas City School of Medicine, contributed greatly to the extensive literature review and subject indexing that were necessary to write this book. Jean Grider has done a remarkable job in putting this manuscript together. She is to be complimented for her perseverance and excellent judgment in coordinating my efforts and those of Mr. Funk and the series editor, Dr. Lee Langley.

This book is dedicated to two superb investigative endocrinologists from different eras, both of whom have been inspirations to me in my studies in neuroendocrinology and in writing this book. They are Dr. Geoffrey Harris, whom I consider the father of neuroendocrinology and whose death prevented him from receiving a Nobel prize, and Dr. Jerome Hershman. Dr. Hershman has not only been a friend as well as my mentor; he gave me the latitude to pursue studies of my own interest and helped me achieve the discipline needed for academic and investigational excellence, which he personifies.

JAMES R. SOWERS

CONTENTS

Series Editor's Foreword — v
Preface — vii
Contents by Author — xvii

Introduction — 1

PART I: EARLY BREAKTHROUGHS THAT LEAD TO THE DEVELOPMENT OF THE SCIENCE OF NEUROENDOCRINOLOGY

Editor's Comments on Papers 1 Through 4 — 4

1. POPA, G., and U. FIELDING: A Portal Circulation from the Pituitary to the Hypothalamic Region — 6
   J. Anat. 65:88-91 (1930)

2. WISLOCKI, G. B., and L. S. KING: The Permeability of the Hypophysis and Hypothalamus to Vital Dyes, with a Study of the Hypophyseal Vascular Supply — 10
   Am. J. Anat. 58:421-423, 468-471, 472 (1936)

3. GREEN, J. D., and G. W. HARRIS: The Neurovascular Link Between the Neurohypophysis and Adenohypophysis — 16
   J. Endocrinol. 5:136-137, 141-144, 145 (1947)

4. GREEN, J. D., and G. W. HARRIS: Observation of the Hypophysio-portal Vessels of the Living Rat — 23
   J. Physiol. 108:359-361 (1949)

Editor's Comments on Papers 5 and 6 — 26

5. BARGMANN, W., and E. SCHARRER: The Site of Origin of the Hormones of the Posterior Pituitary — 28
   Am. Sci. 39:255-259 (1951)

6. SLOPER, J. C.: Hypothalamic Neurosecretion in the Dog and Cat, with Particular Reference to the Identification of Neurosecretory Material with Posterior Lobe Hormone — 33
   J. Anat. 89:301-302, 313-314, 315 (1955)

Contents

	Editor's Comments on Papers 7 and 8	37
7	HARRIS, G. W., and D. JACOBSOHN: Functional Grafts of the Anterior Pituitary Gland *R. Soc. London Proc.* **139**:263-264, 275-276 (1952)	38
8	NIKITOVITCH-WINER, M., and J. W. EVERETT: Functional Restitution of Pituitary Grafts Re-transplanted from Kidney to Median Eminence *Endocrinology* **63**:916-918, 929-930 (1958)	40

PART II: THE HYPOTHALAMIC-HYPOPHYSIAL-ADRENOCORTICAL AXIS

	Editor's Comments on Papers 9, 10, and 11	46
9	de GROOT, J., and G. W. HARRIS: Hypothalamic Control of the Anterior Pituitary Gland and Blood Lymphocytes *J. Physiol.* **111**:335, 342-245 (1950)	48
10	FORTIER, C., G. W. HARRIS, and I. R. McDONALD: The Effect of Pituitary Stalk Section on the Adrenocortical Response to Stress in the Rabbit *J. Physiol.* **136**:344-345, 360 (1957)	53
11	GUILLEMIN, R., and B. ROSENBERG: Humoral Hypothalamic Control of Anterior Pituitary: A Study with Combined Tissue Cultures *Endocrinology* **57**:599, 604-606, 607 (1955)	57

PART III: THE HYPOTHALAMIC-HYPOPHYSIAL-THYROID AXIS

	Editor's Comments on Papers 12 Through 15	64
12	GREER, M. A.: Evidence of Hypothalamic Control of the Pituitary Release of Thyrotrophin *Soc. Exp. Biol. Med. Proc.* **77**:603-608 (1951)	66
13	GANONG, W. F., D. S. FREDRICKSON, and D. M. HUME: The Effect of Hypothalamic Lesions on Thyroid Function in the Dog *Endocrinology* **57**:355, 360-362 (1955)	72
14	HARRIS, G. W., and J. W. WOODS: The Effect of Electrical Stimulation of the Hypothalamus or Pituitary Gland on Thyroid Activity *J. Physiol.* **143**:246-247, 264-273 (1958)	76
15	HALÁSZ, B., L. PUPP, and S. UHLARIK: Hypophysiotrophic Area in the Hypothalamus *J. Endocrinol.* **25**:147, 151-153 (1962)	88
	Editor's Comments on Papers 16 and 17	92
16	BOWERS, C. Y., A. V. SCHALLY, W. D. HAWLEY, C. GUAL, and A. PARLOW: Effect of Thyrotropin-Releasing Factor in Man *J. Clin. Endocrinol. Metab.* **28**:978, 980-982 (1968)	94

Contents

17	FOLKERS, K., F. ENZMANN, J. BØLER, C. Y. BOWERS, and A. V. SCHALLY: Discovery of Modification of the Synthetic Tripeptide-sequence of the Thyrotropin Releasing Hormone Having Activity *Biochem. Biophys. Res. Commun.* 37:123-126 (1969)	98
	Editor's Comments on Papers 18 and 19	102
18	MARTIN, J. B., and S. REICHLIN: Thyrotropin Secretion in Rats after Hypothalamic Electrical Stimulation or Injection of Synthetic TSH-Releasing Factor *Science* 168:1366-1368 (1970)	104
19	BROWNSTEIN, M. J., M. PALKOVITS, J. M. SAAVEDRA, R. M. BASSIRI, and R. D. UTIGER: Thyrotropin-Releasing Hormone in Specific Nuclei of Rat Brain *Science* 185:267-269 (1974)	107

PART IV: THE HYPOTHALAMIC-HYPOPHYSIAL-GONADAL AXIS

	Editor's Comments on Papers 20 Through 24	112
20	HARRIS, G. W.: The Induction of Ovulation in the Rabbit, by Electrical Stimulation of the Hypothalamo-hypophysial Mechanism *R. Soc. London Proc.* 122:374-376, 388-392, 393 (1957)	115
21	SAWYER, C. H., J. E. MARKEE, and W. H. HOLLINSHEAD: Inhibition of Ovulation in the Rabbit by the Adrenergic-Blocking Agent Dibenamine *Endocrinology* 41:395-396, 399-402 (1947)	123
22	BARRACLOUGH, C. A., and C. H. SAWYER: Induction of Pseudopregnancy in the Rat by Reserpine and Chlorpromazine *Endocrinology* 65:563-564, 568, 570-571 (1959)	129
23	BARRACLOUGH, C. A., and R. A. GORSKI: Evidence That the Hypothalamus Is Responsible for Androgen-Induced Sterility in the Female Rat *Endocrinology* 68:68-69, 73-79 (1961)	134
24	SAWYER, C. H., and J. E. MARKEE: Estrogen Facilitation of Release of Pituitary Ovulating Hormone in the Rabbit in Response to Vaginal Stimulation *Endocrinology* 65:614-615, 618-621 (1959)	142
	Editor's Comments on Papers 25 Through 29	147
25	McCANN, S. M., S. TALEISNIK, and H. M. FRIEDMAN: LH-Releasing Activity in Hypothalamic Extracts *Soc. Exp. Biol. Med. Proc.* 104:432-434 (1960)	150
26	CAMPBELL, H. J., G. FEUER, and G. W. HARRIS: The Effect of Intrapituitary Infusion of Median Eminence and Other Brain Extracts on Anterior Pituitary Gonadotrophic Secretion *J. Physiol.* 170:474-475, 484-485 (1964)	154

Contents

27	RAMIREZ, V. D., and C. H. SAWYER: Fluctuations in Hypothalamic LH-RF (Luteinizing Hormone-Releasing Factor) During the Rat Estrous Cycle *Endocrinology* 76:282-283, 286-289 (1965)	157
28	IGARASHI, M., and S. M. McCANN: A Hypothalamic Follicle Stimulating Hormone-Releasing Factor *Endocrinology* 74:446-447, 450-452 (1964)	163
29	HALASZ, B., and R. A. GORSKI: Gonadotrophic Hormone Secretion in Female Rats After Partial or Total Interruption of Neural Afferents to the Medial Basal Hypothalamus *Endocrinology* 80:608-609, 618-622 (1967)	167

Editor's Comments on Papers 30 and 31 — 173

30A	MATSUO, H., Y. BABA, R. M. G. NAIR, A. ARIMURA, and A. V. SCHALLY: Structure of the Porcine LH- and FSH-Releasing Hormone. I. The Proposed Amino Acid Sequence *Biochem. Biophys. Res. Commun.* 43:1334-1339 (1971)	175
30B	BABA, Y., H. MATSUO, and A. V. SCHALLY: Structure of the Porcine LH- and FSH-Releasing Hormone. II. Confirmation of the Proposed Structure by Conventional Sequential Analyses *Biochem. Biophys. Res. Commun.* 44:459-463 (1971)	181
31	BURGUS, R., M. BUTCHER, M. AMOSS, N. LING, M. MONAHAN, J. RIVIER, R. FELLOWS, R. BLACKWELL, W. VALE, and R. GUILLEMIN: Primary Structure of the Ovine Hypothalamic Luteinizing Hormone-Releasing Factor (LRF) *Natl. Acad. Sci. Proc.* 69:278-282 (1972)	186

Editor's Comments on Papers 32 Through 35 — 191

32	SCHALLY, A. V., A. ARIMURA, A. J. KASTIN, H. MATSUO, Y. BABA, T. W. REDDING, R. M. G. NAIR, L. DEBELJUK, and W. F. WHITE: Gonadotropin-Releasing Hormone: One Polypeptide Regulates Secretion of Luteinizing and Follicle-Stimulating Hormones *Science* 173:1036-1038 (1971)	194
33	ARIMURA, A., A. J. KASTIN, A. V. SCHALLY, M. SAITO, T. KUMASAKA, Y. YAOI, N. NISHI, and K. OHKURA: Immunoreactive LH-Releasing Hormone in Plasma: Midcycle Elevation in Women *J. Clin. Endocrinol. Metab.* 38:510-513 (1974)	197
34	PALKOVITS, M., A. ARIMURA, M. BROWNSTEIN, A. V. SCHALLY, and J. M. SAAVEDRA: Luteinizing Hormone-Releasing Hormone (LH-RH) Content of the Hypothalamic Nuclei in Rat *Endocrinology* 96:554-555, 557-558 (1974)	201
35	SOWERS, J. R., M. COLANTINO, J. FAYEZ, and H. JONAS: Pituitary Response to LH-RH in Midtrimester Pregnancy *Obstet. Gynecol.* 52:685-688 (1978)	205

Contents

PART V: HYPOTHALAMIC-HYPOPHYSIAL CONTROL OF GROWTH HORMONE SECRETION

Editor's Comments on Papers 36 Through 41   210

36 REICHLIN, S.: Growth and the Hypothalamus   213
Endocrinology 67:760, 769-773 (1960)

37 ROTH, J., S. M. GLICK, R. S. YALOW, and S. A. BERSON: Secretion of Human Growth Hormone: Physiologic and Experimental Modification   218
Metabolism 12:577-579 (1963)

38 BLACKARD, W. G., and S. A. HEIDINGSFELDER: Adrenergic Receptor Control Mechanism for Growth Hormone Secretion   221
J. Clin. Invest. 47:1407-1408, 1412-1414 (1968)

39 DEUBEN, R. R., and J. MEITES: Stimulation of Pituitary Growth Hormone Release by a Hypothalamic Extract *in Vitro*   225
Endocrinology 74:408-409, 412-414 (1964)

40 FROHMAN, L. A., L. L. BERNARDIS, and K. J. KANT: Hypothalamic Stimulation of Growth Hormone Secretion   229
Science 162:580-582 (1968)

41 WILBER, J. F., and J. C. PORTER: Thyrotropin and Growth Hormone Releasing Activity in Hypophysial Portal Blood   232
Endocrinology 87:807, 810-811 (1970)

Editor's Comments on Papers 42 Through 45   235

42 KRULICH, L., A. P. S. DHARIWAL, and S. M. McCANN: Stimulatory and Inhibitory Effects of Purified Hypothalamic Extracts on Growth Hormone Release from Rat Pituitary *in Vitro*   237
Endocrinology 83:783, 789-790 (1968)

43 BRAZEAU, P., W. VALE, R. BURGUS, N. LING, M. BUTCHER, J. RIVIER, and R. GUILLEMIN: Hypothalamic Polypeptide That Inhibits the Secretion of Immunoreactive Pituitary Growth Hormone   240
Science 179:77-79 (1973)

44 VALE, W., C. RIVIER, P. BRAZEAU, and R. GUILLEMIN: Effects of Somatostatin on the Secretion of Thyrotropin and Prolactin   243
Endocrinology 95:968, 974-977 (1974)

45 BROWNSTEIN, M., A. ARIMURA, H. SATO, A. V. SCHALLY, and J. S. KIZER: The Regional Distribution of Somatostatin in the Rat Brain   248
Endocrinology 96:1456-1461 (1975)

PART VI: HYPOTHALAMIC-HYPOPHYSIAL CONTROL OF PROLACTIN SECRETION

Editor's Comments on Papers 46 Through 49   256

Contents

46	EVERETT, J. W.: Luteotrophic Function of Autografts of the Rat Hypophysis *Endocrinology* 54:685-690 (1954)	259
47	RATNER, A., and J. MEITES: Depletion of Prolactin-Inhibiting Activity of Rat Hypothalamus by Estradiol or Suckling Stimulus *Endocrinology* 75:377-382 (1964)	265
48	GROSVENOR, C. E., S. M. McCANN, and R. NALLAR: Inhibition of Nursing-Induced and Stress-Induced Fall in Pituitary Prolactin Concentration in Lactating Rats by Injection of Acid Extracts of Bovine Hypothalamus *Endocrinology* 76:883-889 (1965)	271
49	JACOBS, L. S., P. J. SNYDER, J. F. WILBER, R. D. UTIGER, and W. H. DAUGHADAY: Increased Serum Prolactin after Administration of Synthetic Thyrotropin Releasing Hormone (TRH) in Man *J. Clin. Endocrinol. Metab.* 33:996-998 (1971)	278

Editor's Comments on Papers 50 Through 53 — 281

50	LU, K.-H., and J. MEITES: Inhibition by L-Dopa and Monoamine Oxidase Inhibitors of Pituitary Prolactin Release; Stimulation by Methyldopa and *d*-Amphetamine *Soc. Exp. Biol. Med. Proc.* 137:480-483 (1971)	284
51	MacLEOD, R. M., and J. E. LEHMEYER: Studies on the Mechanism of the Dopamine-Mediated Inhibition of Prolactin Secretion *Endocrinology* 94:1077, 1082-1085 (1974)	289
52	SOWERS, J. R., H. E. CARLSON, N. BRAUTBAR, and J. M. HERSHMAN: Effect of Dexamethasone on Prolactin and TSH Responses to TRH and Metoclopramide in Man *J. Clin. Endocrinol. Metab.* 44:237-241 (1977)	293
53	RIVIER, C., W. VALE, N. LING, M. BROWN, and R. GUILLEMIN: Stimulation *in vivo* of the Secretion of Prolactin and Growth Hormone by β-Endorphin *Endocrinology* 100:238-241 (1977)	298

PART VII: MORPHOLOGY AND NEUROENDOCRINE ROLE OF HYPOTHALAMIC CATECHOLAMINE NEURONS

Editor's Comments on Papers 54 and 55 — 304

| 54 | CARLSSON, A., B. FALCK, and N.-A. HILLARP: Cellular Localization of Brain Monoamines
Acta Physiol. Scand. 56(suppl. 196):23-27 (1962) | 306 |
| 55 | FUXE, K., and T. HÖKFELT: Further Evidence for the Existence of Tubero-infundibular Dopamine Neurons
Acta Physiol. Scand. 66:245-246 (1966) | 311 |

PART VIII: ENDOGENOUS OPIATE AGONISTS IN THE BRAIN

Editor's Comments on Papers 56 and 57   314

56   LAZARUS, L. H., N. LING, and R. GUILLEMIN: β-Lipotropin as a Prohormone for the Morphinomimetic Peptides Endorphins and Enkephalins   317
Natl. Acad. Sci. Proc. 73:2156–2159 (1976)

57   GUILLEMIN, R., T. VARGO, J. ROSSIER, S. MINICK, N. LING, C. RIVIER, W. VALE, and F. BLOOM: β-Endorphin and Adrenocorticotropin Are Secreted Concomitantly by the Pituitary Gland   321
Science 197:1067–1069 (1977)

Author Citation Index   325
Subject Index   337

About the Editor   343

CONTENTS BY AUTHOR

Amoss, M., 186
Arimura, A., 175, 194, 197, 201, 248
Baba, Y., 175, 181, 194
Bargmann, W., 28
Barraclough, C. A., 129, 134
Bassiri, R. M., 107
Bernardis, L. L., 229
Berson, S. A., 218
Blackard, W. G., 221
Blackwell, R., 186
Bloom, F., 321
Bøler, J., 98
Bowers, C. Y., 94, 98
Brautbar, N., 293
Brazeau, P., 240, 243
Brown, M., 298
Brownstein, M. J., 107, 201, 248
Burgus, R., 186, 240
Butcher, M., 186, 240
Campbell, H. J., 154
Carlson, H. E., 293
Carlsson, A., 306
Colantino, M., 205
Daughaday, W. H., 278
Debeljuk, L., 194
de Groot, J., 48
Deuben, R. R., 225
Dhariwal, A. P. S., 237
Enzmann, J., 98
Everett, J. W., 40, 259
Falck, B., 306
Fayez, J., 205
Fellows, R., 186
Feuer, G., 154
Fielding, U., 6

Folkers, K., 98
Fortier, C., 53
Fredrickson, D. S., 72
Friedman, H. M., 150
Frohman, L. A., 229
Fuxe, K., 311
Ganong, W. F., 72
Glick, S. M., 218
Gorski, R. A., 134, 167
Green, J. D., 16, 23
Greer, M. A., 66
Grosvenor, C. E., 271
Gual, C., 94
Guillemin, R., 57, 186, 240, 243, 298, 317, 321
Halász, B., 88, 167
Harris, G. W., 16, 23, 38, 48, 53, 76, 115, 154
Hawley, W. D., 94
Heidingsfelder, S. A., 221
Hershman, J. M., 293
Hillarp, N.-A., 306
Hökfelt, T., 311
Hollinshead, W. H., 123
Hume, D. M., 72
Igarashi, M., 163
Jacobs, L. S., 278
Jacobsohn, D., 38
Jonas, H., 205
Kant, J. J., 229
Kastin, A. J., 194, 197
King, L. S., 10
Kizer, J. S., 248
Krulich, L., 237
Kumasaka, T., 197

xvii

Contents by Author

Lazarus, L. H., 317
Lehmeyer, J. E., 289
Ling, N., 186, 240, 298, 317, 321
Lu, K.-H., 284
McCann, S. M., 150, 163, 237, 271
McDonald, I. R., 53
MacLeod, R. M., 289
Markee, J. E., 123, 142
Martin, J. B., 104
Matsuo, H., 175, 181, 194
Meites, J., 225, 265, 284
Minick, S., 321
Monahan, M., 186
Nair, R. M. G., 175, 194
Nallar, R., 271
Nikitovitch-Winer, M., 40
Nishi, N., 197
Ohkura, K., 197
Palkovits, M., 107, 201
Parlow, A., 94
Popa, G. T., 6
Porter, J. C., 232
Pupp, L., 88
Ramirez, V. D., 157
Ratner, A., 265
Redding, T. W., 194
Reichlin, S., 104, 213

Rivier, C., 243, 298, 321
Rivier, J., 186, 240
Rosenberg, B., 57
Rossier, J., 321
Roth, J., 218
Saavedra, J. M., 107, 201
Saito, M., 197
Sato, H., 248
Sawyer, C. H., 123, 129, 142, 157
Schally, A. V., 94, 98, 175, 181, 194, 197, 201, 248
Scharrer, E., 28
Sloper, J. C., 33
Snyder, P. J., 278
Sowers, J. R., 205, 293
Taleisnik, S., 150
Uhlarik, S., 88
Utiger, R. D., 107, 278
Vale, W., 186, 240, 243, 298, 321
Vargo, T., 321
White, W. F., 194
Wilber, J. F., 232, 278
Wislocki, G. B., 10
Woods, J. W., 76
Yalow, R. S., 218
Yaoi, Y., 197

HYPOTHALAMIC HORMONES

INTRODUCTION

For centuries psychiatric and neurological conditions were thought to be secondary to endocrine dysfunction: That emotional stress might precipitate diabetes or hyperthyroidism lead to amenorrhea or false pregnancy and that psychiatric symptoms seen in patients with primary endocrine disease were secondary to hormonal effects on the central nervous system. The first experiment of any significance in the entire field of endocrinology, reported 130 years ago, demonstrated a relationship between the brain and hormone secretion. In 1849, Professor A. A. Berthold of Göttingen showed that the testes of cocks required no specific nerve connections to exert masculinizing effects. He found that the functional testes, through the secretion of a substance into the bloodstream, acted on the brain so as to produce a rooster that had wattles, crowed, fought, and took a noticeable interest in hens, whereas, castrated roosters did not display this type of behavior (Berthold, 1849).

The two systems that coordinate and integrate the functions of the body and are responsible for homeostatic adjustments to meet environmental changes are the nervous and the endocrine systems. However, the closeness and intricacy of this relationship and the recognition that neuroendocrine mechanisms, functions involving the interaction of the nervous system and the endocrine system, regulate a wide variety of body mechanisms has only come about in the last forty years.

The science of neuroendocrinology had its real beginning in the late 1940s and yearly 1950s with the studies of G. W. Harris, which stressed the significance of the observation that virtually all blood reaching the adenohypophysis via the hypophysial-portal system has been in contact, via a primary capillary plexus, with the median eminence area of

Introduction

the hypothalamus (Papers 3 and 4). These observations complemented those studies of Bargmann and Scharrer demonstrating neurosecretory cells within the central nervous system (and abundantly in the hypothalamus) to be responsive to classical means of synaptic activation. They were also found to be capable of characterizing specific secretory products that could be borne via the bloodstream to a target organ, specifically from the hypothalamus via the hypophysial-portal system to the adenohypophysis (Paper 5). Although the pioneering work of Harris and his colleagues clearly established the concept of the hypothalamic regulation of adenohypophyseal function (Paper 7 and Harris, 1955), it was not until 1969 that two groups of investigators, after long, laborious, and brilliantly conducted experiments, defined the precise nature of TRH and LH-RH, the first of the hypothalamic regulatory hormones to be elucidated and synthesized, (see Papers 17, 30, 31, and Burgus et al., 1970). Following this, there has been an exponentially expanding knowledge base caused by unprecedented discoveries in this field, which has had unexpected impact on the understanding of normal and pathological hypothalamic-hypophysial function. Since 1969, new hormones and neurotransmitters of the brain have been discovered, new diseases described, and old ones better understood. The discipline of neuroendocrinology has ceased to be merely an academic interest and has become of immediate relevance to the clinician. The investigative and clinical aspects of neuroendocrinology now involve the collaborative efforts of endocrinologists, neurologists, immunologists, biophysicists, physiologists, gastroenterologists, and nephrologists, giving an idea of the importance of the science of neuroendocrinology with respect to all organ systems.

REFERENCES

Berthold, A. A. 1849. Transplantation der hoden. *Arch. Anat. Physiol. Wiss. Med.* 16:42.

Burgus, R., T. F. Dunn, D. Desiderio, D. N. Ward, W. Vale, and R. Guillemin. 1970. Characterization of Ovine Hypothalamic Hypophysiotropic TSH-Releasing Factor. *Nature* **226**:321.

Harris, G. W. 1955. The Function of the Pituitary Stalk. *Johns Hopkins Hosp. Bull.* 97:358.

Part I
EARLY BREAKTHROUGHS THAT LEAD TO THE DEVELOPMENT OF THE SCIENCE OF NEUROENDOCRINOLOGY

Editor's Comments
on Papers 1 Through 4

1   POPA and FIELDING
    A Portal Circulation from the Pituitary to the Hypothalamic Region

2   WISLOCKI and KING
    Excerpts from *The Permeability of the Hypophysis and Hypothalamus to Vital Dyes, with a Study of the Hypophyseal Vascular Supply*

3   GREEN and HARRIS
    Excerpts from *The Neurovascular Link Between the Neurohypophysis and Adenohypophysis*

4   GREEN and HARRIS
    Observation of the Hypophysio-portal Vessels of the Living Rat

The anatomical basis for the control of the adenohypophysis by the hypothalamus was established by the work of Popa and Fielding (Paper 1), Wislocki and King (Paper 2), and Green and Harris (Papers 3 and 4). Popa and Fielding first described a peculiar and important arrangement of vessels connecting the hypophysis to the hypothalamus (the hypophysial-portal circulation). They observed thin-walled vessels on the surface of the human hypophysial stalk, which were found to connect capillary beds in the hypothalamus and the hypophysis. Thus, they were the first to describe the hypophysial-portal system of vessels beginning as capillaries in the median eminence of the tuber cinereum, forming vascular trunks on the hypophysial stalk, and breaking up into the sinusoids of the adenohypophysis. However, despite their very lucid description of the anatomy of the hypophysial-portal system, they expressed the erroneous opinion that blood flow occurred upward from the sinusoids of the adenohypophysis to the floor of the infundibular recess of the third ventricle, carrying colloid material formed in the hypophysis to this region of the hypothalamus.

Wislocki and King (Paper 2) conducted a thorough study of the

Editor's Comments on Papers 1 Through 4

blood supply of the adenohypophysis in monkeys and on the basis of their morphological studies concluded that blood must flow down the hypophysial-portal vessels to the adenohypophysis. They noted that the portal vessels originate in the region of the hypophysial stalk as a plexus surrounding, and in part penetrating, the infundibulum and terminate by uniting to form the sinusoids of the adenohypophysis.

The concept of a neurovascular pathway linking the hypothalamus to the anterior lobe of the hypophysis was set forth by Green and Harris (Paper 3). They demonstrated that the greatest proportion of blood reaching the adenohypophysis has first traversed the portal capillaries lying in the substance of the median eminence. They suggested that humoral substances, later called *releasing factors*, are liberated from nerve endings of hypothalamic nerve tracts into the primary plexus of capillaries of the hypophysial-portal vessels and are carried by these vessels to the adenohypophysis, where they regulate secretions of hormones from the adenohypophysis. They further suggested that nervous stimuli from higher brain centers might cause the liberation of these substances into the capillary sinusoids of the median eminence and that these humoral substances are then transported via the hypophysial-portal system to the adenohypophysis, resulting in stimulation or inhibition of release of adenohypophysial hormones.

Green and Harris (Paper 4) described a method of exposing the hypophysial-portal vessels of living anesthetized rats and microscopic visualization of these vessels. They observed that the direction of blood flow in these vessels is from the median eminence of the tuber cinereum to the adenohypophysis. Their results conclusively confirmed the earlier conclusions of Wislocki and King that the portal blood flow occurs downward from the median eminence. These studies gave further credence to the concept proposed by Green and Harris that the capillary loops in the median eminence and infundibulum form a necessary link in which not only nerve tracts originating in the hypothalamus, but also those from the higher centers of the brain, regulated adenohypophysial activity via humoral relay through the hypophysial-portal vasculature.

A PORTAL CIRCULATION FROM THE PITUITARY TO THE HYPOTHALAMIC REGION

By GREGOR POPA
*Professor of Anatomy, University of Jassy, Roumania,
Rockefeller Foundation Fellow, University College, London,*

AND UNA FIELDING
*Lecturer in Neurology and Demonstrator of Anatomy,
University College, London.*

This communication is of the nature of a preliminary note upon a peculiar and important arrangement of the vessels connecting the pituitary gland to the hypothalamus.

We have observed in the stalk (S) of the human pituitary a system of vessels arranged after the manner of a portal system, which we propose to call the hypophyseo-portal veins (1).

Although we have not been able to demonstrate the presence of any muscular tissue in the walls of these vessels, we refer to them as veins because they carry the blood away from the blood vessels distributed to the pituitary.*

Inferiorly, these vessels collect blood from the pars anterior (A), pars intermedia (I), pars tuberalis and pars posterior (P) of the pituitary. Then they ascend in the stalk (S) as parallel veins (1), which after a short course acquire thick neuroglia sheaths (14). Sometimes one glial sleeve contains several such vessels. There is no surrounding capillary net served by the vessels while they are thus ensheathed, and the tissues of the stalk between the glial cylinders appear to be without blood vessels of any sort.

Superiorly, beneath the infundibular recess of the third ventricle (III) these vessels of the portal system lose their heavy neuroglial wrapping and open out into a network of very fine channels (15). This may be called the secondary distributing net. Long processes from the ependymal cells lining the ventricle contribute to the supporting tissue of these fine vessels. This secondary net is not haphazard in its distribution in the hypothalamic region. Its connection with certain nuclear groups is at present under investigation.

The voluminous blood content of the anterior lobe of the human pituitary is brought to it by arteries (3), one on either side (in some cases more than one) springing from the internal carotid (2). As this bilateral arterial supply approaches the gland the two arteries approximate and supply the posterior lobe. Then each passes in between the glandular and nervous portions. It penetrates into the substance of the anterior lobe on its own side, carrying with it an appreciable amount of connective tissue, and then gives out its blood in all directions to the sinusoids (13).

* Since this paper was written examples of portal vessels with plain muscle in their walls have been found.

A Portal Circulation from Pituitary to Hypothalamic Region

In addition to this bilateral supply from the carotids there are some fine arteries from the circle of Willis which pass along the outside of the stalk and open into the sinusoids of the pars tuberalis. There are some small venous channels corresponding to these arteries.

From the sinusoids of the pars anterior and pars intermedia some blood is returned on either side towards the place of entry of the main arterial stem, and venous channels are formed which drain out by a vein (10) following the course of the entering artery and opening into the cavernous sinus.

The whole of the blood, however, is not taken away by these bilateral venous channels (10) and the small veins of the pars tuberalis mentioned above—as has been stated already, sinusoids of the pars anterior (13), pars intermedia and pars tuberalis help in feeding the portal vessels of the stalk and so deliver blood to the secondary distribution net in the hypothalamus.

The blood which is sent into the posterior lobe by branches from the bilateral arterial supply for the glandular portion, is conveyed away in part by the hypophyseo-portal vessels (1) and in part by the systemic veins (10) following the course of the arterial branches. The accompanying table summarises the results of our observations to date upon the pituitary circulation.

Part of pituitary	Arterial supply	Systemic venous return	Portal system return
Pars anterior and pars intermedia	From carotids: a bilateral supply, usually one on each side, sometimes more than one	Systemic veins to cavernous sinus following the course of the bilateral arteries	Contribute blood to portal vessels
Pars tuberalis	From circle of Willis by small branches around the outside of the stalk	Small systemic veins corresponding to the arteries	Contributes blood to the portal vessels
Pars posterior	By branches from the bilateral supply from the carotids	By small systemic venous branches following the course of the arterial twigs	Contributes blood to the portal vessels by fine channels opening into them below their heavy glial sleeves

Colloid material is found in association with the vessels of this portal system. Sometimes it is found within the vessels (1) and sometimes in the perivascular sleeves (14). It can also be detected among the cells of certain hypothalamic nuclei. The staining reaction of the colloid varies at different levels of the same section; i.e. in the glandular portion it is different in colour from that in the hypothalamic region. These contrasts are being investigated. In the matter of colloid distribution in the hypothalamus our observations so far are confirmatory of those of Remy Collin (see *Archives de Morphologie*, 1928, No. 28). As they pass upward in the stalk the vessels of this portal system do not appear to have plain muscle in their walls,* but their lumina appear to be actively and precisely controlled.

In some hypophyses the contraction is so extreme that there are no patent

* See footnote, page 88.

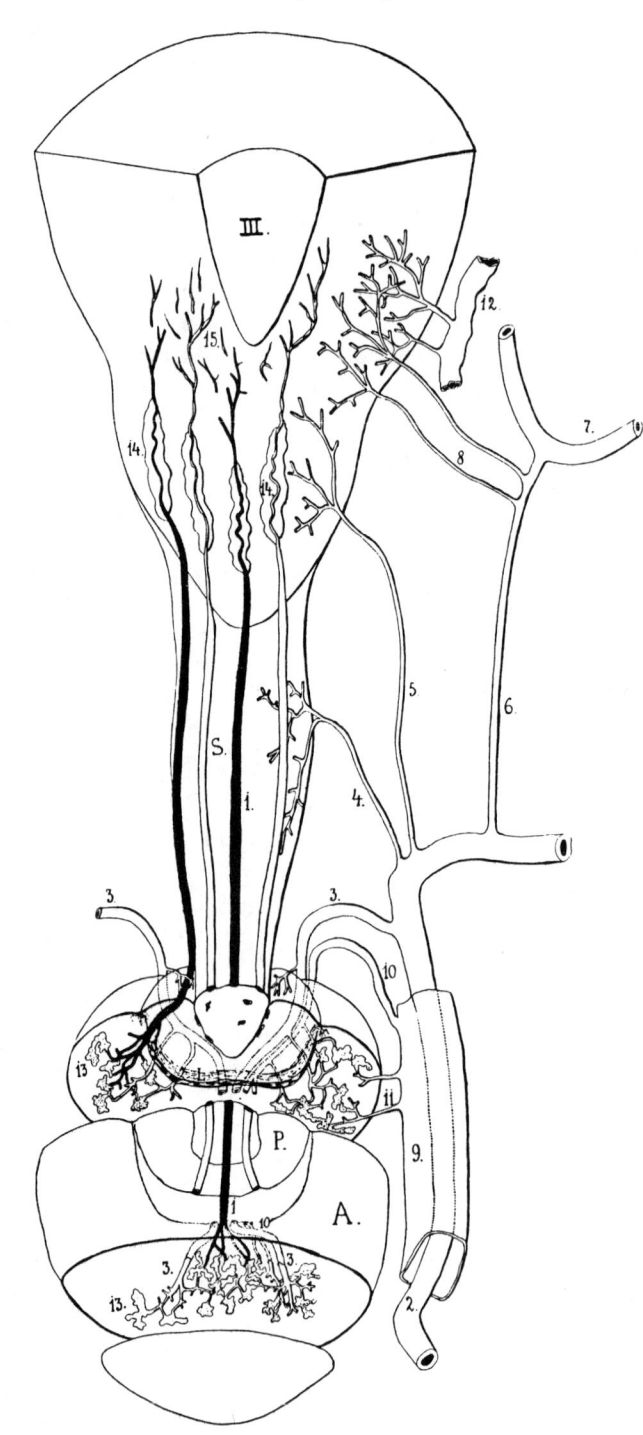

(1) Hypophyseo-portal vessel
(2) Carotid artery
(3) Hypophyseal artery
(4) Small artery for pars tuberalis
(5) Small artery for tuber cinereum
(6) Posterior communicating artery
(7) Posterior cerebral artery
(8) Small arteries for infundibulum
(9) Cavernous sinus
(10) Hypophyseal vein
(11) Small hypophyseal veins
(12) Basal vein
(13) Sinusoids
(14) Heavy glial sheaths of the hypophyseo-portal veins
(15) Secondary distribution net
(A) Pars anterior of pituitary
(P) Pars posterior of pituitary
(I) Pars intermedia of pituitary
(S) Stalk

lumina. In these cases the tissue mass of the posterior lobe and stalk appears almost avascular.

Sometimes it happens that the lowest parts of these channels are widely open, where they communicate with the sinusoids, while the upper parts are constricted to a thread or absolutely closed.

In other hypophyses the hypophyseo-portal vessels are seen through their course as leashes of dilated and engorged channels which spread out superiorly into the very much finer secondary distribution net.

Work is in progress to discover how the lumina of the vessels is regulated.

Our observations indicate that the secondary distribution net is richer beneath the infundibular recess anteriorly than it is posteriorly.

A full statement of the details of our observations, with accompanying microphotographs, is being prepared.

We hope before our next publication to be able to reproduce experimentally the various conditions of the lumina of the portal vessels described above.

The observations here recorded are the result of dissection and the study of serial sections.

THE PERMEABILITY OF THE HYPOPHYSIS AND HYPOTHALAMUS TO VITAL DYES, WITH A STUDY OF THE HYPOPHYSEAL VASCULAR SUPPLY

GEORGE B. WISLOCKI AND LESTER S. KING

Department of Anatomy, Harvard Medical School, Boston, Massachusetts

By the use of the so-called vital dyes of the benzidine series, such as trypan blue and pyrrhol blue, Goldmann came to the conclusion that these dyes do not stain the normal central nervous system, aside from the chorioid plexuses. Moreover he observed that they do not enter the cerebrospinal fluid. In the course of time this concept has become modified to the effect that vital benzidine dyes do penetrate the brain in a few quite localized small areas. The most constant of these in order of their discovery are the posterior lobe of the hypophysis (Schulemann, '12), the tuber cinereum (Rachmanow, '13), the area postrema (Wislocki and Putnam, '20), the epiphysis or pineal body (Macklin and Macklin, '20), the paraphysis (Putnam, '22), and the wall of the optic recess (Behnsen, '27). The areas enumerated stain rather constantly in all species of animals investigated. Behnsen ('27) showed, however, that in young mice, using relatively large doses, much wider areas of the brain may become stained than occurs in the adult. Rachmanow ('13), Behnsen ('27) and Mandelstamm and Krylow ('27) have demonstrated, moreover, that within the more specific areas the vital dyes, besides occurring in occasional macrophages and endothelial cells along the vessels, are deposited within the glial and ependymal cells, and are found also to some extent as free granules among the glial fibers. There is evidence also that actual neurones may at times stain occasionally when they are presumably entirely normal (Mandelstamm and Krylow), whereas at other times a previously imposed injury of the nerve cells appears to have been responsible for the staining. Nevertheless damaged neurones do not invariably store vital dyes, for King ('35), working in this connection, found no vital staining in the neurones of the vagus and hypoglossal nuclei which showed marked chromatolysis following retrograde degeneration.

No unanimity of opinion exists regarding the nature of the staining of certain localities of the brain by vital stains. Rachmanow ('25) looks upon it as a form of special affinity of vegetative centers for such dyes; Behnsen ('27) and others invoke a hypothetical brain barrier more permeable in young animals than in adults, while Mandelstamm and Krylow ('27) and Mandelstamm ('28) attribute the selective staining to special vascularity of the regions plus an added factor of looseness of the brain tissue in these areas, for which, however, they advance little or no strict anatomical evidence.

In view of the uncertainty in this subject, we have reinvestigated what can justly be regarded as the major one of these small areas, namely, the hypophyseal region. The previous workers have been interested solely in the deposition of trypan blue in this and similar areas of the brain. No one has availed himself of the opportunity to use dyes or salts other than trypan blue. Relatively little attention has been paid to the special problems involving the hypophyseal region because previous interest has been centered mainly upon vital staining in the related areas as a whole. Moreover, in order to clarify our observations upon the permeability of the pituitary body, we undertook an investigation of the complex question of the vascular supply to the hypophyseal region, the results of which are reported at some length.

The results of this work are presented under the following headings which set forth the scope of our study:

I. The differential staining of the diencephalic floor with trypan blue.

II. The differential staining of the diencephalic floor by acid dyes in general.

III. The differential staining of the diencephalic floor by Prussian blue. A. Perfusion of Prussian blue reagents. B. Intravitam injection of Prussian blue reagents.

IV. The vascular supply of the hypophysis of the monkey with comparisons with that of man and other mammals.

V. The differential staining of the supraoptic crest.

It should be added that the experiments of Behnsen were all carried out on mice, those of Mandelstamm and Krylow upon rabbits, with results sufficiently variable to indicate the importance of species differences in the way in which vital dyes are deposited and stored in the central nervous system. We chose for our experimental purposes several dissimilar mammals, principally rabbits, cats and monkeys, so that we might in some measure be able to gauge the important factor of species variation.

[*Editor's Note:* Material has been omitted at this point.]

SUMMARY AND CONCLUSIONS

1. Acid dyes, whether readily diffusible or colloidal, injected into living adult animals, stain the hypophysis and a few other small areas of the brain vitally, leaving the bulk of the brain unstained. The staining of the hypophysis involves both the epithelial and neural parts of the organ. The tuber cinereum is unstained excepting that portion, termed the eminentia saccularis, immediately adjacent to and continuous with the stalk. The latter area, by virtue of its vital staining, appears to be essentially a part of the infundibulum. The line of separation of the stained infundibular stalk (including the investing pars tuberalis and eminentia saccularis) from the unstained hypothalamus of the brain proper is rather sharp. The vegetative centers of the hypothalamus are practically devoid of stain.

Colloidal acid dyes, such as trypan blue, become deposited, after repeated intravitam administration, in the endothelial cells and epithelial elements of the anterior lobe. In the neurohypophysis granules lie within the glial cells, as well as free in the interstices of the fibrillar ground work. This aggregation of free extra-cellular dye particles in the tissue interstices of the infundibulum is a specific reaction in certain areas of brain tissue unknown under normal conditions in the fibrillar matrix of the mesenchymal connective tissues.

Basic dyes, which as a class are much more toxic than acid dyes, penetrate the whole central nervous system.

2. The Prussian blue reagents (iron ammonium citrate and potassium ferrocyanide—both acid salts), when perfused through the vascular system of a recently killed animal, stain the hypophysis with intensity and distribution similar to the acid dyes. The combined evidence from the experiments with the Prussian blue reagents and acid dyes demonstrates that the staining of the neurohypophysis is due to the rapid diffusion of these substances into the loose glial tissue of the neural lobe. The Prussian blue reagents confirm the observation made with acid dyes that the dissemination of acid substances is sharply localized to the neurohypophysis, the hypothalamic vegetative centers not becoming stained, either by diffusion from the blood vessels, or by direct spread from the neighboring tissue of the infundibulum. In regard to staining with the Prussian blue reagents (analogous to acid dyes), the eminentia saccularis is allied in its reaction to the infundibulum and not to the tuber cinereum.

3. A study of the blood supply of the hypophysis of the adult rhesus monkey is presented, based upon injected material from which an entirely new concept is derived. Evidence is adduced to demonstrate that the anterior lobe of the hypophysis, analogous to the liver, is supplied by afferent portal veins as well as by afferent arteries. The terminal branches of these two systems unite to form the characteristic sinusoids in the anterior lobe. The portal veins have their origin in the region of the hypophyseal stalk from a plexus surrounding and in part penetrating the infundibular stem. The efferent venous drainage of the anterior lobe is by way of veins, which we have described and illustrated, which leave the lateral poles of the anterior lobe to enter the adjacent cavernous sinuses. The infundibular process is fed and drained, for the most part, independently by arteries and veins entering and leaving its posterior pole.

The hypophyseal stem is the region of origin of the hypophyseal portal veins. It does not itself receive veins from either anterior or posterior lobe. Moreover there are no veins or arteries of any consequence passing from the infundibular stem to the hypothalamic region (vegetative centers) or vice versa. Sheathed veins penetrating the infundibular stalk do not exist; there are, however, penetrating arborizing plexuses, the nature of which is described. In reference to arteries and veins the hypothalamic region has an independent blood supply, identical with that of the brain proper and not derived from the infundibulum. The capillary bed of the hypothalamus differs characteristically from the wide-calibered plexuses enveloping and penetrating the infundibular stalk. The eminentia saccularis, on the score of its vascular supply, is an integral part of the infundibulum and distinct from the tuber cinereum of the hypothalamus. All of the various regions of the hypophysis and adjacent brain are to some degree in communication with one another by virtue of capillary collaterals; but this does not imply arterial or venous anastomoses excepting in so far as such connections have been specifically described in the above account.

Brief investigation of the human hypophysis indicates that what has been ascertained regarding the blood supply in the monkey holds also for man. A discussion of this question is presented in the text.

4. The eminentia saccularis, on anatomical and physiological grounds, is closely allied or identical with the infundibulum of the hypophysis. It should be regarded as a part of the infundibulum and not be considered as belonging to the tuber cinereum from which it differs fundamentally.

5. The evidence obtained regarding the permeability of the infundibulum to acid dyes and salts, as well as the character of the blood supply to the hypophysis, indicates that the pituitary gland is not intimately connected with the surrounding neural centers or other parts of the hypothalamus either by demonstrable interstitial pathways or by vascular connections. The infundibular stalk is, on the other hand,

intimately connected with the anterior lobe of the hypophysis by portal veins, and with the infundibular process by tissue spaces which are readily demonstrated by the Prussian blue reagents.

6. Other small areas of the brain, more particularly the area postrema of the hindbrain and the supraoptic crest of the diencephalon, resemble the infundibulum in regard to their selective staining by acid dyes and the richness and complexity of their blood supply. The nature and similarities of these areas are discussed.

LITERATURE CITED

BEHNSEN, G. 1927 Über die Farbstoffspeicherung im Zentralnervensystem der weissen Maus in verschiedenen Alterszuständen. Zeitsch. f. Zellforsch. u. mikr. Anat., Bd. 4, S. 515–572.

KING, L. S. 1935 Vital staining of the nervous system. I. Factors in the vital staining of neurones. J. Anat., vol. 69, pp. 177–180.

MACKLIN, C. C., AND M. T. MACKLIN 1920 A study of brain repair in the rat by use of trypan blue, with especial reference to the vital staining of the macrophages. Arch. Neur. and Psych., vol. 3, pp. 353–394.

MANDELSTAMM, M. 1928 Weitere Untersuchungen über die Farbenspeicherung im Zentralnervensystems. III. Mitteilung. Zeitschr. f. d. ges. exp. Med., Bd. 62, S. 471–491.

MANDELSTAMM, M., AND L. KRYLOW 1927 Vergleichende Untersuchungen über die Farbenspeicherung im Zentralnervensystem bei Injektionen der Farbe ins Blut und in der Liquor cerebrospinalis. Zeitschr. f. d. ges. exp. Med., Bd. 58, S. 256–275.

PUTNAM, T. J. 1922 The intercolumnar tubercle, an undescribed area in the anterior wall of the third ventricle. Johns Hopkins Hosp. Bull., vol. 38, pp. 181–182.

RACHMANOW, A. 1913 Beiträge zur vitalen Färbung des Zentralnervensystems. Folia Neuro-Biologica, vol. 7, pp. 750–771.

——— 1925 Die vitale Färbung der vegetativen Zentren des Zentralnervensystems. Korsakoffsches J. f. Neur. u. Psychiatrie, Bd. 3–4, S. 5. (Cit. Behnsen.)

SCHULEMANN, W. 1912 Beiträge zur Vitalfärbung. Arch. f. mikr. Anat., Bd. 79, S. 223–246.

WISLOCKI, G. B., AND T. J. PUTNAM 1920 Note on the anatomy of the area postrema. Anat. Rec., vol. 19, pp. 281–287.

THE NEUROVASCULAR LINK BETWEEN THE NEUROHYPOPHYSIS AND ADENOHYPOPHYSIS

BY J. D. GREEN AND G. W. HARRIS

There is little doubt that the secretory activity of the adenohypophysis is to some extent under the control of the nervous system [see Marshall, 1936, 1942; Brooks, 1939]. Two hypotheses have been advanced by various authors to explain this neural control: first, that the glandular cells possess a direct secretor-motor nerve supply, or secondly, that a humoral relay transmits the nervous stimuli from the hypothalamus by means of the hypophysial portal vessels.

The nerve supply of the hypophysis is derived from several sources. A sympathetic supply was first described by Bourgery in 1845. It consists of a few fine twigs passing from the carotid plexus to the pars distalis. The method of termination of these fibres and their function remain doubtful. Possibly they end on gland cells and are secretomotor, but more probably they end on blood vessels and are vasomotor. It is certain, however, that they do not subserve many of the nervous influences acting on the adenohypophysis. For example, coitus still excites ovulation in the rabbit and pseudopregnancy in the rat [Vogt, 1931, 1933; Haterius, 1933] after cervical sympathectomy. Other autonomic pathways that have been suggested, such as a supply via the greater superficial petrosal nerve [Hinsey & Markee, 1933], have likewise been shown to be unessential for the ovulation response in the rabbit [Vogt, 1942].

The major nerve supply to the hypophysis arises in the hypothalamus and passes to the gland through the hypophysial stalk. This supply has been described in all vertebrates studied from cyclostomes to mammals [for references see Fisher, Ingram & Ranson, 1938]. However, the number of fibres which pass from the hypothalamico-hypophysial tract to the pars distalis is uncertain. Some workers have described numerous fibres passing from the neural lobe into the adenohypophysis [Truscott, 1944], possibly ending in pericellular nets around the glandular cells [Pines, 1925; Brooks & Gersh, 1941]. The majority of workers find these fibres to be few in number. Rasmussen [1938], after a careful study in a variety of forms, found large areas of the adenohypophysis to be free of nerve fibres.

The possibility of a neurohumoral transmission of stimuli has been tentatively suggested on many occasions since the classical work of Popa & Fielding [1930, 1933], in which they first described a system of portal vessels linking the hypothalamus with the hypophysis. Wislocki & King [1936] and Wislocki [1936, 1937] confirmed the presence of these vessels in the hypophysial stalk but differed in their views on the extent of the system and direction of blood flow in it. The descriptions of the systemic circulation of the hypophysis given by various authors are in more general agreement. The pars distalis is supplied by small branches (the superior hypophysial arteries) derived from the internal carotid artery. These run caudo-ventrally (in most forms) into the anterolateral region of the gland. The venous drainage of the pars distalis is by short trunks into the surrounding dural venous sinuses, though in some cases communication with the basal vein would appear to be present [Wislocki, 1937]. The infundibular process receives its arterial supply posteriorly. Small twigs from both internal carotid arteries run medially, may anastomose to some extent in the midline, and enter the posterior pole of the gland as the inferior hypophysial arteries. The venous drainage of the infundibular process is into the adjacent venous sinuses. The blood systems of the pars distalis and infundibular process appear to be separate and independent, the pars intermedia being in circulatory association with the infundibular process. According to Stevens [1937], the pars tuberalis and pars distalis are the most vascular parts of the hypophysis, with the infundibular process and the pars intermedia being vascular in that order.

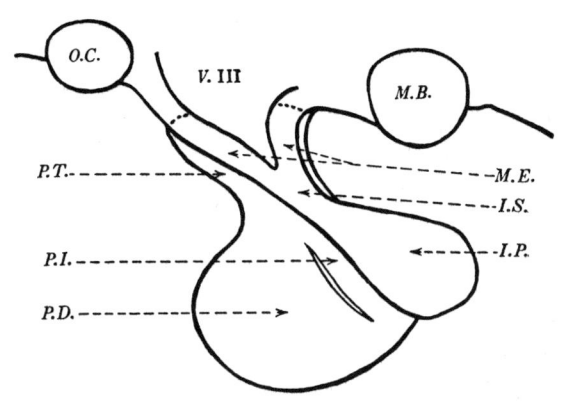

Fig. 1. Diagram to illustrate the terms used for the different parts of the hypophysis. The median eminence is differentiated from the hypothalamus proper. The neurohypophysis comprises: *M.E.* median eminence; *I.S.* infundibular stem; *I.P.* infundibular process; and the adenohypophysis: *P.T.* pars tuberalis; *P.I.* pars intermedia; *P.D.* pars distalis. (*M.B.* mammillary body; *O.C.* optic chiasma; *V.* III, third ventricle.)

The experimental evidence available indicates that neural control of the adenohypophysis is mediated in some way from the hypothalamus through the hypophysial stalk [Harris, 1937; Haterius & Derbyshire, 1937; Brooks, 1938; and others]. The present work is an investigation of the nervous and vascular connexions which may be involved in this transmission.

The terminology used for the various subdivisions of the hypophysis will be that proposed by Rioch, Wislocki & O'Leary [1939]. Since the clarity of the following account depends largely on the precision with which these terms are used, they are given below and illustrated in Fig. 1.

Adenohypophysis Lobus glandularis { Pars distalis (anterior lobe)
                                     Pars tuberalis
                                     Pars intermedia } Posterior lobe
Neurohypophysis Lobus nervosus (neural lobe) Infundibular process
                 Infundibulum (neural stalk) { Infundibular stem
                                                Median eminence of tuber cinereum

(Neural stalk + associated sheath of lobus glandularis = hypophysial stalk).

[*Editor's Note:* Material has been omitted at this point. Also, Plates 1, 2, and 3 have not been reproduced.]

DISCUSSION

Our anatomical observations will be discussed first, followed by their possible functional significance.

Nerve fibres passing from the infundibular stem and process into the pars intermedia have been described by Gemelli [1906], Cajal [1911], Tello [1912], Croll [1928], Rasmussen [1938], Truscott [1944], and many others. The presence of these fibres we can confirm, although they appeared few in number. Hair [1938], Brooks & Gersh [1941], and Truscott [1944] were able to demonstrate a similar nerve supply for the pars distalis, although Hair (cat) and Brooks & Gersh (rat) admit that the number of fibres passing to the pars distalis is not large. Our results are in agreement with Rasmussen [1938], who was unable to find any convincing nerve supply to the glandular cells of the pars distalis. There are two technical difficulties in reaching a conclusion regarding the presence or absence of nerve fibres in the pars distalis. First, impregnation of the nerve fibres with silver salts is often unsatisfactory. Croll [1928] suggested the reason might be failure of penetration of the fixative or silver salt, but found that increasing the time allowed for penetration did not improve the results. It might also be pointed out that even when thin (5μ) sections are stained on the slide, an increased number of stained nerve fibres does not appear. The second difficulty is the lack of a specific stain for nervous tissue, so that connective tissue may be confused with nerve fibres and pericellular nets. Although it is impossible to exclude, on anatomical data, a direct nervous influence of the hypothalamus on the secretion of the pars distalis, we feel this is sufficiently improbable to warrant investigation of alternative pathways.

The existence of a portal circulation of the hypophysis, as first described by Popa & Fielding [1930, 1933] for man, has been confirmed in a variety of animals. Regarding the precise extent of this system and the direction of blood flow within the portal vessels two views are current. On the one hand, Popa & Fielding maintain that the upper system of capillaries extends far into the hypothalamus, that the direction of flow in the vessels is upwards, and that the blood is collected by the lower system of capillaries from both lobes of the gland. On the other, Wislocki & King [1936] believe the upper limit of the portal system does not extend beyond the expanded lower end of the tuber cinereum (known as the median eminence), which is functionally part of the neurohypophysis. They claim the direction of blood flow to be downwards, all the blood entering the pars distalis. In general our results confirm those of Wislocki as to the extent of the portal system, the presence of a plexus in the pars tuberalis, and the presence of capillary loops or tufts in the median eminence and infundibular stem.

The vascular pattern of the median eminence varies in detail in different forms. In the rat the loops are concentrated in the midline anteriorly; in the dog discrete capillary loops are arranged more uniformly (as depicted by Wislocki [1937] for the cat), in the guinea-pig and rabbit the pattern is similar to that of the carnivores though the loops are less regular in shape, whilst in the monkey Wislocki & King [1936] described more branching of the vessels, which they call 'vascular tufts'. We have been unable to find a detailed account of human material injected with indian ink, but the microphotograph published by Wislocki [1936, Fig. 11] seems to show, as he stated, an arrangement similar to that of the monkey.

We shall not discuss here the problem of the direction of blood flow in the portal vessels, but one of us (J.D.G.) hopes to present the results of some experimental work on this subject at a later date.

It might be suggested that the pattern of the portal vessels is only an expression of the complex embryological development of the hypophysis, and lacks any underlying functional significance. This view would appear unlikely from a consideration of the relative vascularity of the hypothalamus, neural stalk and process. In our material one very striking feature was the great vascularity of the median eminence (and infundibular stem in man), as compared with adjacent neural tissue (Pl. 3, figs. 14, 15). The vascular nature of the median eminence of the rabbit is well shown in Pl. 2, fig. 10. It would seem that these vessels are more extensive than the nerve fibres and general neurohypophysial tissue require, so that they may have an additional function.

One hypothesis that has been tentatively suggested at intervals [Harris, 1937; Hinsey, 1937; Brooks, 1938; Taubenhaus & Soskin, 1941] to explain the neural control of the adenohypophysis in the absence of a well-marked nerve supply is a humoral transmission of stimuli from the neurohypophysis to the pars distalis. The anatomical evidence available suggests that this transmission may occur from the median eminence through the portal system of vessels to the pars distalis. Some other evidence which has accumulated in favour of this view is summarized below.

(a) Ovulation in the rabbit normally occurs 10 hr. after coitus. If hypophysectomy is performed within 1 hr. of coitus ovulation does not occur, but if more than 1 hr. is allowed to elapse ovulation occurs normally [Fee & Parkes, 1929]. It seems that 1 hr. is necessary for the secretion of sufficient gonadotrophic hormone to produce follicular rupture. The explanation may be that stimulation of the hypophysis is normally effected by a slow humoral mechanism.

(b) Markee, Sawyer & Hollinshead [1946] have shown that ovulation in the rabbit is more easily elicited by electrical stimulation of the hypothalamus than of the hypophysis. One of us (G.W.H.) can confirm this in a limited number of rabbits stimulated in the conscious state by the remote-control method. (Further work is in progress.) If the adenohypophysis is devoid of a direct secretomotor nerve supply it is possibly not excited by direct electrical stimulation.

(c) The different effects recorded after section of the hypophysial stalk [Harris, 1937; Hinsey, 1937; Brooks, 1938] may be due to variations in regeneration of the portal vessels.

(d) The results of Dempsey [1939], Dey [1943], and Leininger & Ranson [1943], indicating that a greater disturbance of the oestrous cycle in the guinea-pig may follow a lesion in the median eminence than section of the hypophysial stalk, may be due to the former producing a complete irreparable denervation of the median eminence, whilst stalk section allows the possibility of vascular repair.

(e) In some animals—the whale, porpoise, sea-cow, armadillo, Indian elephant [Wislocki & Geiling, 1936; Geiling, Voss & Oldham, 1940; Oldham, McCleery & Geiling, 1938; Oldham, 1938; Wislocki, 1939]—the infundibular lobe is separated from the pars intermedia, or pars distalis if the intermedia is lacking, by a connective tissue septum derived from the capsule. This makes it difficult to visualize a neural pathway from the infundibular process to the pars distalis. However, from a study of the literature, it appears that these animals have a pars tuberalis in contact with the median eminence and probably a portal system of vessels.

(f) Taubenhaus & Soskin [1941] state that the pars distalis of the rat may be stimulated by local application of a mixture of prostigmine and acetylcholine. They adduce this fact as evidence for the theory of humoral control of the adenohypophysis.

Sufficient evidence is not available to prove neurohumoral control of the adenohypophysis, but we feel this theory has much to support it.

It is of interest to speculate about the nervous pathways by which the hypothalamus might influence the capillary loops in the median eminence and infundibular stem, and so form the first link in a neurovascular chain. The nerve fibres entering the tuber cinereum, apparently destined to supply the neurohypophysis, have been described as arising in the following regions and nuclei in the hypothalamus: the supraoptic nucleus, paraventricular nucleus, anterior nucleus, ventromedial nucleus, ventral periventricular nucleus, ventral hypothalamic nucleus pars centralis [Young, 1936], scattered cells in the tuberal region, and perhaps in the mammillary region [see Fisher et al. 1935; Ingram, 1939]. Lesions placed in the hypophysial stalk or median eminence cause a clear-cut retrograde degeneration in only the supraoptic and paraventricular nuclei [Rasmussen, 1939; Frykman, 1942], but it is possible that some of the scattered cells and more loosely knit nuclei in the hypothalamus also undergo some degeneration. At the moment it cannot be decided which of the above nuclei, if any, are linked with the portal vessels. It is possible to state, however, that the capillary loops in the median eminence are surrounded by large numbers of nerve fibres derived from various hypothalamic nuclei, which in turn are connected with the thalamic and subthalamic centres, and so with the cerebral cortex and other regions of the nervous system.

As to the nature of the hypothetical humoral substance transmitted via the portal vessels there is little evidence. Two possibilities are the hormone(s) of the neurohypophysis (since the median eminence has been shown to be part of the secretory neurohypophysis [Magoun, Fisher & Ranson, 1939] and acetylcholine or related compounds. This latter suggestion receives some support from the work of Taubenhaus & Soskin [1941]. Excitation of the neurohypophysis probably entails a cholinergic mechanism at some point on the neural pathway [Pickford, 1939], thus making it difficult to obtain direct evidence of a similar mechanism for the adenohypophysis.

SUMMARY

1. The anatomy of the nervous and vascular connexions between the neurohypophysis and adenohypophysis is described.
2. The nervous connexions are scanty in the rabbit, monkey, and man.
3. The vascular connexions are prominent in the rat, guinea-pig, rabbit, dog and man. They are described with particular reference to the capillary loops found in the median eminence and infundibular stem, and the hypophysial portal vessels.
4. Nerve fibres from the hypothalamico-hypophysial tract are intimately associated with the capillary loops.
5. It is suggested that the central nervous system regulates the activity of the adenohypophysis by means of a humoral relay through the hypophysial portal vessels.

It is a pleasure to record our thanks to Prof. H. A. Harris for his ever-willing advice and encouragement, to Dr F. W. Gunz for his help in obtaining human material, to Mr J. A. F. Fozzard for his skilful microphotography, and also to Messrs J. Cash and R. Smith for their valuable aid in the preparation of the histological material.

REFERENCES

Bourgery, J. M. [1845]. *C.R. Acad. Sci., Paris*, **20**, 1014.
Brooks, C. McC. [1938]. *Amer. J. Physiol.* **121**, 157.
Brooks, C. McC. [1939]. *Res. Publ. Ass. Nerv. Ment. Dis.* **20**, 525.
Brooks, C. McC. & Gersh, I. [1941]. *Endocrinology*, **28**, 1.
Cajal, S. R. y. [1911]. *Histologie du système Nerveux*, French edition, **2**, 489. Paris: Maloine.
Croll, M. M. [1928]. *J. Physiol.* **66**, 316.
Dempsey, E. W. [1939]. *Amer. J. Physiol.* **126**, 758.
Dey, F. L. [1943]. *Anat. Rec.* **87**, 85.
Fee, A. R. & Parkes, A. S. [1929]. *J. Physiol.* **67**, 383.
Fisher, C., Ingram, W. R. & Ranson, S. W. [1935]. *Arch. Neurol. Psychiat., Chicago*, **34**, 124.
Fisher, C., Ingram, W. R. & Ranson, S. W. [1938]. *Diabetes Insipidus*. Ann Arbor: Edward.
Frykman, H. M. [1942]. *Endocrinology*, **31**, 23.
Geiling, E. M. K., Voss, B. J. & Oldham, F. K. [1940]. *Endocrinology*, **27**, 309.
Gemelli, A. [1906]. *Anat. Anz.* **28**, 613.
Hair, G. W. [1938]. *Anat. Rec.* **71**, 141.
Harris, G. W. [1937]. *Proc. Roy. Soc.* B, **122**, 374.
Haterius, H. O. [1933]. *Amer. J. Physiol.* **103**, 97.
Haterius, H. O. & Derbyshire, A. J. [1937]. *Amer. J. Physiol.* **103**, 97.
Hinsey, J. C. [1937]. *Cold Spr. Harb. Symp. Quant. Biol.* **5**, 269.
Hinsey, J. C. & Markee, J. E. [1933]. *Proc. Soc. Exp. Biol., N.Y.*, **31**, 270.
Ingram, W. R. [1939]. *Res. Publ. Ass. Nerv. Ment. Dis.* **20**, 195.
Leininger, C. R. & Ranson, S. W. [1943]. *Anat. Rec.* **87**, 77.
Magoun, H. W., Fisher, C. & Ranson, S. W. [1939]. *Endocrinology*, **25**, 161.
Markee, J. E., Sawyer, C. H. & Hollinshead, W. H. [1946]. *Endocrinology*, **38**, 345.
Marshall, F. H. A. [1936]. The Croonian Lecture. *Philos. Trans.* B, **226**, 423.
Marshall, F. H. A. [1942]. *Biol. Rev.* **17**, 68.
Oldham, F. K. [1938]. *Anat. Rec.* **72**, 265.
Oldham, F. K., McCleery, D. P. & Geiling, E. M. K. [1938]. *Anat. Rec.* **71**, 27.
Pickford, M. [1939]. *J. Physiol.* **95**, 226.
Pines, J. L. [1925]. *Z. ges. Neurol. Psychiat.* **100**, 123.
Popa, Gr. T. & Fielding, U. [1930]. *J. Anat., Lond.*, **65**, 88.
Popa, Gr. T. & Fielding, U. [1933]. *J. Anat., Lond.*, **67**, 227.
Rasmussen, A. T. [1938]. *Endocrinology*, **23**, 263.
Rasmussen, A. T. [1939]. *Res. Publ. Ass. Nerv. Ment. Dis.* **20**, 245.
Rioch, D. McK., Wislocki, G. B. & O'Leary, J. L. [1939]. *Res. Publ. Ass. Nerv. Ment. Dis.* **20**, 3.
Stevens, H. M. [1937]. *Anat. Rec.* **67**, 377.
Taubenhaus, M. & Soskin, S. [1941]. *Endocrinology*, **29**, 958.
Tello, J. F. [1912]. *Trab. Lab. Invest. biol. Univ. Madr.* **10**, 145.
Truscott, B. L. [1944]. *J. Comp. Neurol.* **80**, 235.
Vogt, M. [1931]. *Arch. exp. Path. Pharmak.* **162**, 197.
Vogt, M. [1933]. *Arch. exp. Path. Pharmak.* **170**, 72.
Vogt, M. [1942]. *J. Physiol.* **100**, 410.
Wislocki, G. B. [1936]. *Res. Publ. Ass. Nerv. Ment. Dis.* **17**, 48.
Wislocki, G. B. [1937]. *Anat. Rec.* **69**, 361.
Wislocki, G. B. [1939]. *Anat. Rec.* **74**, 321.
Wislocki, G. B. & Geiling, E. M. K. [1936]. *Anat. Rec.* **66**, 17.
Wislocki, G. B. & King, L. S. [1936]. *Amer. J. Anat.* **58**, 421.
Young, M. W. [1936]. *J. Comp. Neurol.* **65**, 295.

OBSERVATION OF THE HYPOPHYSIO-PORTAL VESSELS
OF THE LIVING RAT

By J. D. GREEN AND G. W. HARRIS

From the Physiological Laboratory, University of Cambridge

(*Received* 13 *July* 1948)

The hypophysio-portal circulation was first described by Popa & Fielding (1930). They believed the blood in it flowed from the hypophysis to the hypothalamus. Wislocki & King (1936) and Wislocki (1938) suggested, on indirect evidence, that the blood flow is from the median eminence of the tuber cinereum to the pars distalis. Since Wislocki & King's work there has been much uncertainty as to the direction of flow in this system of vessels. Available evidence regarding the blood flow may be summarized: (1) histological appearance of the vessels (Wislocki & King, 1936; Green, 1948a); (2) observations on glands in which the vessels had been incompletely filled with india ink (Green & Harris, 1947); (3) the site of arrest of fat emboli within the system (Morato, 1939); (4) slow injection of india ink in dead animals with observation of filling of the vessels (Green, 1948a); (5) india ink injections made into the aorta of anaesthetized rats with intact, hemisected or transected pituitary stalks, followed by immediate decapitation. Observations on the filling of the vessels with ink indicated the blood flow to be towards the pars distalis (Harris, 1948); (6) direct observation of the direction of blood flow in the living animal.

Clearly the last type of evidence is the most satisfactory, but so far such observations have been confined to Amphibia. Houssay, Biasotti & Sammartino (1935) observed the direction of flow in *Bufo arenarum*, and Green (1947) has likewise seen the flow in the hypophysial vessels of anaesthetized amphibians (*Rana catesbiana*, *Ambystoma tigrinum*, *Triturus torosus* and *Necturus*). Recently (Green, 1948b) it has been found possible to expose the hypophysis in *Rana catesbiana* under procaine anaesthesia and observe the course of blood flow for many hours. Since the operation is nearly bloodless and the animals are conscious, it is felt that conditions are almost ideal. As far as is known, no observations have been made on the circulation in living mammals.

METHODS

Rats were used since they possess long hypophysio-portal vessels, in a horizontal plane, which are readily approached and easily observed. Adult animals were anaesthetized with ether and tracheotomized. The facial artery and vein were ligated near the angle of the jaw and clamped dorsal to the angle of the mouth. The lower jaw was divided on either side through the angle and removed. As soon as haemostasis had been secured the soft palate was incised and removed except for a narrow rim. The periosteum of the skull was stripped beneath the sphenoid and anterior part of the basiocciput. The bone was then picked away with a dental scaling pick. A transverse venous sinus lies in the sphenoid beneath the stalk. This was opened and packed with beeswax. As soon as a clean field had been obtained the cancellous bone was scraped away until the shiny inner table could be seen. The remaining bone was then carefully picked away under a binocular dissecting microscope to expose the dura. The dura was pricked and the hole extended by tearing. For observation of the vessels an ordinary microscope was used ($\frac{2}{3}$ objective and × 9 eyepiece, with oblique illumination from above).

RESULTS

A satisfactory exposure of the portal vessels was secured in twelve rats. It was seen that the median eminence of the tuber cinereum and pituitary stalk are clearly demarcated from the surrounding hypothalamus by their extreme vascularity. The rich capillary network of the median eminence extends into the pituitary stalk and collects to form the large portal trunks which may be observed to fan out into the sinusoids of the pars distalis. In all twelve rats the blood flow was seen to be from the median eminence towards the pars distalis. Under the $\frac{2}{3}$ objective the red blood corpuscles within the vessels were readily observed. In many cases the animals were in excellent condition and only lightly anaesthetized. A few, however, showed signs of surgical shock and an occasional vessel appeared thrombosed. These signs of damage were not associated with any change in direction of flow. The blood stream in the vessels appeared comparable in rate to that in the hypothalamic veins. The flow shows no signs of pulsation and is always of a uniform character. All the large vessels of the hypophysial stalk appear to carry blood caudally to the pars distalis from the dense capillary plexus of the median eminence. They cannot in any sense be regarded as T-shaped branches from the carotid artery.

DISCUSSION

These observations accord well with the concept of neurovascular control of the pars distalis (Harris, 1944; Green & Harris, 1947). Histological evidence indicates that a hypophysio-portal circulation is a constant feature in vertebrates from the Salientia to the Primates (Green, 1948c), even in those species in which the pars distalis is separated from the neurohypophysis by a dural septum (Harris, 1947; Green, 1948b).

It is felt that the above data provide the most direct and satisfactory evidence that the vessels of the hypophysial stalk are true portal vessels carrying blood from the median eminence of the tuber cinereum to the pars distalis.

SUMMARY

1. A method of exposing the hypophysio-portal blood vessels of the living rat is described.

2. The direction of the blood flow in these vessels is from the median eminence of the tuber cinereum to the pars distalis.

REFERENCES

Green, J. D. (1947). *Anat. Rec.* **99**, 21.
Green, J. D. (1948a). *Anat. Rec.* **100**, 273.
Green, J. D. (1948b). Unpublished observation.
Green, J. D. (1948c). Proc. Anat. Soc., *J. Anat., Lond.* (in the Press).
Green, J. D. & Harris, G. W. (1947). *J. Endocrinol.* **5**, 136.
Harris, G. W. (1944). Thesis for M.D. degree, Cambridge University.
Harris, G. W. (1947). *Nature, Lond.*, **159**, 874.
Harris, G. W. (1948). Unpublished observation.
Houssay, B. A., Biasotti, A. & Sammartino, R. (1935). *C.R. Soc. Biol., Paris*, **120**, 725.
Morato, M. J. X. (1939). *Anat. Rec.* **74**, 297.
Popa, G. T. & Fielding, U. (1930). *J. Anat., Lond.*, **65**, 88.
Wislocki, G. B. (1938). *Res. Publ. Ass. nerv. ment. Dis.* **17**, 48.
Wislocki, G. B. & King, L. S. (1936). *Amer. J. Anat.* **58**, 421.

Editor's Comments
on Papers 5 and 6

5   BARGMANN and SCHARRER
The Site of Origin of the Hormones of the Posterior Pituitary

6   SLOPER
Excerpts from *Hypothalamic Neurosecretion in the Dog and Cat, with Particular Reference to the Identification of Neurosecretory Material with Posterior Lobe Hormone*

    Studies conducted by Bargmann and Scharrer (Paper 5) and Sloper (Paper 6) clearly demonstrated that neurons of the hypothalamus are capable of synthesizing peptide hormones that alter hypophysial function. Bargmann and Scharrer (Paper 5) provided the first evidence that neurons of the hypothalamus can synthesize and liberate hormones. They made use of a basic dye, chrome alum hematoxylin (CAH), preceded by acid permanganate oxidation, to stain neurosecretory material in neuronal cell bodies of the supraoptic (SON) and paraventricular (PVN) nuclei in beaded nerve fibers in the hypophyseal tract and in dense masses in the infundibular process. They thus proposed the presence of a neurosecretory pathway, based on the concept that the peptide hormones oxytocin and vasopressin are synthesized in hypothalamic nuclei, packaged into neurosecretory vesicles, and transported along axons to nerve terminals in the neurohypophysis, where they are released into the systemic circulation by appropriate physiological stimuli.

    Sloper (Paper 6), using a variety of staining techniques, corroborated Bargmann and Scharrer's observation that neurons of the hypothalamo-hypophysial system synthesize vasopressin and oxytocin and that these substances are transported down the axons of these neurons to nerve terminals in the neurohypophysis. He further showed that a protein rich in cystine, proposed to be a hormone or hormone precursor, characterized Bargmann and Scharrer's neurosecretory material (NSM). This disclosure disposed of the view prevalent at that time that NSM was a glycoprotein carrier substance that could not, by virtue of its cytochemical properties, represent the posterior hypophysial hormones. He also suggested that these materials represent cystine-rich octapeptides, which display oxytocic, vasopressor and antidiuretic properties in agreement with DuVigneaud and co-workers, who had elucidated and reported the structures of oxytocin and antidiuretic hormones in 1953.

THE SITE OF ORIGIN OF THE HORMONES OF THE POSTERIOR PITUITARY

By WOLFGANG BARGMANN and ERNST SCHARRER

EXTRACTS of the pars nervosa of the pituitary gland exhibit vasopressor, antidiuretic, and oxytocic activities. Although it is generally assumed that these principles are produced in the pars nervosa, recent reviewers have not been unmindful of the unsatisfactory nature of the evidence, both cytological and experimental, on which this assumption is based. "The cells of the pars nervosa are few and have little in common with secreting cells elsewhere in the body to suggest for them a secretory function" [19].

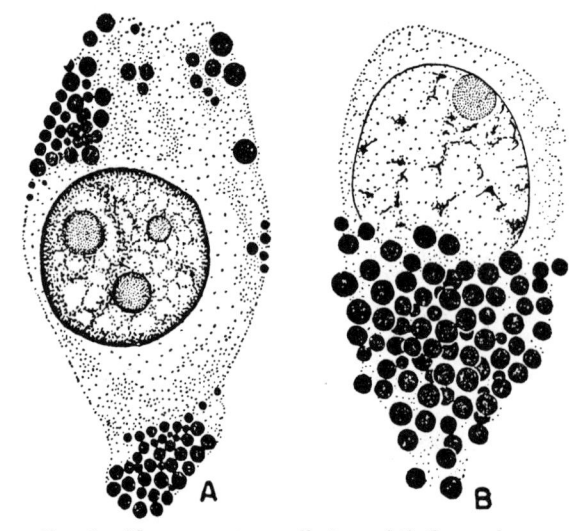

FIG. 1. Neurosecretory cells from (A) the nucleus preopticus of the toad, *Bufo americanus*, and (B) the nucleus paraventricularis of the monkey, *Cebus capucinus*. (Redrawn from E. and B. Scharrer [30].)

Thus the question arises as to where, if not in the pars nervosa, the hormones do originate. Recent observations indicate that they are produced by nerve cells in the hypothalamus; if this is true the pars nervosa functions as a place of storage rather than a site of production of hormones. The cytological and experimental evidence supporting this concept will be briefly reviewed in this paper.

The observation of a secretory activity of nerve cells (neurosecretion) in the hypothalamus, first reported for the nucleus preopticus of various species of teleost fishes, has in the course of years been extended to include the nucleus preopticus of amphibians, and the homologous nuclei supraopticus and paraventricularis of reptiles, birds, and mammals. The secretory activity of these cells compares, so far as its cytological aspects are concerned, with that of other gland cells such as those of the exocrine pancreas. In early stages of the secretory cycle the cells contain many small granules. The granules grow and coalesce to form larger inclusions of a colloidlike material which in many cases become so numerous that they occupy large areas of the cell body (Fig. 1).

In sections stained with Heidenhain's Azan or Masson's trichrome the colloid masses may be traced for some distance in the tracts descending toward the hypophysis. More recently the application of the chrome alum-hematoxylin-phloxine method, recommended by Gomori for the staining of the beta granules of the islets of Langerhans, not only permitted the demonstration of neurosecretory activity in animals in which the methods used before did not reveal its existence as in birds, but showed also with great clarity the pathway along which the neurocolloid reaches the pars nervosa.

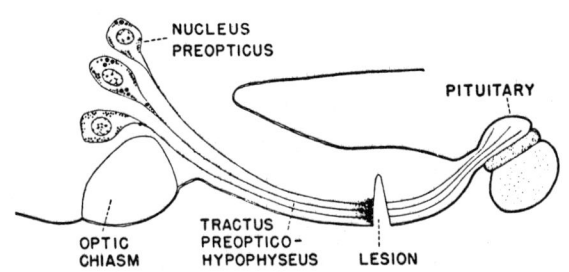

FIG. 2. Diagrammatic illustration of Hild's experiment [14]. The stainable material produced by nerve cells of the preoptic nucleus of the frog accumulates at the lesion, where its passage along the fibers of the tractus preoptico-hypophyseus is halted.

There is evidence that the stainable material elaborated by the neurosecretory cells is actually transported from the hypothalamic nuclei to the posterior lobe of the hypophysis. When, for instance in the frog, the stalk of the pituitary is cut (Fig. 2), this material within a few days accumulates in the tract proximal to the site of interruption of the axons. Furthermore, in snakes, when the pituitary is replaced by fibrin foam, the colloid from the hypothalamic nuclei is lodged in the nonliving material in a way similar to that seen normally in the posterior lobe of the pituitary. The concept of a transportation of the material produced by the neurosecretory cells from the hypothalamus to the neurohypophysis does not require the assumption of special forces. The peripheral movement of axoplasm provides a mechanism by which the neurosecretory material may well be carried from the site of its origin to the site of storage. Although this explanation seems satisfactory it cannot be considered as final, and further investigation is necessary.

The axons of the neurosecretory cells terminate in the pituitary stalk and in the pars nervosa. In mammals the endings frequently appear as bulbous swellings which are known as Herring bodies. These terminal bulbs contain granules which stain deep blue in Gomori preparations the same way that the colloid along the nerve fibers is stained. Herring bodies occur not only at the nerve endings but also along the fibers (Fig. 3). In addition to the granules contained in the Herring bodies, colloid is also lodged in the delicate fibrous network of the pars nervosa, particularly in the neighborhood of blood vessels, and near the border of the pars intermedia. Here it is not possible to determine with certainty whether the stainable material is still attached to the nerve fibers.

Provided it can be shown that the active principles of the pars nervosa are associated with the stainable material elaborated by the neurosecretory cells of the hypothalamus, these cytological observations suggest the solution of the problem of origin of the pars nervosa properties.

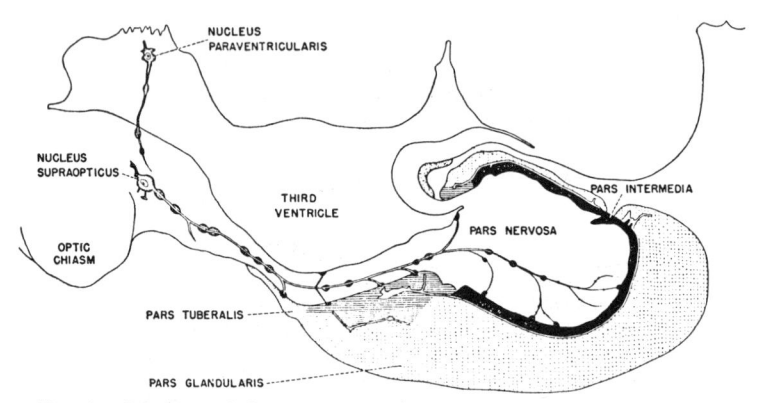

FIG. 3. Diagram of the mammalian hypothalamic-hypophyseal system. The products of the secretory activity of nerve cells in the hypothalamus are transferred to the neurohypophysis by way of the tractus supraopticohypophyseus. (From Bargmann [2].)

The presence of the posterior lobe hormones in the hypothalamus was demonstrated as early as 1924 and has been confirmed by experimental and clinical observations. Quantitative data concerning the antidiuretic activity of the nucleus supraopticus have been obtained in the dog; it has been found to amount to 15–25 per cent of that contained in the neurohypophysis. With respect to the oxytocic principle, the two nuclei paraventriculares of one dog contained 0.22 Voegtlin unit, the two nuclei supraoptici 0.3 Voegtlin unit, the neurohypophysis 6.5 Voegtlin units. The stainable material was found present in the extracts of isolated nuclei supraoptici and paraventriculares, but was absent in the extracted tissues.

In view of these results it should be possible to influence the neurosecretory process by subjecting animals to extreme conditions of retention and excretion of water. This is actually the case. In rats dehydration results not only in loss of antidiuretic potency of the posterior lobe, but also in marked depletion of stainable material in the hypothalamic-hypophyseal system. On the other hand, excessive water intake causes an accumulation of the secretory product in the hypothalamic nuclei, the hypothalamo-hypophyseal tracts, and the pars nervosa. Evidently increased demand for the antidiuretic principle in dehydrated animals parallels the disappearance of the stainable material. Conversely, the stainable material accumulates when excess of water is available for the elimination of waste products and there is consequently less need for the antidiuretic hormone.

Other observations point in the same direction. Thus the chromatolytic reaction of the cells of the supraoptic and paraventricular nuclei of rats acutely overloaded with sodium chloride indicates a functional relationship between the neurosecretory cells of the hypothalamus and the excretion of excess salt. Similarly, the decrease of stainable material within the hypothalamic-hypophyseal system of rats made diabetic with alloxan may be related to the diabetic polyuria.

The experiments of Ranson and his co-workers, who do not agree with the concept outlined here, support it nevertheless with impressive evidence. By placing bilateral lesions in different parts of the hypothalamic-hypophyseal system diabetes insipidus could be caused in cats and monkeys. "In general the intensity of the diabetes insipidus is proportional to the degree of interruption of the supraoptico-hypophyseal tracts. It may be added that more than half the fibers must be bilaterally interrupted before any increase in the fluid exchange can be observed" [22]. Ranson and his co-workers interpret these results to mean that the neural portion of the hypophysis ceases to produce the antidiuretic hormone once it is effectively cut off from its innervation. However, as the same and other investigators have shown, lesions in the supraoptico-hypophyseal tracts also result in the atrophy and disappearance of cells of the supraoptic nuclei and, to a lesser extent, of the paraventricular nuclei. In the light of the observations reported above with regard to the secretory activity of these cells, it would appear that the amount of available antidiuretic hormone in the animals with experimental diabetes insipidus was diminished to the extent to which the neurosecretory cells and their pathway were destroyed.

The phenomenon of neurosecretion has also been described in invertebrate animals, including worms, mollusks, and arthropods. In insects, both the brain and the corpus cardiacum, an analogue of the neurohypophysis, furnish a chromatophorotropic hormone, and the brain has been identified as the site of origin of hormones controlling postembryonic development. Thus in invertebrates and vertebrates the experimental evidence agrees with the cytological observations on which the concept of the dual role of neurosecretory cells as neurons and glandular elements was originally based. This concept seems now to be firmly established [24].

Many problems remain to be studied. With regard to vertebrates the available data apply only to neurosecretory cells in the hypothalamus and their relationship to the pars nervosa of the pituitary; nothing is known about corresponding relationships of these cells to other endocrine organs. Neither do we have any information concerning the significance of neurosecretory centers other than those in the hypothalamus. Such centers have been described in lower vertebrates in different parts of the central nervous system, and additional ones may yet be found. Still less is known about the role of neurosecretory processes in the peripheral autonomic system.

In summary, morphological and experimental evidence strongly suggests that the pars nervosa of the vertebrate hypophysis stores, but does not produce, the stainable material which it contains. This material originates in the neurosecretory cells of the nuclei supraopticus and paraventricularis in the higher vertebrates and the homologous nucleus preopticus in the lower vertebrates; it passes to the pars nervosa by way of the hypothalamo-hypophyseal tracts. There is evidence that this stainable material carries the antidiuretic, oxytocic, and vasopressor principles from the site of origin in the hypothalamic nuclei to the place of storage in the pars nervosa.

REFERENCES

This article is based on the published papers cited below. Editorial policy of the *American Scientist* does not permit specific references throughout the text.

1. ABEL, J. J. *Bull. Johns Hopkins Hosp.*, *35*, 305, 1924.
2. BARGMANN, W. *Z. Zellforsch.*, *34*, 610, 1949.
3. BARGMANN, W. Unpublished paper.
4. BARGMANN, W., and HILD, W. *Acta Anat.*, *8*, 264, 1949.
5. BARGMANN, W., HILD, W., ORTMANN, R., and SCHIEBLER, Th. H. *Acta Neuroveg.*, *1*, 1950.
6. DRAGER, G. A. *Anat. Rec.*, *106*, 267, 1950.
7. GOMORI, G. *Am. J. Path.*, *17*, 395, 1951.
8. HANSTRÖM, B. *Lunds Univ. Årsskr. N.F. Avd. 2*, *44*, No. 10, 1948.
9. HANSTRÖM, B. *Lunds Univ. Årsskr. N.F. Avd. 2*, *46*, No. 3, 1950.
10. HARRIS, G. W. *Physiol. Rev.*, *28*, 139, 1948.
11. HECHST, B. *Arch. Psychiat.*, *91*, 319, 1930.
12. HICKEY, R. C., HARE, K., and HARE, R. S. *Anat. Rec.*, *81*, 319, 1941.
13. HILD, W. *Z. Zellforsch.*, *35*, 33, 1950.
14. HILD, W. *Z. Anat.* (in press).
15. HILD, W., and ZETLER, G. *Experientia* (in press).
16. HILLARP, N.-Å. *Acta Endocrinol.*, *2*, 33, 1949.
17. KRATZSCH, E. Unpublished data.
18. MELVILLE, E. V., and HARE, K. *Endocrinology*, *36*, 332, 1945.
19. O'CONNOR, W. J. *Biol. Rev.*, *22*, 30, 1947.
20. ORTMANN, R. *Klin. Wschr.*, *28*, 449, 1950.
21. PALAY, S. L. *J. Comp. Neur.*, *82*, 129, 1945.
22. RANSON, S. W., and MAGOUN, H. W. *Ergebn. Physiol.*, *41*, 56, 1939.
23. SATO, G. *Arch. Exp. Path. u. Pharmakol.*, *131*, 45, 1928.
24. SCHARRER, B. Hormones in insects. Chap. IV in *Hormones, Physiology, Chemistry, and Applications*, ed. by G. Pincus and K. V. Thimann; Vol. I, New York, 1948; pp. 121-158.
25. SCHARRER, B., and SCHARRER, E. *Biol. Bull.*, *87*, 242, 1944.
26. SCHARRER, E. *Z. Vergl. Physiol.*, *7*, 1, 1928.
27. SCHARRER, E. *Z. Vergl. Physiol.*, *11*, 767, 1930.
28. SCHARRER, E. *Z. Vergl. Physiol.*, *17*, 491, 1932.
29. SCHARRER, E., and SCHARRER, B. *Biol. Rev.*, *12*, 186, 1937.
30. SCHARRER, E., and SCHARRER, B. *Res. Publ. Ass. Nerv. Ment. Dis.*, *20*, 170, 1940.
31. SCHARRER, E., and SCHARRER, B. *Physiol. Rev.*, *25*, 171, 1945.
32. SMITH, S. W. Unpublished data.
33. TRENDELENBURG, P. *Klin. Wschr.*, *7*, 1679, 1928.
34. WARING, H., and LANDGREBE, F. W. Hormones of the posterior pituitary. Chap. VIII in *Hormones, Physiology, Chemistry, and Applications*, ed. by G. Pincus and K. V. Thimann; Vol. II, New York, 1950; pp. 427-514.
35. WEISS, P. *Biol. Bull.*, *87*, 160, 1944.

6

Copyright © 1955 by Cambridge University Press

Reprinted from pages 301–302, 313–314, and 315 of
J. Anat. 89:301–316 (1955)

HYPOTHALAMIC NEUROSECRETION IN THE DOG AND CAT, WITH PARTICULAR REFERENCE TO THE IDENTIFICATION OF NEUROSECRETORY MATERIAL WITH POSTERIOR LOBE HORMONE

By J. C. SLOPER

Bernhard Baron Institute of Pathology, London Hospital

The site of formation of the hormones of the posterior lobe of the pituitary has long been disputed. Thus they are held by some to be secreted by the pituicytes of the infundibular process (Gersh, 1939) and by others by the neurones of the supraoptic and paraventricular nuclei, whence they are passed along axones to the infundibular process (Scharrer & Scharrer, 1937). This second theory, although quite compatible with the known behaviour of neurones (Zuckerman, 1954) because of technical difficulties gained little credence until Bargmann (1949) showed that with Gomori's (1939) chrome-haematoxylin technique a stainable material could readily be demonstrated in mammals as well as other vertebrates, the distribution of which favoured the theory of hypothalamic secretion. This so-called 'neurosecretory material' (N.S.M.) is characteristically aggregated in the cytoplasm of the neurones of the supraoptic and paraventricular nuclei, whence it passes along their axones in the form of fibres, often beaded like 'strings of pearls'. According to Laqueur (1954), in the dog at least, there is a direct pathway from paraventricular as well as supraoptic nucleus to infundibular process. There and in the infundibular stem, large aggregations of stainable material are seen, which may be identified with Herring bodies: but in the infundibular process the greater part of this stainable material is diffusely and finely distributed, particularly at the periphery. Two remarkable claims are made for Gomori's stain, namely first that the material in the cytoplasm of the cell-body of the neurone is identical with that spreading down its axone: and second that this material is extremely limited in its distribution.

Since Bargmann's original observations much has been published in favour of hypothalamic neurosecretion (Scharrer & Scharrer, 1954), in particular by Hild (1951), who demonstrated the accumulation of N.S.M. above the cut pituitary stalk, and by Hild & Zetler (1951) who isolated oxytocic, vasopressor and antidiuretic substances from the hypothalamus as well as from the infundibular process. It is probable that these substances are present in differing proportions in the two sites, an observation which suggests either secretion at both sites, or alternatively secretion at one site, with chemical modification at the other (Vogt, 1953). The fact that there is a close similarity between the formulae of two cyclic octapeptides recently published by Du Vigneaud and his colleagues (Du Vigneaud, Ressler, Swan, Roberts, Katsoyannis & Gordon, 1953; Du Vigneaud, Lawler & Popenhoe, 1953), the one with oxytocic and the other with vasopressor-antidiuretic activity, supports the second view.

The purpose of this work is the re-examination of Bargmann's theory, with a view to its corroboration and modification in the light of these recent advances. Observations have been confined to the dog and cat. First the relative distribution of certain enzymes has been studied in the supraoptic and paraventricular nuclei as compared with the infundibular process, on the hypothesis that secretion should be accompanied by particularly marked cellular activity in one site or the other. Secondly, the specificity of the stains used for the demonstration of N.S.M. has been reassessed. Thirdly, the histochemistry of N.S.M. has been investigated. It will be shown that, although N.S.M. is claimed to be a complex and variable glycolipoprotein (Schiebler, 1951, 1952a), a bearer-substance, akin to thyroid colloid, and readily separable from posterior-lobe hormone (Hild & Zetler, 1952-3), this substance is more probably a protein, representing the hormone itself.

[*Editor's Note:* Material has been omitted at this point.]

CONCLUSIONS

Our observations corroborate Bargmann's theory of neurosecretion, and indicate a variety of techniques applicable to the physiological and pathological investigation of the neurohypophysis. Thus, with regard to the relative distribution of enzymes in this region, it is likely that the study of esterases and of acid phosphatases will be rewarding.

With regard to the specificity of the stains used for the demonstration of N.S.M., this is limited: for Nissl substance, and granules probably akin to lipofuscin or 'glycolipid' inclusions, are also stained in varying degree by the chrome-haematoxylin and aldehyde-fuchsin techniques. On the other hand, it has been confirmed that no material in the hypothalamus or in its immediate vicinity has the morphology and intensity of staining of N.S.M. Further evidence in favour of the homogeneity of N.S.M. was obtained by the development of a third staining method, the phosphotungstic acid–Congo red technique, for its demonstration.

Since the chemical basis for these techniques is obscure, diverse histochemical tests were applied to discover the nature of N.S.M. It became clear that there was no great concentration of lipid or carbohydrate throughout the distribution of this material, an observation which accorded well with its loss after incubation in trypsin, and its persistence in paraffin sections after the alcoholic extraction of lipids. The alcoholic extraction of fresh unfixed tissues removed a certain amount of stainable material, but N.S.M. could still be demonstrated in large amounts in the infundibular process. In short, contrary to general opinion, N.S.M. lacked the properties of a carbohydrate or lipid.

It remained to find a histochemical technique for the identification of N.S.M., and this was achieved with a method which probably demonstrates high concentrations of cystine. Since certain recently described substances with high oxytocic and antidiuretic activity are also rich in cystine, it is possible that the material demonstrated in sections was the hormone itself.

SUMMARY

1. Current views on the formation of oxytocin, vasopressin and antidiuretic hormone are discussed.

2. In the cat the relative distribution of esterase and acid phosphatase in the hypothalamus as opposed to the infundibular lobe of the pituitary is compatible with hypothalamic neurosecretion.

3. In the dog and cat the chrome-haematoxylin and aldehyde-fuchsin techniques are shown to be of limited specificity when used for the demonstration of 'neurosecretory' material (N.S.M.) in the hypothalamus and neurohypophysis.

4. A different staining method, the phosphotungstic acid–Congo red technique, also demonstrates N.S.M.; the common affinity of these three different techniques for N.S.M. corroborates the view that N.S.M. is a single substance.

5. Histochemical evidence indicates that N.S.M. is not a glycolipoprotein, but is a protein rich in cystine. It is suggested that this material may represent certain cystine-rich octapeptides which show marked oxytocic vasopressor and antidiuretic activity.

I am particularly grateful to Mr Kenneth Swettenham for his technical assistance. Thanks are also due to Prof. Dorothy Russell, Prof. R. J. Harrison and Dr Bourne for help in the preparation of this paper; to Messrs May and Baker for the gift of tetrazolium salts; to Messrs Hopkins and Williams for the synthesis of dihydroxy-dinaphthyldisulphide and to Mr A. L. Gallup for the photography.

REFERENCES

BARGMANN, W. (1949). Über die neurosekretorische Verknüpfung von Hypothalamus und Neurohypophyse. *Z. Zellforsch.* **34**, 610–634.

DU VIGNEAUD, V., LAWLER, H. C. & POPENHOE, E. A. (1953). Enzymatic cleavage of glycinamide from vasopressin and a proposed structure for this pressor-antidiuretic hormone of the posterior pituitary. *J. Amer. chem. Soc.* **75**, 4880–4881.

DU VIGNEAUD, V., RESSLER, C., SWAN, J. M., ROBERTS, C. W., KATSOYANNIS, P. G. & GORDON, J. (1953). The synthesis of an octapeptide amide with the hormonal activity of oxytocin. *J. Amer. chem. Soc.* **75**, 4879–4880.

GERSH, I. (1939). The structure and function of the parenchymatous glandular cells in the neurohypophysis of the rat. *Amer. J. Anat.* **64**, 407–443.

GOMORI, G. (1939). A differential stain for cell types in the pancreatic islets. *Amer. J. Path.* **15**, 497–499.

HILD, W. (1951). Experimentell-morphologische Untersuchungen über das Verhalten der 'Neurosekretorischen Bahn' nach Hypophysenstieldurchtrennungen, Eingriffen in den Wasserhaushalt und Belastung der Osmoregulation. *Virchows Arch.* **319**, 526–546.

HILD, W. & ZETLER, G. (1951). Über das Vorkommen der Hypophysenhinterlappenhormone im Zwischenhirn. *Arch. exp. Path. Pharmak.* **213**, 139–153.

HILD, W. & ZETLER, G. (1952–3). Über die Funktion des Neurosekrets im Zwischenhirn-Hypophysensystem als Trägersubstanz für Vasopressin, Adiuretin und Oxytocin. *Z. ges. exp. Med.* **120**, 236–243.

LAQUEUR, C. (1954). *Recent Progress in Hormone Research*, **10**, p. 233, edited by Pincus, G. New York.

SCHARRER, E. & SCHARRER, B. (1937). Über Drusen-Nervenzellen und neurosekretorische Organe bei Wirbeltiere und Wirbellosen. *Biol. Rev.* **12**, 185–216.

SCHARRER, E. & SCHARRER, B. (1954). *Neurosekretion. Handbuch der mikroskopischen Anatomie des Menschen*, **6**, part 5, 953–1066. Edited by Möllendorf, W. Berlin.

SCHIEBLER, T. H. (1951). Zur Histochemie des neurosekretorischen hypothalamisch-neurohypophysären Systems. *Acta Anat.* **13**, 233–255.

SCHIEBLER, T. H. (1952a). Die chemischen Eigenschaften der neurosekretorischen Substanz in Hypothalamus und Neurohypophyse. *Exp. Cell. Res.* **3**, 249–250.

VOGT, M. (1953). Vasopressor, antidiuretic, and oxytocic activities of extracts of the dog's hypothalamus. *Brit. J. Pharmacol.* **8**, 193–200.

ZUCKERMAN, S. (1954). The secretions of the brain. Relation of hypothalamus to pituitary gland. *Lancet*, **1**, 789–795.

Editor's Comments on Papers 7 and 8

7   HARRIS and JACOBSOHN
    Excerpts from *Functional Grafts of the Anterior Pituitary Gland*

8   NIKITOVITCH-WINER and EVERETT
    Excerpts from *Functional Restitution of Pituitary Grafts Retransplanted from Kidney to Median Eminence*

Harris and Jocobsohn (Paper 7) and Nikitovitch-Winer and Everett (Paper 8) carried out elegant studies that provided conclusive evidence of hypothalamic neural control of adenohypophysial function and showed that this control is mediated via the hypophysial-portal vascular system. Harris and Jacobsohn performed a study to determine whether adenohypophysial tissue vascularized by the hypophysial-portal system functioned differently from that vascularized by the systemic circulation. They found that adenohypophysial tissue transplanted under the median eminence in hypophysectomized rats not only became highly vascularized but also rendered the animals essentially normal with respect to estrus cycles, pregnancy, and lactation and maintenance of normal thyroid and adrenal size. Contrarily, in hypophysectomized rats in which hypophysial grafts were transplanted in the subarachnoid space under the temporal lobe, there was no ability to regain the regulation of sex cycles and normal thyroid or adrenal size, even though the transplant was well vascularized and viable. Thus, this study demonstrated that only when the adenohypophysis receives its blood supply from the median eminence is the adenohypophysis able to exert its role in maintaining normal target gland morphology and function.

Functional grafts of the anterior pituitary gland

By G. W. Harris and Dora Jacobsohn

Physiological Laboratory, University of Cambridge, and Physiological Department, University of Lund, Sweden

A study has been made of pituitary grafts placed into hypophysectomized adult rats under the median eminence of the tuber cinereum, under the temporal lobe of the brain and into the hypophysial capsule. Good union was obtained in all three sites, the grafts becoming richly vascularized and remaining viable for long periods. Grafts placed under the median eminence acquired vascular connexions with the primary plexus of the hypophysial portal vessels, whereas those under the temporal lobe of the brain and in the hypophysial capsule were not supplied by the portal system. Grafts placed under the temporal lobe of the brain and in the hypophysial capsule had greatly diminished, if any, function, but many of those placed under the median eminence of female rats had normal function as judged by (a) oestrous cycles, pregnancy, milk secretion (milk withdrawal from the nipple by the young was impossible, owing to neural lobe deficiency as shown by replacement therapy), (b) ovarian and adrenal weight and histology, (c) thyroid histology. Anterior pituitary tissue obtained from immature donors grafted into adult recipients showed hastened development. Similar tissue obtained from adult male donors grafted into adult female recipients was capable of maintaining normal oestrous cycles and pregnancy. A few experiments using male recipients indicated similar results concerning structure and function of the grafts. These results offer strong support to the view that the secretion of anterior pituitary hormones is under hypothalamic control, mediated by the hypophysial portal vessels.

Introduction

It has long been known that functional transplants (autotransplants and homotransplants in inbred strains) of the majority of endocrine glands may be obtained; as examples from the many accounts in the literature may be quoted: testis, Berthold (1849), Moore (1939); ovary, Marshall & Jolly (1907, 1908), Goodman (1934); thyroid, Loeb (1930), Marine & Rosen (1934); parathyroids, Halsted (1909); adrenal cortex, Ingle, Higgins & Nilson (1938), Eversole, Edelmann & Gaunt (1940). There are no indications in the literature that transplants of the adrenal medulla or posterior pituitary gland maintain normal activity. This may be explained by the fact that these endocrines are functionally dependent on their nerve supply.

The available data concerning the anterior pituitary gland indicate that this gland, which appears to lack a secretomotor innervation, loses its functional capacity after transplantation into hypophysectomized animals (as reported and reviewed by Westman & Jacobsohn 1940; Harris 1948; Cheng, Sayers, Goodman & Swinyard 1949; McDermott, Fry, Brobeck & Long 1950a, b). Of the earlier workers only Hill & Gardner (1935, 1936), May (1935, 1937) and Greep (1936) claim normal function for transplanted anterior pituitary tissue. Hill & Gardner (1935, 1936) used two mice that were later found to be incompletely hypophysectomized, and May

(1935, 1937) used four rats and noted that anterior pituitary function continued after removal of the graft from one of his hypophysectomized animals. Greep (1936) placed the transplanted tissue into the pituitary capsule of hypophysectomized rats. With such a procedure it is difficult to control the completeness of hypophysectomy. In 1942 the position was summarized by Ingle & Griffiths as follows: 'Viable grafts of anterior lobe tissue may be obtained but no method has been established whereby such grafts can be made to maintain a normal level of functional activity.'

It is clear that the anterior pituitary gland is under neural control (Harris 1948), and there is much evidence that such control is mediated by the hypophysial portal vessels (Harris 1950a, b). If the normal stimulus to anterior pituitary activity is transmitted by this vascular system, then it is possible that the failure of anterior pituitary transplants to maintain normal function is due to the fact that portal blood vessels no longer supply the glandular tissue. Therefore in the present work we have investigated the functional activity of anterior pituitary grafts placed in a position whereby they might become revascularized by the hypophysial portal vessels.

[*Editor's Note:* Material has been omitted at this point.]

REFERENCES

Berthold, A. A. 1849 *Arch. Anat. Physiol. wiss. med.* p. 42.
Cheng, C. P., Sayers, G., Goodman, L. S. & Swinyard, C. A. 1949 *Amer. J. Physiol.* **159**, 426.
Eversole, W. J., Edelmann, A. & Gaunt, R. 1940 *Anat. Rec.* **76**, 271.
Goodman, L. 1934. *Anat. Rec.* **59**, 223.
Greep, R. O. 1936 *Proc. Soc. Exp. Biol., N. Y.,* **34**, 754.
Halsted, W. S. 1909 *J. Exp. Med.* **11**, 175.
Harris, G. W. 1948 *Physiol. Rev.* **28**, 139.
Harris, G. W. 1950a *J. Physiol.* **111**, 347.
Harris, G. W. 1950b *Brit. Med. Bull.* **6**, 345.
Hill, R. T. & Gardner, W. U. 1935 *Proc. Soc. Exp. Biol., N. Y.,* **32**, 1382.
Hill, R. T. & Gardner, W. U. 1936 *Proc. Soc. Exp. Biol., N. Y.,* **34**, 78.
Ingle, D. J. & Griffiths, J. Q. 1942 *The rat in laboratory investigation,* p. 383. Ed. by J. Q. Griffiths & E. J. Farris. Philadelphia: J. B. Lippincott Co.
Ingle, D. J., Higgins, G. M. & Nilson, H. W. 1938 *Amer. J. Physiol.* **121**, 650.
Loeb, L. 1930 *Physiol. Rev.* **10**, 547.
McDermott, W. V., Fry, E. G., Brobeck, J. R. & Long, C. N. H. 1950a *Proc. Soc. Exp. Biol., N. Y.,* **73**, 609.
McDermott, W. V., Fry, E. G., Brobeck, J. R. & Long, C. N. H. 1950b *Yale J. Biol. Med.* **23**, 52.
Marine, D. & Rosen, S. H. 1934 *Amer. J. Physiol.* **107**, 677.
Marshall, F. H. A & Jolly, W. A. 1907 *Trans. Roy. Soc. Edinb.* **45**, 589.
Marshall, F. H. A. & Jolly, W. A. 1908 *Quart. J. Exp. Physiol.* **1**, 115.
May, R. M. 1935 *C. R. Soc. Biol., Paris,* **120**, 867.
May, R. M. 1937 *C. R. Soc. Biol., Paris,* **124**, 920.
Moore, C. R. 1939 *Sex and internal secretions,* p. 353. Ed. by E. Allen. London: Ballière, Tindall and Cox.
Westman, A. & Jacobsohn, D. 1940 *Acta path. microbiol. scand.* **17**, 328.

8

Copyright © 1958 by J. B. Lippincott Company

Reprinted from pages 916–918 and 929–930 of *Endocrinology* 63:916–930 (1958)

FUNCTIONAL RESTITUTION OF PITUITARY GRAFTS RE-TRANSPLANTED FROM KIDNEY TO MEDIAN EMINENCE[1]

MIROSLAVA NIKITOVITCH-WINER[2] AND JOHN W. EVERETT

Department of Anatomy, Duke University School of Medicine, Durham, North Carolina

ABSTRACT

The present study is based on the fact that rat pituitaries autografted on the kidney lose power to maintain ovarian follicles and interstitium, although luteotropic function is retained or enhanced. In 62 adult, cycling rats the pars distalis was autotransplanted to the kidney immediately after parapharyngeal hypophysectomy. In the definitive experimental group of 14 rats (MEm-1) the grafts were re-transplanted after 3 to 4 weeks via the transtemporal route into close relation to the median eminence. Estrous cycles returned spontaneously in 13 animals 8 to 68 days later; 7 rats became pregnant. Ovaries, uteri and vaginae were histologically normal save for reduced numbers of follicles and corpora lutea. In another group of 10 rats (MEm-2) grafts were re-transplanted under the median eminence 2 to 3 weeks after the first operation. These were each "primed" later with a short sequence of FSH and LH injections, a treatment of little benefit. Gonadotropin secretion became evident at 11 to 66 days; 3 rats cycled while 4 became persistent-estrous; none was fertile.

In 21 control animals (group TL) in which the graft was re-transplanted from kidney to a site under the temporal lobe and in 17 rats (group Ky) in which the grafts remained on the kidney, there was no sign of return of FSH and/or LH secretion during experimental periods of 30 to 105 days.

Adrenals and thyroids were studied histologically, ACTH was evaluated functionally by adrenal hypertrophy after unilateral adrenalectomy, and TSH was evaluated by thyroid uptake of I^{131}. While residual stimulation of adrenals and thyroids was evident in control groups TL and Ky, there was significant improvement in group MEm-1. Group MEm-2 was not studied.

In the MEm group all grafts were closely adherent to the median eminence. Results clearly demonstrate that the extreme functional deficiencies observed when the pars distalis is removed to sites distant from the hypothalamus are caused by the loss of hypothalmic influences, stimuli that are probably mediated by the hypophysial portal vessels. This is true with respect to secretion of ACTH, TSH, FSH and LH.

TRANSPLANTATION of the pars distalis of the adenohypophysis to sites remote from the hypothalamus in hypophysectomized female rats results in atrophy of the ovarian follicular apparatus and interstitial

---

[1] Supported in part by a grant from the Committee on Research in Problems of Sex, National Academy of Sciences—National Research Council. Additional support was given by the Research council of Duke University.

[2] Present address: Institute of Physiology, University of Lund, Sweden.

tissue, as well as in marked reduction in thyroid and adrenocortical stimulation (1, 2, 3). Somatotropin secretion is probably retained in diminished amount. Luetotropin secretion, on the other hand, is spared and may possibly be increased (3, 4, 5), with the result that recently formed corpora lutea existing at the time of hypophysial transplantation will be stimulated to full activity. This will be indefinitely maintained.

Accompanying the apparent losses of FSH and LH activities and the deficiencies in TSH and ACTH output, there are pronounced changes in cytology of the pars distalis graft. The predominant cell types that can be recognized in routinely stained material (3, 4, 6) are judged to be small chromophobes and modified acidophiles. Recent investigation with the aldehyde-fuchsin (AF), periodic acid-Schiff (PAS) and other techniques indicate that occasional minute beta and delta basophiles are retained for long periods (7), and that the acidophiles are characteristically orangeophilic in Azan preparations (6).

Not only does one find these qualitative changes in cytology in the transplanted gland, but there is also a predictable quantitative loss of parenchyma caused by the massive central infarction (7). The healthy parenchyma of the graft derives from a relatively thin shell of tissue not involved in the infarct.

The several functional deficiencies mentioned could be ascribed to the extensive quantitative loss, perhaps in combination with unrecognized damage in the remaining parenchyma consequent to manipulation of the gland and to its temporary deprivation of blood supply. The cytologic changes could be thought of as an expression of such damaging action. Other facts, however, do not agree with that view and indicate that a close neurovascular relationship of the pars distalis to the hypothalamus is required for normal gland activities. The present study emphatically supports that contention by demonstrating the return of reasonably normal functions and cytology after the re-transplantation of a long-established renal autograft of pars distalis to a site immediately under the median eminence.

These experiments are based on those of Greep (8), and Harris and Jacobsohn (2). Greep found reproductive functions well preserved in hypophysectomized rats if the hypophyses were simply replaced in their original sites. The impossibility of histologic control, however, lent unavoidable uncertainty to the interpretation of the result. Harris and Jacobsohn eliminated this fault by introducing the transplant directly beneath the median eminence via the trans-temporal route, immediately after parapharyngeal hypophysectomy. The hypophysial capsule thus could be searched later on for remnants. These authors used post-partum mothers as recipients in most cases, transplanting 5 to 11 pituitaries from members of the animal's own litter into each host. While such grafts placed under the temporal lobe of the brain failed to sustain ovarian function, those under the median eminence usually became functional in a short time. Not only did estrous cycles return, but many rats experienced normal pregnancy with spontaneous parturition. With respect to thyroid and adrenal function, the somewhat limited data reported indicate "normal" maintenance by grafts under the median eminence, but complete or partial atrophy in the temporal lobe controls. Here was substantial demonstration that some influence mediated by the median eminence, presumably chemical and transmitted by hypophysial portal vessels, is essential for most normal functions of the pars distalis.

Our findings agree with this and go further by showing that an animal's own hypophysis, after losing its ability to support ovarian functions other than progestational when the gland is removed from the influence of the tuber cinereum, will regain them when this influence is restored. Analogous restoration of thyroid and adrenal function is also documented. Preliminary experiments of this kind were reported last year (9, 10) in a group of 13 rats among which 5 resumed estrous cycles and 3 became pregnant. That work has now been amplified, and most of the grafts of the experimental and control series have been studied cytologically. The cytologic features are described elsewhere (7).

Experimental plan. The general plan remains unchanged, one group of animals receiving re-transplants under the median eminence, another receiving re-transplants under the temporal lobe, and a third group retaining the grafts in the renal capsule. There were a few minor modifications. Estrogen priming was omitted, but in part of the median eminence group a brief priming with extrinsic FSH and LH was administered—unnecessarily, it seems. The definitive median eminence group was not primed in any way. In all but one animal of that group, the graft was left on the kidney for a full month before re-transplantation. Finally, any possible complications that might have been introduced by persisting functional corpora lutea were avoided by carrying out the initial transplantations to the renal capsule during proestrus (5).

[*Editor's Note:* Material has been omitted at this point.]

DISCUSSION

Circumstances which distinguish the results of re-transplantation from those of direct transplantation of the fresh gland to the median eminence region immediately after hypophysectomy are (a) that the gland is twice insulted—severely so, in fact (7), and (b) that while in the kidney the gland undergoes an apparent functional de-differentiation with accompanying cytologic regression. It is all the more surprising and significant, therefore, to have encountered the high degree of functional restoration in the large proportion of animals in the median eminence groups.

This improved frequency of success in contrast to the small number in the preliminary experiments (9, 10) may be ascribed to greater uniformity achieved in placing the graft and, possibly, to the fact that special effort was made to strip off encapsulating connective tissue. In several failures of the preliminary series histologic examination of the graft and adjacent brain had disclosed a considerable sheet of connective tissue which might well have constituted a partial barrier.

The priming treatments proved to be of little value, either the small amounts of estrogen used in the preliminary series or the FSH-LH injections in group MEm-2. One may properly assume that in all animals in which cycling was restored this took place entirely spontaneously. The FSH-LH treatment appears to have been deleterious in one respect, seemingly having brought about persistent estrus in several cases. The reason is not apparent.

There was a detectable amount of functional recovery in even the four members of groups MEm-1 and MEm-2 that failed to cycle. Ovarian stimulation was evidenced by interstitial-cell repair in local areas, occasional theca luteinization and moderate estrogenic stimulation of the vagina and uteri. There was little indication of increased follicle development, however. The reason is not evident why these ovaries were not better stimulated, for the grafts were very well placed. There is a possibility of hypothalamic damage in the one failure of group MEm-1; the graft was imbedded in a cleft in the tuber.

Inspection of serial sections of the grafts disclosed no greater volume of parenchyma after re-transplantation under the median eminence than one usually finds in established grafts in the renal capsule. In fact, the trend was in the other direction. By contrast with the normal gland, the amount of parenchyma in even the best examples of the median eminence series was clearly rather small. This quantitative deficiency affords a ready explanation for the fact that ovarian weights, numbers of follicles and corpora lutea in each set, thyroid uptake of I^{131}, adrenal weight and adrenal hypertrophy after hemiadrenalectomy were all less than in the normal rat. Only thyroid weights were equivalent. However, one must admit that the initial atrophy of the target tissues may have contributed to the end result by impairing their ability to respond.

Grafts under the temporal lobe were characteristically smaller than those on the kidney or under the median eminence. In this respect, they constitute less satisfactory controls than those left on the kidney. Nevertheless, several were shown to be competent sources of luteotropin, a fact which attests to their vitality, and there was no cytologic restoration to suggest changes in function from that prevailing in the kidney site.

It should now be fully evident that the extreme deficiencies observed when the pars distalis is removed to sites distant from the hypothalamus result from the loss of hypothalamic influences. The observations contribute additional strong evidence of humoral mediation of these stimuli, on the basis of the well documented opinion that the hypophysial portal circulation constitutes the principal link between median eminence and pars distalis (1, 15). The rapid onset of renewed gonadotropic function in a few animals of the median eminence series agrees with the known rapidity of regeneration of these portal venues (11).

Greater vigor of TSH and ACTH secretion in the median eminence groups, compared with controls bearing grafts on the kidney or under the temporal lobe, demonstrates that for even these functions the rat pars distalis depends importantly on hypothalamic stimuli. Our findings agree with others in this respect (16) and, on the other hand, with the numerous observations that a residual secretion of TSH and ACTH can proceed without close linkage of the pars distalis with the hypothalamus. Comparable residual secretion of FSH and LH, although not denied by this study, is clearly below levels that can be detected by the present methods

REFERENCES

1. Harris, G. W.: Neural Control of the Pituitary Gland. Edward Arnold, Ltd., London. 1955.
2. Harris, G. W. and Dora Jacobsohn: *Proc. Roy. Soc., London* **B139**: 263. 1952.
3. Everett, J. W.: *Endocrinology* **54**: 685. 1954.
4. Everett, J. W.: *Endocrinology* **58**: 786. 1956.
5. Nikitovitch-Winer, M. and J. W. Everett: *Endocrinology* **62**: 522. 1958.
6. Sanders, A. and E. G. Rennels: *Anat. Rec.* **127**: 360. 1957.
7. Nikitovitch-Winer, M. and J. W. Everett: (Manuscript in preparation).
8. Greep, R. O.: *Proc. Soc. Exper. Biol. and Med.* **34**: 754. 1936.
9. Nikitovitch-Winer, M. and J. W. Everett: *Fed. Proc.* **16**: 94. 1957.
10. Nikitovitch-Winer, M. and J. W. Everett: *Nature (London)* **180**: 1434. 1957.
11. Harris, G. W.: *J. Physiol.* **111**: 347. 1950.
12. Elftman, H.: *Stain Technol.* **32**: 25. 1957.
13. Everett, J. W.: *Anat. Rec.* **124**: 287. 1956.
14. Meyer, R. K., M. R. N. Prasad and R. L. Cochrane: *Anat. Rec.* **130**: 339. 1958.
15. Benoit, J. and I. Assenmacher: *J. de Physiol.* **47**: 427. 1955.
16. Sayers, G., E. S. Redgate and P. C. Royce: *Ann. Rev. Physiol.* **20**: 243. 1958.

ERRATUM

Page 917, line 3 should read: "amount. Luteotropin secretion, . . ."

Part II
THE HYPOTHALAMIC-HYPOPHYSIAL-ADRENOCORTICAL AXIS

Editor's Comments
on Papers 9, 10, and 11

9   de GROOT and HARRIS
    Excerpts from *Hypothalamic Control of the Anterior Pituitary Gland and Blood Lymphocytes*

10 FORTIER, HARRIS, and McDONALD
    Excerpts from *The Effect of Pituitary Stalk Section on the Adrenocortical Response to Stress in the Rabbit*

11 GUILLEMIN and ROSENBERG
    Excerpts from *Humoral Hypothalamic Control of Anterior Pituitary: A Study with Combined Tissue Cultures*

The first study demonstrating that adenohypophysial secretion of adrenocorticotropic hormone (ACTH) is under hypothalamic control was that of deGroot and Harris (Paper 9). They observed that electrical stimulation of the posterior median eminence and mammary body led to increased ACTH release in rabbits, indirectly determined by production of lymphopenia. They further demonstrated that placement of lesions in the posterior median eminence, mammary body, and portal vasculature (zona tuberalis) abolished the lymphopenic response to stress in rabbits. They noted that the lymphopenia associated with electrical stimulation of the median eminence and mammary body was similar temporally and in magnitude to that associated with emotional stress. Contrarily, electrical stimulation of other regions of the hypothalamus, of the pars and zona tuberalis, pars distalis, and pars intermedia of the hypophysis and infundibulum did not elicit a lymphopenic response. These results indicated that adenohypophysial secretion of ACTH is under hypothalamic neural control mediated via hypophysialportal vessel connection with the adenohypophysis. They emphasized the importance of avoiding incidental emotional stress while conducting studies of control of adrenocortical function.

Fortier, Harris, and McDonald (Paper 10) performed another important physiological study of the effects of hypophysial stalk section on the adrenocortical response to stress using lymphopenia and adrenal ascorbic acid depletion as indicators of ACTH release from the adeno-

Editor's Comments on Papers 9, 10, and 11

hypophysis. The effects of stalk resection were determined in rabbits subjected to a large variety of physically and emotionally stressful stimuli. Plates were placed between the sectioned ends of portal vasculature; nevertheless, varying degrees of portal vessel regeneration occurred. In those animals in which there was significant portal vessel regeneration, a normal lymphopenic response to stress occurred. In the animals in which little or no portal regeneration developed, the lymphopenic response to stress was abolished. They concluded that there was a good correlation between regeneration of the hypothalamo-hypophysial neurovascular connections and the return of the ACTH response to stressful stimuli acting through the CNS. They also noted a direct correlation between ovarian and genital tract atrophy and lack of regeneration of portal vessels. This study further elucidated the dependence of intact hypothalamo-hypophysial connections on ACTH and gonadotropin secretion, as noted in earlier studies conducted by Harris and others.

The fact that a chemical substance capable of releasing an adenohypophysial hormone could be extracted from the hypothalamic infundibulum was demonstrated by Guillemin and Rosenberg (Paper 11). In this study they showed that crude hypothalamic extracts induced the release of ACTH from cultured adenohypophysial tissue. They further demonstrated that acetylcholine, epinephrine, norepinephrine, and 5-hydroxytrytophane were not releasing factors for ACTH. They proposed that there exists a hypothalamic-hypophysial mediator involved in ACTH secretion that is not a central biogenic amine. The work of these investigators as well as that of Schally and his co-workers, in attempting to identify a corticotropin releasing factor (CRF), established the in-vitro hypophysial tissue system as an invaluable bioassay tool for the study of hypothalamic-hypophysial releasing agents. This early work, aimed at obtaining CRF active extracts from median eminence tissue, paved the way toward development of the more sophisticated methodology that eventually allowed Guillemin and Schally to identify and elucidate the structure of thyrotropin-releasing and luteinizing-releasing hormone. Guillemin and Rosenberg described the three orders of evidence to ascertain endocrine activity: demonstration of a deficiency syndrome following extirpation of the endocrine tissue, correction of the deficit subsequent to replacement therapy and purification and isolation of the corresponding hormonal principles and demonstration of their activity.

HYPOTHALAMIC CONTROL OF THE ANTERIOR PITUITARY GLAND AND BLOOD LYMPHOCYTES

By J. DE GROOT AND G. W. HARRIS

From the Physiological Laboratory, University of Cambridge

(*Received* 6 *December* 1949)

It has been shown that the secretion of the anterior pituitary gland is essential to the development of an acute lymphopenia following emotional stress (Dougherty & White, 1944; Colfer, de Groot & Harris, 1950). The probable sequence may be represented: emotional stress (nervous system)—adenohypophysis—adrenal cortex—lymphopenia. It was decided: (*a*) to stimulate various regions of the hypothalamus and pituitary gland electrically, to see whether secretion by the anterior pituitary with a resultant lymphopenia could be so induced; and (*b*) to place lesions in different parts of the hypothalamus and pituitary to see whether the lymphopenia that follows emotional stress in normal rabbits could be blocked. In this way it was hoped to obtain evidence relevant to hypothalamic control of pituitary secretion and the anatomical pathways by which any such control was mediated.

Although the lymphopenia that follows anterior pituitary secretion is the most rapid and easily observed indicator of such activity available, care must be taken in using this reaction that the animal is not subjected to incidental emotional stress in the course of the experiment. Therefore, in order to stimulate the hypothalamus and pituitary gland electrically in the unanaesthetized *quiescent* rabbit, it became necessary to use a specialized technique.

[*Editor's Note:* Material has been omitted at this point.]

DISCUSSION

The lymphopenic response has been found of great value in the present study in indicating anterior pituitary activity. When using this response it is essential to work without anaesthesia and with quiescent animals. For this purpose the method of electrical stimulation used was very satisfactory. Incidental emotional stress during the course of an experiment may produce a lymphopenia which repetition of the experiment shows was not due to the electric stimulation. A single positive response in an animal is not significant, whereas a single negative result is highly significant. We should also like to stress the importance of being able to repeat an experiment many times on any individual animal. This allows the elimination of many variable factors (changes in diet, external temperature, phase of sex cycle and so on), and enables definite conclusions to be drawn from the study of fewer animals than would otherwise be possible.

It has been shown that emotional stress produces a lymphopenia in the normal, but not in the hypophysectomized rabbit (Colfer *et al.* 1950). The mechanism by which the nervous system causes anterior pituitary secretion (of probably the adrenocorticotrophic hormone) and so a lymphopenia has received little attention in the past. The observation of Mikkelsen & Hutchens (1948), that electric shock therapy in man is followed by a lymphopenia 3 hr. later, made it seem likely that some part of the neural mechanism underlying the response would be excitable to electric stimulation. This is so, for localized stimulation of the posterior part of the tuber cinereum or mammillary body has been found to produce a lymphopenic response similar to that following emotional stress. The evidence indicates that transverse lesions in the posterior part of the tuber cinereum or mammillary body, or lesions in the zona tuberalis of the pituitary gland, abolish the response to emotional stress. It is felt that the evidence derived from study of the lesions is not so clear cut as that derived from the study of stimulation. However, both lines of approach indicate the same conclusions.

The stimulus from hypothalamus to hypophysis does not pass by way of the cervical sympathetic system, as shown by the fact that cervical sympathectomy does not abolish the lymphopenia following stimulation of the tuber cinereum. The tubero-hypophysial tract of nerve fibres runs through the posterior wall of the tuber cinereum (Fisher, Ingram & Ranson, 1935) and is possibly concerned with the transmission of the stimulus. The most likely anatomical pathway involved between hypothalamus and adenohypophysis is the hypophysial stalk. Following Rioch, Wislocki & O'Leary (1940), the term hypophysial stalk is taken to include the neural stalk together with its sheath of portions of the glandular lobe. There are two possible pathways between hypothalamus and the anterior pituitary gland in the hypophysial stalk: either the hypothalamo-hypophysial nerve tract, or the hypophysial portal vessels contained in the pars and zona tuberalis (see Text-fig. 2).

Transmission of stimuli to anterior pituitary cells by means of the hypothalamo-hypophysial nerve fibres seems unlikely. Most workers find that nerve fibres passing from neurohypophysis to adenohypophysis are very scanty in number, if present at all. A few fibres have been described, however (see Harris, 1948c), as passing from the supraoptico-hypophysial tract in the median eminence to the pars and zona tuberalis, and from the infundibular stem and process to the pars intermedia. It appears unlikely that either of these sets of fibres is concerned in the lymphopenic response for the following reasons: (i) stimulation of the supraoptico-hypophysial tract in the median eminence (B, in Text-fig. 2) or the infundibular stem (C) does not evoke a lymphopenia; (ii) stimulation of the zona tuberalis (D) does not evoke a lymphopenia; (iii) interruption of the infundibular stem (C) does not prevent a lymphopenic response following emotional stress.

Transmission of stimuli to anterior pituitary cells by means of a humoral agent carried from the median eminence to the pars distalis via the hypophysial portal vessels seems probable. It has been suggested (Harris, 1944; Green & Harris, 1947) that the hypothalamus may influence anterior pituitary secretion by a two-link chain: nerve fibres passing from the hypothalamus to the median eminence where they liberate a humoral transmitter into the hypophysial portal vessels, which in turn carry the substance to the pars distalis. This theory is in accordance with the facts noted in the present work. Electrical stimulation of the posterior part of the tuber cinereum evokes a lymphopenia, possibly through stimulation of nerve fibres which are passing to the primary plexus of the portal vessels in the median eminence. The fact that a lymphopenia is not produced by electrical stimulation of the pars distalis, pars intermedia, pars or zona tuberalis of the pituitary gland may be because the adenohypophysis lacks a secreto-motor nerve supply and is humorally controlled. Again lesions of the zona tuberalis block the lymphopenia which normally follows emotional stress (even though electrical stimulation of this structure does not evoke the response), and this may be due to the fact that all the portal vessels traverse the zona tuberalis in passing to the main part of the pars distalis (Harris, 1947a).

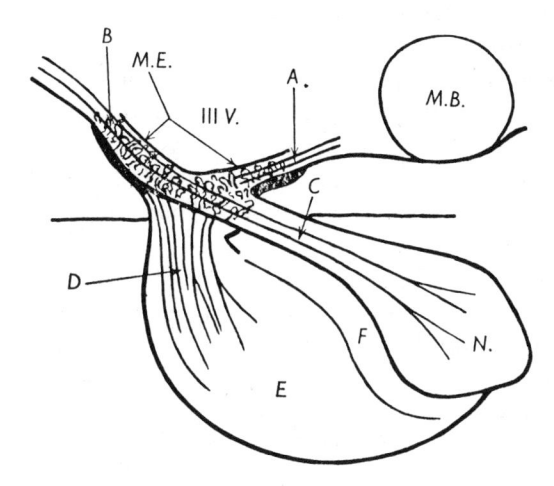

Text-fig. 2. Diagram of a sagittal section through the hypothalamus and pituitary gland of a rabbit, to illustrate the anatomy and to summarize the results obtained. *A*, posterior wall of the tuber cinereum containing the tuberohypophysial tract (stimulation evokes lymphopenia; most lesions here block lymphopenic response to emotional stress); *B*, anterior wall of the tuber cinereum containing the supraopticohypophysial tract (stimulation negative); *C*, infundibular stem (stimulation negative; lesions do not abolish lymphopenic response); *D*, zona tuberalis containing the trunks of the portal vessels and possibly some nerve fibres from the supraopticohypophysial tract (stimulation negative; lesions block lymphopenic response to emotional stress); *E*, main part of pars distalis (stimulation negative; subtotal lesions do not block lymphopenic response); *F*, pars intermedia; *M.B.*, mammillary body; *M.E.*, median eminence, surrounded by the very vascular collar of pars tuberalis, and containing the primary plexus of the hypophysial portal vessels; *N.*, neural lobe of the hypophysis; III *V.*, third ventricle.

It is of interest that the evidence indicates the hypophysial portal vessels as the pathway underlying humoral control of the secretion of gonadotrophic hormone(s) in the rabbit (Harris, 1948b) and in the rat (Harris, 1950). The work of Markee and his colleagues (Markee, Sawyer & Hollinshead, 1948; Sawyer, Markee & Townsend, 1949; Sawyer, Everett & Markee, 1949; Everett, Sawyer & Markee, 1949) indicates that an adrenergic substance humorally excites the secretion of gonadotrophic hormone(s), and that the action of this substance may be blocked by sympatholytic drugs, such as dibenamine. It would be of interest to see whether sympatholytic drugs also blocked the lymphopenic response to emotional stress.

SUMMARY

1. Electrical stimulation of the posterior region of the tuber cinereum or of the mammillary body, of unanaesthetized, unrestrained rabbits resulted in a lymphopenia, which was similar in time relations and magnitude to that following an emotional stress stimulus. Cervical sympathectomy did not abolish this response. Electrical stimulation of certain other regions in the hypothalamus (including the supraopticohypophysial tract), of the pars and zona tuberalis, pars distalis, pars intermedia and infundibular stem of the pituitary gland did not elicit the response.

2. The lymphopenic response which follows an emotional stress stimulus in normal rabbits was abolished by lesions in the zona tuberalis (two cases), and, in most cases, was abolished or diminished by transverse lesions in the posterior region of the tuber cinereum or in the mammillary body. Similar lesions in the pars distalis and pars intermedia, and lesions which interrupt the infundibular stem, were compatible with normal responses.

3. The conclusion is drawn that anterior pituitary secretion (of probably the adrenocorticotrophic hormone) is under neural control via the hypothalamus and the hypophysial portal vessels of the pituitary stalk.

We are grateful to Mr L. Hatton for the radiography and microphotography involved in this work, and to Mr R. R. W. Dye for valuable technical assistance and for his care of the animals. Our thanks are also due to Mr L. Herbert, of the Research Laboratories of the British Thompson-Houston Company, Ltd., Rugby, for advice on the ignitron circuit.

REFERENCES

Chaffee, E. L. & Light, R. U. (1934). *Yale J. Biol. Med.* **7**, 83.
Colfer, H. F., de Groot, J. & Harris, G. W. (1950). *J. Physiol.* **111**, 328.
Dougherty, T. F. & White, A. (1944). *Endocrinology*, **35**, 1.
Everett, J. W., Sawyer, C. H. & Markee, J. E. (1949). *Endocrinology*, **44**, 234.
Fisher, C., Ingram, W. R. & Ranson, S. W. (1935). *Arch. Neurol. Psychiat., Chicago*, **34**, 124.
Green, J. D. & Harris, G. W. (1947). *J. Endocrinol.* **5**, 136.
Harris, G. W. (1937). *Proc. Roy. Soc.* B, **122**, 374.
Harris, G. W. (1944). Thesis for M.D. degree. Cambridge University.
Harris, G. W. (1947a). *J. Anat., Lond.*, **81**, 343.
Harris, G. W. (1947b). *Philos. Trans.* B, **232**, 385.
Harris, G. W. (1948a). *J. Physiol.* **107**, 412.
Harris, G. W. (1948b). *J. Physiol.* **107**, 418.
Harris, G. W. (1948c). *Physiol. Rev.* **28**, 139.
Harris, G. W. (1950). *J. Physiol.* **111**, 347.
Jacobsohn, D. & Westman, A. (1940). *Acta Physiol. Scand.* **1**, 71.
Markee, J. E., Sawyer, C. H. & Hollinshead, W. H. (1948). *Rec. Progr. Horm. Res.* **2**, 117.
Mikkelsen, W. P. & Hutchens, T. T. (1948). *Endocrinology*, **42**, 394.
Rioch, D. McK., Wislocki, G. B. & O'Leary, J. L. (1940). *Res. Publ. Ass. nerv. ment. Dis.*, **20**, 3.
Sawyer, C. H., Everett, J. W. & Markee, J. E. (1949). *Endocrinology*, **44**, 218.
Sawyer, C. H., Markee, J. E. & Townsend, B. F. (1949). *Endocrinology*, **44**, 18.

THE EFFECT OF PITUITARY STALK SECTION ON THE ADRENOCORTICAL RESPONSE TO STRESS IN THE RABBIT

BY C. FORTIER,* G. W. HARRIS AND I. R. McDONALD†

From the Department of Neuroendocrinology, Institute of Psychiatry, Maudsley Hospital, London

(*Received* 10 *December* 1956)

It is now generally agreed that the hypothalamus exerts a controlling influence over the release of adrenocorticotrophic hormone (ACTH) from the anterior pituitary gland. Electrical stimulation of various hypothalamic regions have been found to result in a lymphopenia or eosinopenia (de Groot & Harris, 1950; Hume & Wittenstein, 1950; Hume, 1953; Porter, 1953, 1954) in the rabbit, dog, cat and monkey. Also, hypothalamic lesions have been found to abolish the adrenocorticotrophic response to stressful or noxious stimuli (de Groot & Harris, 1950; Hume & Wittenstein, 1950; Hume, 1953; McCann, 1953; Laqueur, McCann, Schreiner, Rosemberg, Rioch & Anderson, 1953; Porter, 1953, 1954) in the rabbit, dog, rat, cat and monkey. However, it is uncertain whether the hypothalamus and its connexions with the adenohypophysis are necessary for the mediation of the ACTH response to all types of stressful stimuli. Several groups of workers (Cheng, Sayers, Goodman & Swinyard, 1949b; McDermott, Fry, Brobeck & Long, 1950b; Fortier, 1951) have found that intra-ocular pituitary transplants in the hypophysectomized rat may be stimulated to release ACTH by unilateral adrenalectomy and by injection of histamine or adrenaline. Fortier (1951) found that such rats did not show an ACTH response after exposure to loud sounds or forced immobilization, and on these grounds divided stresses into two groups: (1) neurotropic stresses (such as loud sounds and forced immobilization), those that elicit ACTH discharge by an action solely through the central nervous system; and (2) systemic stress (such as administration of adrenaline), which may act by producing chemical or metabolic changes in the general blood stream as well as by

* Present address: Bluebird Neurological Research Laboratories, Methodist Hospital, Texas Medical Center, Houston, Texas, U.S.A.

† Present address: Physiology Department, University of Melbourne, Carlton N3, Victoria, Australia.

an action through the nervous system. The anatomical pathway by which the hypothalamus influences anterior pituitary secretion of ACTH appears to be the hypophysial portal vessels, which pass from the tuber cinereum down the pituitary stalk to the anterior lobe. Electrolytic lesions placed in these vessels in the zona tuberalis of the rabbit's pituitary were found to abolish the lymphopenic response to emotional stress (de Groot & Harris, 1950); the return of the lymphopenic response to stress in the pituitary stalk-sectioned mouse was found to be correlated with regeneration of the portal vessels between the stalk ends (de Groot, 1952); and the maintenance of a normal adrenal cortex in the hypophysectomized rat bearing a pituitary transplant was observed to be dependent on the vascularization of the grafted tissue by the portal vessels (Harris & Jacobsohn, 1952). Recent studies made with the electron-microscope show *no* nerve fibres in relation to parenchymal cells within the confines of the pars distalis of the pituitary (M. G. Farquhar & J. F. Rinehart, personal communication; S. L. Palay, personal communication); such a finding is compatible with the above thesis. The factors controlling anterior pituitary activity have recently been reviewed (Harris, 1955).

In order to define further the control exerted by the hypothalamus over pituitary-adrenal function, and the mechanism whereby this control is exerted, a study has been made of the effect, on the adrenocorticotrophic response to different stimuli, of dividing the pituitary stalk in the rabbit. The stimuli used consisted of procedures calculated to produce (1) predominantly nervous or emotional excitation without physical damage (restraint, exposure to cold), or (2) tissue trauma or metabolic disturbances (laparotomy, injection of adrenaline). A fall in blood lymphocytes at the third hour after the beginning of the stressful procedure was taken as a criterion of adrenal cortical activation. As a further test of the adrenocorticotrophic response to trauma, the adrenal ascorbic acid concentration of the right adrenal gland was compared with that of the left gland which had been surgically removed one and a half hours previously.

[*Editor's Note:* Material has been omitted at this point.]

SUMMARY

1. The pituitary stalk was divided in 42 rabbits, using a fronto-temporal approach. A waxed-paper plate was inserted between the cut ends in 29 of these animals. Groups of these rabbits were used for investigating (a) the effects of a variety of stress stimuli in activating the pituitary-adrenal axis, and (b) the effect of pituitary stalk section on pituitary volume, adrenal gland weight and ovarian activity and weight. The results of these observations were compared with similar observations in 37 normal rabbits and 25 hypophysectomized animals.

2. Examination of thick serial sections through the pituitary region of the stalk-sectioned rabbits revealed that regeneration of the hypophysial portal vessels had occurred to a marked extent in 'simple stalk-sectioned' animals, and to a slight and variable degree in 'stalk-sectioned animals with plates.'

3. Stalk section followed by little or no regeneration of the portal vessels reduced or abolished the lymphopenic response to restraint and exposure to cold, but exerted little effect on the response to injection of adrenaline or laparotomy or on the adrenal ascorbic acid depletion following unilateral adrenalectomy. These findings support the view that environmental stimuli may be divided into two types: those that affect ACTH secretion solely by an action through the central nervous system, and those that act also by affecting the composition of the blood in the systemic circulation.

4. A correlation was found between the incidence of portal vessel regeneration and the recurrence of the lymphopenic response to the stress of restraint.

5. A significant degree of adrenal atrophy was observed to follow pituitary stalk section in all animals.

6. Ovarian atrophy following stalk section was limited to those cases in which portal vessel regeneration was effectively prevented. The 6 animals in which the greatest degree of portal vessel regeneration occurred showed ovaries of normal weight, and 2 of these animals showed the usual reflex response of ovulation consequent on coitus. Marked atrophy of the ovaries and genital tract was observed in those animals subjected to stalk section in which little or no portal vessel regeneration occurred.

7. These findings are discussed in the light of previous studies on the effect of stalk section, pituitary transplantation and hypothalamic lesions.

REFERENCES

Cheng, C. P., G. Sayers, L. S. Goodman, and C. A. Swinyard. 1949b. Discharge of Adrenocorticotrophic Hormone from Transplanted Pituitary Tissue. *Am. J. Physiol.* **159**:426–432.

de Groot, J. 1952. *The Significance of the Portal System.* M.D. thesis, Univ. Amsterdam, Van Goreum and Co.

de Groot, J., and W. Harris. 1950. Hypothalamic Control of the Anterior Pituitary and Blood Lymphocytes. *J. Physiol.* **111**:335–346.

Fortier, C. 1954. Dual Control of Adrenocorticotrophin Release. *Endocrinology* **49**:782–788.

Harris, G. W. 1955. *Neural Control of the Pituitary Gland.* London: Edward Arnold Ltd.

Harris, G. W., and D. Jacobsohn. 1952. Functional Grafts of the Anterior Pituitary Gland. *R. Soc. London Proc.*, ser. B, **139**:263–276.

Hume, D. M. 1953. The Neuroendocrine Response to Injury: Present Status of the Problem. *Ann. Surg.* **138**:548–557.

Hume, D. M., and G. J. Wittenstein. 1950. The Relationship of the Hypothalamus to Pituitary-Adrenocortical Function. *Proc. 1st Clin. ACTH Conf.*, J. R. Mote, ed. pp. 134–146.

Laqueur, G. L., S. M. McCann, L. H. Schreiner, E. Rosemberg, D. M. Rioch, and E. Anderson. 1953. Alterations of Adrenal-cortical and Ovarian Acitivity Following Hypothalamic Lesions. *Endocrinology* **57**:44–54.

McCann, S. M. 1953. Effects of Hyophalamic Lesions on the Adrenal Cortical Response to Stress in the Rat. *Am. J. Physiol.* **175**:13–20.

McDermott, W. V., E. G. Fry, J. R. Brobeck, and C. N. H. Long. 1950b. Release of Adreno-corticotrophic Hormone by Direct Application of Epinephrine to Pituitary Grafts. *Soc. Exp. Biol. N. Y. Proc.* **73**:609–610.

Porter, R. W. 1953. Hypothalamic Involvement in the Pituitary-Adrenocortical Response to Stress Stimuli. *Am. J. Physiol.* **172**:515–519.

Porter, R. W. 1954. The Central Nervous System and Stress-Induced Casinopenia. *Recent Prog. Hormone Res.* **10**:1–18.

HUMORAL HYPOTHALAMIC CONTROL OF ANTERIOR PITUITARY: A STUDY WITH COMBINED TISSUE CULTURES

ROGER GUILLEMIN[1] AND BARRY ROSENBERG

Department of Physiology, Baylor University College of Medicine, Texas Medical Center, Houston, Texas

THE current concepts of hypothalamo-pituitary relationships are based on the results of numerous *in vivo* experiments (Harris, 1951; Fortier, 1951; McCann, 1953; Hume, 1949; Benoit and Assenmacher, 1953). The possibility of investigating this problem by simple *in vitro* techniques was particularly challenging in view of a number of findings which suggested the necessity of some hypothalamic factor, so far overlooked, for the release of pituitary hormones *in vitro*. Indeed, conflicting results are to be found in the literature regarding possible secretion of hormones by the various endocrines in tissue cultures. If we consider the anterior lobe of the pituitary, it has been reported as able to produce gonadotrophins (Rosenberg, 1954), or growth hormone (Gaillard, 1948; Martinovitch, 1953) whereas other investigators concluded that it could not secrete gonadotrophins (Cutting and Lewis, 1938) or any hormone whatever (Anderson and Haymaker, 1935). It appears from a study of this literature that, whenever hormonal production has been found at all, it has always been early (4-5 days) after explantation of the tissue; older cultures of the anterior pituitary, though producing a good outgrowth, yield negative results in hormonal assays. To test the hypothesis of the necessity of of a hypothalamic factor for pituitary activation *in vitro*, we therefore decided 1) to study the release of one hormone (ACTH) in cultures of the adenohypophysis as a function of time; 2) to investigate whether the ACTH secretion could be modified by adding to the tissue cultures of the pituitary, fragments of hypothalamic tissue. A simple "direct" assay procedure for hypothalamic hypophysiotropic activity was contemplated along the same lines, should any specific effect due to the hypothalamic tissue be demonstrable.

[1] Scholar of the John and Mary R. Markle Foundation.

[*Editor's Note:* Material has been omitted at this point.]

DISCUSSION

The results of these *in vitro* experiments are best interpreted in terms of a humoral (as opposed to a neural) mechanism. To ascertain endocrine activity, the classical rules of endocrinology require three orders of evidence: a) demonstration of a deficiency syndrome following extirpation of the alleged endocrine tissue; b) correction of the deficit subsequent to replacement therapy (auto or homo-graft, administration of crude extracts); c) purification and isolation of the corresponding hormonal principles and demonstration of its (or their) activity. There is considerable evidence nowadays for a "deficiency syndrome" in the function of the adenohypophysis following destruction of the hypothalamus in the otherwise intact animal (Harris, 1951, 1954; Hume, 1949; Ganong and Hume, 1954; McCann, 1953; Anand, 1954). On the other hand, restoration of normal pituitary function after "replacement therapy" with hypothalamic extracts and isolation of corresponding stimulatory principles have been advanced on questionable evidence. The difficulties inherent to both phases of the problem, in working with the whole animal, are numerous for reasons of techniques and perhaps unsurmountable for reasons of logic (cf. Fortier's theory of a dual control for ACTH release; Fortier, 1952). The *in vitro* experiments reported here, have shown: a) that the pituitary "deficiency syndrome" is easily demonstrable; b) that it is corrected by introduction of hypothalamic tissues in the *in vitro* pituitary system. Furthermore, specificity of action of the hypothalamic tissue can be reasonably inferred from the data obtained with control tissues and the bioassays of the various fluids for epinephrine, acetylcholine, histamine, etc. Regarding the role of these various autonomic substances as possible mediators for pituitary ACTH release, the failure to demonstrate them with our methods in the *in vitro* system is in keeping with the conclusions reached by entirely different methods *in vivo* (Guillemin, 1954, 1955).

Such an *in vitro* technique or some modification of it, may prove to be of value as a possible bioassay in the isolation of hypothalamic neuro-humoral substances related to pituitary functions.

The literature on *in vitro* cultivation of nervous cells and nervous tissue is extensive (see bibliography in Murray and Kopech, 1953). There is no doubt that nervous cells, even the highly specialized cells of adult organisms, can be maintained *in vitro* for any length of time. The recent study with similar techniques of the dynamic changes produced in the cells of the nucleus supra-opticus by hypo- and hyper-tonic solutions (Hild, 1954) is another example of the adequacy of the tissue culture method for elements of the central nervous system.

The "amounts of ACTH activity" found in these experiments, though we never attempted to quantitate our assays, are in agreement with Sayers and Sydnor (1954) if we compare their dilution factors of the whole pituitary in some of their assays and the amount of tissues used in tissue culture techniques. The fact that ACTH was found at all in our conditions (incubation for several days with tissues, at $37.5-38°$ C., in an absolutely neutral medium) may be more surprising in view of the alleged susceptibility of ACTH to proteolytic enzymes especially at non-acid pH. It may be that the nutrient fluid used in these experiments, known for years by tissue culturists to be the optimal medium, is effective because of its high content in inhibitors of proteolytic ferments.

It was of interest to note the dissociation between morphology and function of the hypophysial outgrowth. Outgrowth from the primary explant and differentiation from the early undifferentiated "fibroblast-like" cells to the classical types of pituitary cells can take place *in vitro* in complete absence of any hypothalamic principle as repeatedly seen by the numerous investigators who over the past 25 years, have grown pituitary *in vitro* (see bibliography in Murray and Kopech, 1953). Interestingly enough, ACTH activity was never found, when the combined cultures with hypothalamic tissue were performed before the 12th to 15th day of the *in vitro* pituitary life, that is, before any differentiated "adult" cells were present in the outgrowth. Similarly, ACTH activity in the fluids was not different from the controls when combined cultures of pituitary and hypothalamus were initiated and studied from day zero to 12 (Guillemin, unpublished).

Another point which was of considerable surprise to us, was the complete absence in pituitary tissue cultures of the vacuolated cells generally related to castration, thyroidectomy, or adrenalectomy. Indeed, when pituitaries of castrated, thyroidectomized or adrenalectomized rats, shown to contain the corresponding "ectomy cells," were placed in tissue cultures, the cells of the outgrowth never showed these characteristics and cells of the explant reverted to normal (Rosenberg, unpublished). It would thus seem that, for their appearing after removal of gonads, adrenals or thyroid the respective "ectomy-cells" need, along with the absence of the peripheral hormone, a constant hypothalamic stimulation. This could not have been properly studied by the particular technique used in this experiment with only 4 days of combined culture with hypothalamus. The data recently reported by Bogdanove and Halmi (1953) on the lack of appearance of thyroidectomy cells in rats treated with propylthiouracyl after hypothalamic lesions, would confirm this hypothesis. Our observations, however, do not clarify the locus of action of the peripheral hormones in their regulatory influence on the pituitary which could be trans-hypothalamic or directly hypophysial. Our experiments do not explain either, whether the hypothalamic hypophysiotropic activity is exerted on synthesis of ACTH by the pituitary tissue, on its release or on both phenomena.

The absence of cytolysis of the pituitary outgrowth after combined culture with anterior hypothalamus, posterior hypothalamus and median eminence is remarkable in view of the constancy of the pituitary tissue lysis when brain cortex, spleen or liver were cultured along with it. As mentioned before, this tissue lysis was first noticed under phase microscopy and subsequently confirmed by staining. Possible artifacts due to a bad fixation, for instance, are therefore eliminated. It is tempting to assume that this structural and ecological compatibility of hypothalamic and pituitary tissues might be correlated with their physiological interrelationship (Blount, 1930). The same compatibility has been reported with the tissue of the posterior lobe of the pituitary (Gaillard, 1937).

We did not attempt in these experiments to elucidate the role of vasopressin in the release of ACTH by the pars distalis, a role recently given considerable importance by various investigators (Mirsky et al., 1953; McCann and Brobeck, 1954). But the latter school of thought will have to account for the fact that ACTH was released in a system in which no posterior lobe activity was demonstrated (by assays for vasopressor and oxytocic hormones) and no ACTH was found when vasopressor or oxytocic activity was demonstrated in the fluid of combined cultures of pars distalis and nuclei of anterior hypothalamus. We have already presented further evidence of this fact when pure arginine-vasopressin, kindly given by Dr. V. du Vigneaud, did not release ACTH in the *in vitro* pituitary (Guillemin, 1955; Guillemin and Hearn, 1955).

SUMMARY

Dog and rat anterior pituitary has been cultured in roller tubes. ACTH activity in the fluid medium (Sayers test) was found only in the first 4 day old sample. No ACTH activity was demonstrable in 8, 12, 15, 19, 22, 31 day old samples in spite of excellent growth and differentiation of the pituitary outgrowth. When explants of hypothalamus or median eminence were added to the pituitary cultures from day 15 to 19 or 22 to 26, ACTH activity was re-initiated. No ACTH activity was found in control hypothalamus cultures nor when pituitary was grown from day 15 to 19 or 22 to 26 with explants of brain cortex, spleen, liver. At the level of sensitivity of the bioassays utilized, histamine, acetylcholine, adrenaline, nor-adrenaline, serotonin, oxytocin and vasopressin could not be demonstrated in the fluids of combined cultures of pituitary plus hypothalamus where ACTH activity was found. It is postulated that there exists some hypothalamic hypophysiotropic mediator involved in ACTH release, which is different from the above mentioned substances. The *in vitro* pituitary is proposed as an ideal bioassay for study of hypothalamic hypophysiotropic principles.

REFERENCES

ANDERSON, E. AND W. HAYMAKER: *Proc. Soc. Exp. Biol. and Med.* **33**: 313. 1935.
ANAND, B. K., P. RAGHUNATH, S. DUA AND S. MOHINDRA: *Indian J. Med. Res.* **42**: 231. 1954.
BENOIT, J. AND I. ASSENMACHER: *Arch. Anat. Microsc. et Morph. Exper.* **42**: 334. 1953
BLOUNT, R. F.: *Proc. Nat. Acad. Sci.* **16**: 218. 1930.
BOGDANOVE, E. M. AND N. S. HALMI: *Endocrinology* **53**: 274. 1953.
CUTTING, W. C. AND M. R. LEWIS: *Arch. Exp. Zellforsch.* **21**: 523. 1938.
FORTIER, C.: *Endocrinology* **49**: 782. 1951.
GAILLARD, P. J.: *Acta Neerland. Morphol. Normal Path.* **1**: 3. 1937.
GANONG, W. F. AND D. M. HUME: *Endocrinology* **55**: 474. 1954.
GUILLEMIN, R.: *Ciba Foundation Colloquia on Endocrinology.* **8**: 647, J. & A. Churchill, London, 1954.
GUILLEMIN, R.: *Endocrinology* **56**: 248, 1955.
GUILLEMIN, R.: *Texas Rep. Biol. and Med.* **13**: No. 3, 1955 (in press).
GUILLEMIN, R. AND W. R. HEARN: *Proc. Soc. Exper. Biol. and Med.* **89**: 365. 1955.
HARRIS, G. W.: *Brit. Med. J.* **627**: Sept. 15. 1951.
HARRIS, G. W.: *Ciba Foundation Colloquia on Endocrinology.* **8**: 531. J. & A. Churchill, London, 1954.
HILD, W.: *Texas Rep. on Biol. and Med.* **12**: 474. 1954.
HUME, D. M.: *J. Clin. Investigation.* **28**: 790. 1949.
MARTINOVITCH, P. N.: *J. Exper. Cell Res.* **4**: 490. 1953.
McCANN, S. M.: *Amer. J. Physiol.* **175**: 13. 1953.
McCANN, S. M. AND J. R. BROBECK: *Proc. Soc. Exper. Biol. and Med.* **87**: 318. 1954.
MIRSKY, A. R. MILLER AND M. STEIN: *Psychosom. Med.* **15**: 574. 1953.
MURRAY, M. R. AND G. KOPECH: *A Bibliography on the Research in Tissue Cultures.* Academic Press, New York, 1953.
ROSENBERG, B.: Thesis for B.Sc. degree, Univ. of Texas Medical Branch, Galveston, 1954.
SAYERS, G. AND K. L. SYDNOR: *Endocrinology.* **55**: 621. 1954.

[*Editor's Note:* The citations for Fortier 1952 and Galliard 1948 were not included in the original publication.]

Part III
THE HYPOTHALAMIC-HYPOPHYSIAL-THYROID AXIS

Editor's Comments
on Papers 12 Through 15

12 GREER
Evidence of Hypothalamic Control of the Pituitary Release of Thyrotrophin

13 GANONG, FREDRICKSON, and HUME
Excerpts from *The Effect of Hypothalamic Lesions on Thyroid Function in the Dog*

14 HARRIS and WOODS
Excerpts from *The Effect of Electrical Stimulation of the Hypothalamus or Pituitary Gland on Thyroid Activity*

15 HALÁSZ, PUPP, and UHLARIK
Excerpts from *Hypophysiotrophic Area in the Hypothalamus*

The existence of a hypothalamic factor regulating thyrotropin (TSH) release from the adenohypophysis was first demonstrated by Greer (Paper 12), who produced lesions in the median eminence of the hypothalamus, resulting in a decrease in circulating TSH and thyroid hormone levels. He found that bilateral symmetrical electrolytic lesions located between the paraventricular nuclei and the median eminence prevented the thyroidal goitrogenic response to thiouracil. On the basis of previously established information that thiouracil induces goiter formation by causing thyroxine deficiency with resultant TSH hypersecretion, Greer concluded that the hypothalamic lesions interfered with the normal feedback regulation of TSH in reponse to lowering of the blood thyroid hormone level. In these studies he introduced modern techniques of placing electrolytic hypothalamic lesions.

Ganong et al. (Paper 13) provided additional physiological evidence that TSH secretion is under hypothalamic control by noting marked thyroid depression in dogs following placement of lesions in the anterior median eminence region. They showed that placement of discrete hypothalamic lesions resulted in selective impairment of secretion of a specific hypophysial trophic hormone without substantially interfering with others, a result difficult to explain simply on the basis of interference with hypophysial-portal blood flow. These results indicated that the decrease in thyroid function was related to a reduction in release of a hypothalamic releasing factor rather than interference with the blood supply to the hypophysis. None of the lesioned dogs showed significant adrenocortical atrophy, and gonadal atrophy did not correlate with thyroid dysfunction. Thus they convincingly demonstrated that TSH secretion and thyroidal function could be independently impaired by selective discrete lesioning of the anterior hypothalamus without impairing anterior trophic hormone release for other target organs.

Harris and Woods (Paper 14) were able to localize more precisely hypothalamic sites responsible for thyrotropin release from the adenohypophysis. They found that electrical stimulation at the anterior portion of median eminence near the supraoptico-hypophysial tract region for periods of twenty-four to seventy-two hours in conscious unanesthetized rabbits increased thyroid function, as evidenced by accelerated thyroidal ^{131}I release and increased protein-bound ^{131}I. Stimulation of more posterior and superior regions of the hypothalamus, as well as the hypophysis, did not elicit thyroid activation. These studies, along with those of Greer and Ganong, indicated that the area of the anterior median eminence, anterior to the ventromedial nucleus, is involved in TSH secretion. These investigators also observed that glucocorticoids have an inhibitory influence on the thyroid-stimulating effects of hypothalamic stimulation and suggested that glucocorticoids act by suppressing hypophysial secretion of TSH, which has subsequently been documented. They were also able to demonstrate that the transplanted thyroid is still stimulatable upon hypothalamic stimulation, indicating that a humoral factor is involved.

Halász et al. (Paper 15) further characterized the hypophysial function of the hypothalamus by transplanting hypophysial fragments into various parts of the brain. Only in the basal tuberal regions were transplants functional in the stimulation of the thyroid, and only there did transplants contain morphologically normal basophils. The area of the hypothalamus in which hypophysial transplants showed thyrotroph differentiation and resulted in increased thyroidal activity was termed the *hypophysiotrophic area*. It was concluded that the material carried by the portal circulation from the hypothalamus to the *hypophysis* is not simply a synaptic mediator discharged by nerve terminals into the portal circulation but a true neurosecretory substance produced by neurons in the hypothalamus. Thus, on the basis of physiological studies employing hypothalamic lesions, electrical stimulation, and intrahypothalamic hypophysial transplants, these investigators were to identify an anatomical region whose neuronal input controlled basal TSH release.

12

Copyright © 1951 by the Society for Experimental Biology and Medicine
Reprinted from *Soc. Exp. Biol. Med. Proc.* 77:603-608 (1951)

Evidence of Hypothalamic Control of the Pituitary Release of Thyrotrophin.* (18862)

MONTE A. GREER.[†] (Introduced by E. B. Astwood.)

From the Ziskind Research Laboratories, New England Center Hospital and the Department of Medicine, Tufts College Medical School, Boston.

Although it has been postulated for many years that the hypothalamus in some manner regulates the secretion of thyrotrophin by the hypophysis, clear-cut experimental evidence demonstrating this phenomenon has not yet been presented(1). The present investigation was designed to provide a maximal stimulus for thyrotrophin release by feeding animals with hypothalamic lesions a diet containing propylthiouracil. In addition to thyroid size and histologic evidence of activity the iodide-concentrating capacity of the thyroid glands was determined, since this had previously been shown to be the most sensitive index of endo-

---

* This work was aided in part by grants to Dr. E. B. Astwood from the American Cyanamid Co. and the U. S. Public Health Service.

† U. S. Public Health Service Postdoctoral Research Fellow of the National Cancer Institute.

1. Harris, G. W., *Physiol. Rev.*, 1950, v28, 139.

TABLE I. Data of Rats with Hypothalamic Lesions. T/S I¹³¹ ratio refers to the concentration of I¹³¹ in comparable quantities of thyroid tissue and serum.

Rat	Initial body wt	Final body wt	Thyroid wt, mg	Thyroid wt, mg/100 g body wt	T/S I¹³¹ ratio	Pituitary damage	Thyroid hyperplasia	Hypothalamic lesions
CR-1	251	277	14.3	5.2	22.3	Severe	Absent	Paraventricular to middle of ventromedian n. Extends through ventral surface hypothalamus bilaterally and more extensive rt. side.
CR-2	256	279	13.7	4.9	128	None	,,	Suprachiasmatic to middle of ventromedian n. Extends across midline, more extensive on rt.
CR-3	239	256	14.1	5.5	247	,,	,,	Paraventricular to middle of ventromedian n.
CR-4	223	224	10.4	4.6	81	Small infarct left lobe	,,	Middle to caudal end of ventromedian n.
CR-5	221	234	10.75	4.6	258	None	,,	Beginning of paraventricular to ventromedian n. Extends across midline.
CR-6	258	249	16.4	6.6	215	,,	,,	Lesion very small, extending across midline at ventral surface of hypothalamus just behind suprachiasmatic n.
CR-7	255	223	19.1	8.6	433	,,	Moderate	Paraventricular to ant. half ventromedian n. Lesions displaced to left.
CR-8	258	258	13.5	5.2	147	,,	Absent	Paraventricular to anterior ventromedian n. Extends through surface of hypothalamus on left, 1 mm from surface on rt.
CR-9	246	252	20.15	8	395	,,	,,	Suprachiasmatic to anterior paraventricular n.

genous thyrotrophin activity available (2,3).

Materials and methods. Male and female Sprague-Dawley rats of the Harvard and Charles River strains were used. Hypothalamic lesions were produced in animals weighing 230-300 g by a modified Krieg stereotaxic instrument (4). Lesions were placed from 6 to 7 mm anterior to the ear plugs and 1 mm on each side of the midline. A varnished steel needle or copper wire with only the tip bare was used as the localizing electrode. After insertion through burr-holes in the dorsum of the skull, this was lowered until it encountered the base of the skull, when it was raised a distance of 0.5-1.0 mm. A direct current of 2.5-8.0 ma was applied for 15-30 seconds on each side. Ether was found to be a more satisfactory anesthetic than barbiturates.

After allowing one to 3 weeks for recovery from the operation to take place, the animals were given a diet of 0.03% propylthiouracil in mink chow and killed at the end of 10 days. The thyroids were dissected and weighed. The head was then removed and all excess tissue including the bony dorsum of the skull trimmed away, leaving the brain and base of the skull with the pituitary intact. All tissues were fixed in 10% formalin. After several days of fixing, 10 μ serial sections were made of the hypothalamic area, every tenth section

2. VanderLaan, J. W., and VanderLaan, W. P., *Endocrinology*, 1947, v40, 403.
3. VanderLaan, W. P., and Greer, M. A., *Endocrinology*, 1950, v47, 36.
4. Krieg, W. J. S., *Quart. Bull. Northwestern Univ. Med. School*, 1946, v20, 199.

TABLE II. Data of Control Rats.

Rat	Final body wt	Thyroid wt, mg	mg/100 g body wt	T/S I131 ratio
1	296	41.4	14	456
2	290	34.15	11.8	298
3	278	29	10.4	232
4	286	44.1	15.4	283
5	307	50.9	16.6	242
6	260	28.2	10.9	285
7	315	35.3	11.2	261
8	296	34.75	11.7	270
9	262	25.2	9.6	283
10	275	35.8	13	343
11	251	31.2	12.4	239
12	271	44.55	16.4	290

being mounted. The pituitary and thyroid were sectioned separately, coronal pituitary sections at 10 μ being used in order to visualize both lateral lobes of the pars anterior adequately. The brain sections were stained with 1% toluidine blue for 6 hours while pituitary and thyroid were stained with hematoxylin and eosin. When determining the iodide-concentrating ability of the thyroid, one lobe was used for determination of radioactivity, the other being fixed in formalin.

The iodide-concentrating capacity of the thyroid was determined as previously described(3). Ten mg of propylthiouracil were injected subcutaneously 30-60 minutes before the injection of a 5 μc tracer dose of I^{131}. One to 2 hours later the animals were killed and the concentration of I^{131} per unit of thyroid tissues compared to the concentration in an equivalent amount of serum. This I^{131} was present only as inorganic iodide since the previous injection of propylthiouracil had effectively blocked all protein binding of iodine.

Results. Preliminary experiments in 19 rats had indicated that lesions in the rostral and tuberal mid-hypothalamic areas were most likely to give positive results. Accordingly, an attempt was made to place the lesions within the area bounded by the optic stalk and the infundibulum. Eleven animals were operated upon, of which 2 died a few days postoperatively. Twelve control animals of approximately the same weight were treated similarly except for the production of hypothalamic lesions. The results are summarized in Tables I and II.

It can be seen that a marked difference existed in the thyroid response to thiouracil feeding between the intact and operated animals. Whereas the thyroid weights of the control animals varied from 9.6 to 16.6 mg per 100 g body weight, averaging 12.8 mg, those of the hypothalamic animals ranged from 4.6 to 8.6, averaging 5.9 mg. The thyroids of the operated animals thus apparently did not undergo any appreciable hypertrophy with thiouracil administration, averaging less than half the size of the controls. In fact, they would seem to be even slightly smaller than the thyroids of untreated, intact rats in this laboratory, which usually weigh 7-8 mg per 100 g body weight.

Microscopic examination of the thyroid tissue revealed an atrophic, flat to low cuboidal epithelium in all operated animals except CR-7. In this one instance there was a moderate hyperplasia, although not nearly as intense as in the unoperated animals. The thyroids of the control group, on the other hand, all showed the usual marked hyperplastic changes seen in thiouracil-treated animals.

Perhaps the most surprising finding of the investigation was the marked increase in the iodide-concentrating capacity of the thyroid tissue in the absence of any anatomic evidence of hyperfunction. The thyroid:serum iodide ratio was well above the normal value of 25:1 in all but one animal and in most instances was fully as high as in the control thiouracil-treated animals. The one exception, CR-1, had a large infarct affecting both lateral lobes

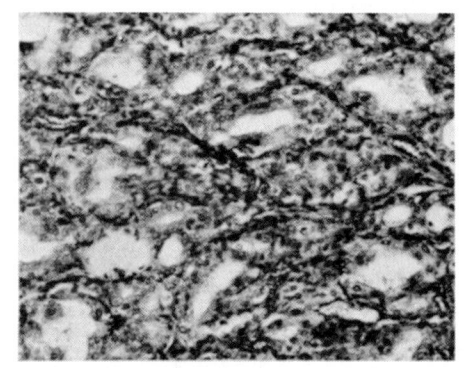

FIG. 1. Typical example of thyroid hyperplasia seen in control rats after 10 days of thiouracil feeding. Notice marked increase in cell height and diminution of colloid. H & E, × 160.

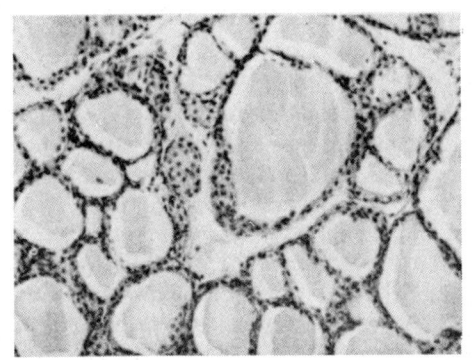

FIG. 2. Thyroid of CR-2. Atrophic appearance with large, colloid-filled follicles. Note flat, atrophic epithelium. H & E, × 160.

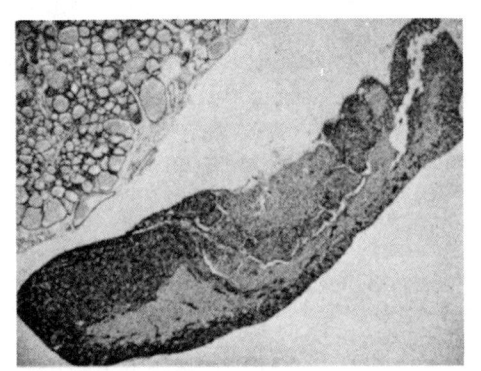

FIG. 3. Coronal section of pituitary of CR-1 showing large infarct affecting both lobes of pars anterior. H & E, × 26.

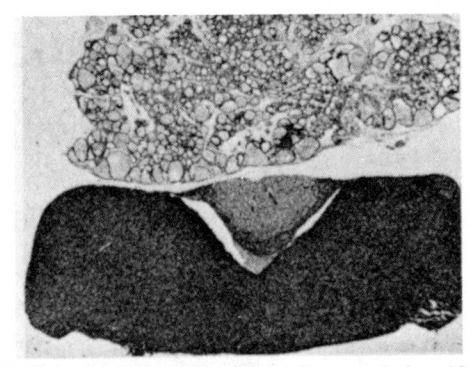

FIG. 4. Coronal section of pituitary and thyroid of CR-8 showing intact pituitary and atrophic thyroid. H & E, × 12.

of the anterior hypophysis, as previously mentioned, and CR-4 had a small infarct in the left lobe of the pars anterior.

The hypothalamic lesions were of small to moderate size and were all located in approximately the area intended. The most anterior lesions were just behind the suprachiasmatic nucleus and the most posterior extended to the caudal portion of the ventromedian nucleus. The lesions in CR-1 with the large pituitary infarct extended through the ventral surface of the hypothalamus from the paraventricular to the middle of the ventromedian nuclei and that on the right side was more extensive. The largest lesions were in CR-2 and extended

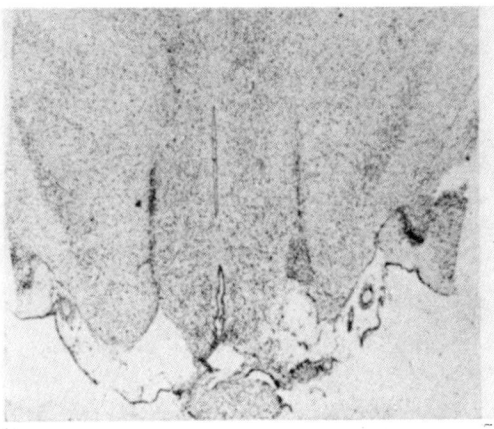

FIG. 5. Coronal section through hypothalamus of CR-4 illustrating bilateral lesions through caudal part of ventromedian nuclei. The infundibular stalk is in the lower midline. H & E, ×10.

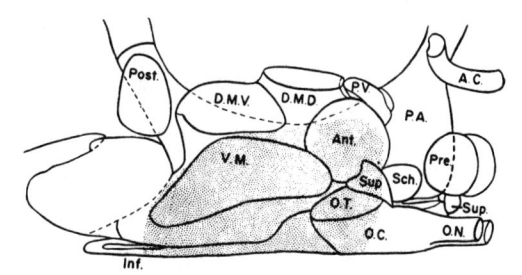

FIG. 6. Scheme of hypothalamus, modified from Krieg. Area of lesions indicated by stippling. A.C., anterior commissure; Ant., nucleus hypothalamicus anterior; D.M.V., D.M.D., ventral and dorsal portions of dorsomedian hypothalamic nucleus. Inf., infundibulum; O.C., optic chiasm; O.N., optic nerves; O.T., optic tract; P.A., nucleus hypothalamicus periventricularis, anterior region; P.V., paraventricular nucleus; Pre., preoptic nucleus; Post., posterior hypothalamic nucleus.

of the anterior hypophysis, but nevertheless maintained a normal thyroid iodide concentration.

The pituitary glands appeared perfectly normal in all but 2 animals. CR-1 had a large infarct destroying most of both lateral lobes from the suprachiasmatic to the middle of the ventromedian nuclei. The lesions in this animal fused in the mid-line in the region of the anterior portion of the ventromedian nucleus, but did not extend through the ventral surface of the hypothalamus. The smallest lesion was in CR-6, extending across the ventral hypothalamic surface through the mid-line, just behind the suprachiasmatic nucleus. In CR-7, the only animal to show any evidence of hyperplasia of the thyroid epithelium, there was a displacement of the lesions to the left so that they were not bilaterally symmetrical. This was the only animal in which symmetrical lesions were not placed.

Discussion. It is evident that the animals with hypothalamic lesions did not show the usual goitrogenic response to propylthiouracil administration. Since the pituitaries of all but two animals were completely intact and only that of CR-1 showed severe damage, it is extremely unlikely that the absence of thyroid hypertrophy was due to pituitary injury. All animals had a final body weight equal to or greater than that at the time of operation. The one exception was CR-7, whose weight fell from 255 to 223 g. As described above, this was the only animal which showed moderate hyperplastic changes in the thyroid. The weight gain, although not marked, may in part have been due to lesions in the region of the ventromedian nucleus, since Brobeck(5) has established that damage to this area produces obesity.

It is difficult to explain the marked dichotomy between thyroid size and iodide-concentrating ability. An intact pituitary has been shown to be essential for both the goitrogenic response(6) and the increase in thyroid iodide concentration(3) following thiouracil administration. In this investigation it is evident that the usual increase in iodide concentration has occurred without concomitant anatomical evidence of hyperplasia. There has been some previous experimental evidence that these two features may be distinct in that the thyroid:serum iodide ratio falls much more rapidly following hypophysectomy in rats chronically treated with propylthiouracil than does thyroid size or cell height(3).

It seems reasonable to postulate that the hypothalamic lesions in some manner prevented the usual augmentation of thyrotrophin secretion in thiouracil-treated rats. Whether this was qualitative, quantitative, or both is not clear from the data available. It does seem evident that some pituitary thyrotrophin was being formed, since there was a marked increase in thyroid iodide concentration which would not occur in the absence of the hypophysis. Two possibilities might be suggested: (1) The pituitary is unable to secrete enough thyrotrophin to stimulate cellular hyperplasia of the thyroid but is able to secrete the smaller amount needed to increase the thyroid iodide concentration; (2) Two different thyrotrophins are secreted by the pituitary, one causing cellular hyperplasia and the other an increase in thyroid function. In the presence of hypothalamic lesions similar to those described above, the pituitary is able to secrete only the latter hormone. With the presently available evidence, it is impossible to state which, if either, of these theories is correct. Even the animal with severe pituitary damage was able to maintain a normal thyroid iodide concentration, so that in none of the animals was hypophyseal function completely absent. Normal animals fed a thiouracil diet for a comparable time immediately following hypophysectomy almost invariably have a thyroid:serum ratio below 10:1 and frequently closely approaching 1:1(7).

These experiments do not determine the nature of the hypothalamic influence on the pituitary. This may be either neural or humoral, but since most investigators have found only a very scanty nerve supply to the pars anterior(1) and since it is established that the hypophyseal portal system carries blood to the pituitary down the hypophyseal stalk(8), it would seem more probable that the influence might be humoral. Whether the hypothalamic area damaged exerts a primary influence on

---

5. Brobeck, J. R., *Physiol. Rev.*, 1946, v26, 541.
6. Astwood, E. B., Sullivan, J., Bissell, A., and Tyslowitz, R., *Endocrinology*, 1943, v32, 210.
7. Greer, M. A., *Endocrinology*, 1949, v45, 178.
8. Barrnett, R. J., and Greep, R. O., *Science*, 1951, v113, 185.

the pituitary or only transmits tracts from other centers is also not clear.

The results of certain investigators with pituitary stalk-sectioned rats is compatible with the data obtained in this investigation. Brolin(9) found that the usual marked hypertrophy and hyperplasia of pituitary basophiles following thyroidectomy did not occur in stalk-sectioned rats and Greep and Barrnett observed a markedly decreased goitrogenic response following 2-3 weeks of thiouracil feeding in intact, stalk-sectioned rats(10). The latter authors, however, found that a marked infarction of the pituitary, similar to that seen in rat CR-1 of the present investigation, was produced by their technic of sectioning. Brolin did not state whether or not pituitary damage had been produced.

Summary. Bilateral, symmetrical, electrolytic lesions in the hypothalamus between the suprachiasmatic and caudal ventromedian nuclei prevented the goitrogenic response of the rat to thiouracil feeding. The iodide-concentrating capacity of the thyroid, however, increased to approximately the same extent as that of intact rats similarly treated. It appears that hypothalamic lesions of this type impair the secretion of thyrotrophin by the pituitary. It is not known whether this interference with thyrotrophin secretion is qualitative or quantitative, nor whether hypothalamic control is exerted by neural or hormonal mechanisms. The available evidence points to the secretion of a hypothalamic hormone, however.

I am indebted to Dr. E. B. Astwood for helpful advice and criticisms during the course of this investigation.

9. Brolin, S. E., *Acta Physiol. Scand.*, 1947, v14, 233.

10. Greep, R. O., and Barrnett, R. J.; Personal communication.

Received June 2, 1951. P.S.E.B.M., 1951, v77.

THE EFFECT OF HYPOTHALAMIC LESIONS ON THYROID FUNCTION IN THE DOG[1,2]

W. F. GANONG,[3] D. S. FREDRICKSON,[4] AND D. M. HUME[5]

Laboratory for Surgical Research, Harvard Medical School, and the Surgical Service, Peter Bent Brigham Hospital, Boston, Massachusetts

IT HAS been suspected for some time that the thyroid was at least in part under the control of the nervous system (Uotila, 1940). However, it remained for Greer (1952) to show that anterior hypothalamic lesions in rats prevent the usual thyroid hypertrophy upon the administration of propylthiouracil. Because his animals also showed normal thyroid-serum iodide ratios, he postulated the existence of two thyrotrophic hormones. Bogdanove and Halmi (1953) have since confirmed these results, but feel that they can be interpreted as due only to a decrease in the amount of thyrotrophin released in response to propylthiouracil administration. No studies are at present available on the effect of hypothalamic lesions on the thyroid in animals that have not been treated with propylthiouracil. In the course of other investigations on the relationship of the hypothalamus to the anterior lobe of the pituitary, the following studies were carried out in dogs. It was felt that they were of interest because they show the effect of hypothalamic destruction on thyroid function in the absence of any modifying agents.

[*Editor's Note:* Material has been omitted at this point.]

Received April 11, 1955.

[1] This work was supported by a grant in aid from the Commonwealth Fund.

[2] These studies were conducted under Atomic Energy Commission Authorization #29940.

[3] U.S.P.H. Research Fellow of the National Institute of Neurologic Diseases and Blindness.

[4] Present Address: National Heart Institute, National Institute of Health, Bethesda, Maryland.

[5] Scholar of the American Cancer Society.

[6] Quaker Oats Co., Chicago, Illinois.

DISCUSSION

It is true that hypothalamic lesions which affect pituitary function in the dog are located in the median eminence and of necessity damage at least part of the portal hypophysial vasculature. It is possible, therefore, that the present results can be explained by pituitary damage secondary to encroachment on this source of pituitary blood supply. An experimental approach to rule out this factor is difficult, and at present, there are no conclusive data that pituitary dysfunction alone cannot explain the observed results. However, for a number of reasons, this seems an unlikely explanation.

In the first place, in all animals with depressed radioactive iodine uptakes, there were at least some portal hypophysial vessels remaining intact. Furthermore, not only did all animals have large amounts of grossly and histologically normal pituitary tissue present, but the small amount of pituitary damage sometives present bore no relation to the presence or absence of end organ deficits. Pituitary cell counts have not been done but it can be stated that eosinophiles and basophiles are both present in what appear to be roughly normal numbers. Another point of considerable interest is the fact that none of these animals showed adrenocortical atrophy histologically, and in only one of them was the adrenal weight less than that of the normal, unstressed dog. This observation has previously been reported in another series of animals from this laboratory (Ganong and Hume, 1954).

Section of the portal hypophysial blood vessels without damage either to the median eminence or the pituitary would provide an excellent experimental approach to this problem. Unfortunately, however, it is impossible to draw conclusions from the rather confusing literature (Uotila, 1940; Harris, 1948) because of a number of factors. In the first place, Harris and Jacobsohn (1952) have pointed out that the portal hypophysial vessels regrow with great ease. Therefore, in all studies in which their regrowth was not prevented by insertion of a large plate of some inert material, the results must be regarded as inconclusive. Furthermore, injection of the vessels with a material such as india ink, which permits their visualization, and serial section of the hypothalamo-pituitary region is essential if one is to conclude that the vessels are indeed completely interrupted. Many people have studied the problem of stalk section in the dog, but none have been able to perform the operation without considerable trauma to the pituitary area, and, in many instances, to the median eminence.

Similarly, the results of transplantation of the anterior pituitary to the eye or other locations remote from the diencephalon (Cheng, Sayers, Goodman, and Swinyard, 1949; McDermott, Fry, Brobeck, and Long, 1951; Harris and Jacobsohn, 1952) are difficult to interpret physiologically, because no matter how well vascularized these grafts may be, it has not

73

been proved that the observed results are not due to a decrease in the amount of functioning pituitary tissue.

Another approach to this problem is to study the animal in whom increasingly large amounts of pituitary tissue have been removed. From studies of this nature in the past (Aschner, 1912) it is now well accepted that one-third or less of the anterior lobe will support the thyroid, gonads and adrenals in the presence of a normal hypothalamus. On the other hand, the problem of what happens to the pituitary target glands with removal of more than two-thirds but less than all of the hypophysis has received little attention. Smith's classic work on the rat (1932) showed that instead of uniform, graded depression of thyroid, gonads and adrenals, the gonads atrophied while the thyroid and adrenals remained histologically normal when nine-tenths of the pituitary was absent. Keller and his colleagues (Keller, 1948; Keller, Lawrence and Blair, 1945) have similarly found that in the dog, as increasingly large amounts of pituitary tissue are removed, gonadal depression is first to appear, and adrenocortical last, adrenocortical function being supported by very small remnants of pituitary tissue. This problem has also been studied in the human, and here, isolated end organ deficits have been reported (Paschkis and Cantarow, 1951; Myers, Maddock, Leach and Klein, 1952). Sheehan and Summers (1949) point out, however, that valid conclusions can be drawn only from autopsied cases, since only in this manner can concurrent hypothalamic damage be ruled out. When this is done, the usual sequence of endocrine atrophy in man with increasing pituitary failure is gonads, thyroids, and lastly adrenals (Sheehan and Summers, 1949; Peters, German, Mann and Welt, 1954).

A study of the effect of subtotal hypophysectomy in the dog is now in progress in this laboratory. Preliminary data, based on 16 dogs, indicate that gonadal function is depressed one month after removal of three-fourths of the anterior lobe. Depression of thyroidal function also occurs after removal of four-fifths of the pars distalis while some adrenocortical function persists unless the removal is complete. It would be reasonable, therefore, to expect gonadal depression alone, or gonadal and thyroidal, or gonadal, thyroidal and adrenal, in that sequence if results in the lesion animals were due to pituitary damage. The dogs in the present study do not follow this pattern. Four had isolated loss of normal adrenocortical stress responses with no other abnormality, while two had thyroidal and adrenocortical deficiency combined. Obviously, more work must be done on this point before definitive conclusions are possible. However, it is clear that the end organ deficits in the dogs with hypothalamic lesions do not correlate with the spectrum of hypopituitarism.

On the other hand, a rough correlation was noted between the part of the hypothalamus destroyed and the particular endocrine deficit seen. Anterior median eminence destruction produced thyroid atrophy, destruction of the anterior and middle median eminence loss of the eosinopenic response to stress, and caudal median eminence lesions gonadal atrophy. These localizations are consistent enough to suggest further investigation.

SUMMARY

1. Thyroidal uptake of radioactive iodine and thyroid weight and histology have been analyzed in 23 dogs with hypothalamic lesions and correlated with the eosinopenic response to stress, adrenal weight and histology, and gonadal weight and histology.

2. Five dogs showed definite depression of thyroidal I^{131} uptake, and histologic evidence of thyroidal atrophy. In these animals, lesions were localized to the region in and just above the anterior end of the median eminence. Thyroid function and histology were normal in animals with lesions elsewhere, including the posterior and middle portion of the median eminence.

3. There was no consistent correlation between thyroid depression and depressions of other pituitary controlled endocrines in the dogs with hypothalamic lesions. Rather, the type of endocrine picture produced correlated roughly with the site of the hypothalamic destruction.

Acknowledgments

Special thanks are due Miss Hildegard Junker, Miss Faith Bebchick, and Miss Ethel Hitchcock for technical assistance.

REFERENCES

ASCHNER, B.: *Pflüger's Arch. f.d. ges. Physiol.* **146**: 1. 1912.
BOGDANOVE, E. M. AND N. S. HALMI: *Endocrinology* **53**: 274. 1953.
CHENG, C., G. SAYERS, L. S. GOODMAN AND C. A. SWINYARD: *Am. J. Physiol.* **159**: 426. 1949.
DEGROOT, J. AND G. W. HARRIS: *Ciba Colloq. on Endoc., Vol. IV*, 108, J. & A. Churchill Ltd., London, Eng., 1952.
FREDRICKSON, D. S., W. F. GANONG AND D. M. HUME: *Proc. Soc. Exp. Biol. and Med.*, in press.
GANONG, W. F. AND D. M. HUME: *Endocrinology* **55**: 474. 1954.
GREER, M.: *J. Clin. Endocrinol.* **12**: 1259. 1952.
HARRIS, G. W.: *Physiol. Rev.* **28**: 139. 1948.
HARRIS, G. W. AND D. JACOBSOHN: *Proc. Roy. Soc., London, S. B.*, **139**: 263. 1952.
HUME, D. M.: *Ann. Surg.* **138**: 548. 1953.
KELLER, A. D.: *Texas Rep. Biol. and Med.* **6**: 275. 1948.
KELLER, A. D., W. E. LAWRENCE AND C. B. BLAIR: *Arch. Path.* **40**: 789. 1945.
MCCANN, S. M.: *Am. J. Physiol.* **171**: 746. 1952.
MCDERMOTT, W. V., E. G. FRY, J. R. BROBECK, AND C. N. H. LONG: *Yale J. Biol. & Med.* **23**: 52. 1951.
MYERS, G. B., W. O. MADDOCK, R. B. LEACH AND S. P. KLEIN: *Tr. A. Am. Phys.* **66**: 72. 1951.
PASCHKIS, K. E. AND A. CANTAROW: *Ann. Int. Med.* **34**: 669. 1951.
PETERS, J. P., W. I. GERMAN, E. B. MANN AND L. G. WELT: *Metabolism* **3**: 118. 1954.
SHEEHAN, H. C. AND V. K. SUMMER: *Quart. J. Med.* **18**: 318. 1949.
SMITH, P. E.: *Anat. Rec.* **52**: 191. 1932.
UOTILA, U. U.: *A. Research Nerv. and Ment. Dis., Proc.*, **29**: 580. 1940.

14

Copyright © 1958 by the Physiological Society, London

Reprinted from pages 246–247, 264–273 of *J. Physiol.*
143:246–274 (1958)

THE EFFECT OF ELECTRICAL STIMULATION OF THE HYPOTHALAMUS OR PITUITARY GLAND ON THYROID ACTIVITY

BY G. W. HARRIS AND J. W. WOODS*

From the Department of Neuroendocrinology, Institute of Psychiatry, Maudsley Hospital, London, S.E. 5

(*Received* 6 *March* 1958)

It is clear that the central nervous system influences the activities of the ovary, adrenal cortex and thyroid gland. Brown-Grant, Harris & Reichlin (1954a) found that procedures calculated to give rise to emotional stress in rabbits (painful stimuli and restraint) result in a prompt and marked decrease of thyroid activity, and that sudden changes in the conditions of environmental lighting, whether from light to dark or vice versa, also result in temporary inhibition of the thyroid. The findings of von Euler & Holmgren (1956b), that hypophysectomized rabbits bearing pituitary transplants do not respond to environmental cold with an increase in thyroid activity and do not respond to the stress of 24 hr anaesthesia with thyroid inhibition, also indicate a neural mechanism underlying these reactions.

It is likely that the means whereby the central nervous system affects thyroid activity involves the hypothalamus and hypophysial portal vessels of the pituitary stalk. Brown-Grant, Harris & Reichlin (1957) found that simple stalk section in the rabbit was followed by regeneration of the portal vessels and a return of the thyroid inhibitory response to the stress of restraint or injection of stilboestrol, whereas stalk section with the placement of a plate between the hypothalamus and pituitary gland was associated with a permanent loss of the thyroidal responses to restraint and stilboestrol. These findings are compatible with those of von Euler & Holmgren (1956b) mentioned above. The inhibition of secretion of the thyrotrophic hormone (TSH) by the anterior pituitary which follows a rise in concentration of thyroxine in the blood may be independent of the hypothalamus, since direct injection of thyroxine into the pars distalis of the pituitary, but not into the hypothalamus

* Present address: Department of Physiology, The Johns Hopkins University School of Medicine, 710 N. Washington Street, Baltimore, Md., U.S.A.

(von Euler & Holmgren, 1956a), results in inhibition of thyroid activity, and administration of thyroxine to the effectively stalk-sectioned rabbit also results in thyroidal inhibition (Brown-Grant et al. 1957). On the other hand, the observations of Greer (1951, 1952) and Bogdanove & Halmi (1953), that certain hypothalamic lesions may prevent the hypertrophy of the thyroid that follows the administration of goitrogenic drugs, indicate that a decreased blood concentration of thyroid hormone requires the mediation of the hypothalamus in order to result in an increased discharge of TSH. The findings of Reichlin (1957), that compensatory hypertrophy of the thyroid does not occur in the presence of anterior hypothalamic damage, is also in accord with this view.

The hypothalamus appears necessary, not only to effect certain reflex changes in thyroid activity in response to environmental stimuli, but also to maintain thyroid activity under conditions of a constant environment. Several procedures have been used to isolate, completely or partially, the pituitary gland from the central nervous system. Pituitary transplantation (von Euler & Holmgren, 1956b), pituitary stalk section (Brown-Grant et al. 1957), and destruction of the anterior part of the median eminence (Ganong, Frederickson & Hume, 1955), or of the anterior hypothalamus (D'Angelo & Traum, 1956) have all been found to result in reduced thyroid function. The converse experiment of applying electrical stimulation to the hypothalamus and observing any change in thyroid activity has rarely been attempted. No increase in oxygen consumption of rabbits was seen by J. D. Green & G. W. Harris (unpublished), following prolonged stimulation of the hypothalamus, but definite conclusions were not drawn from this owing to the limitations of the method for measuring metabolic rate in rabbits. Histological signs of increased thyroid activity in rats and rabbits were reported by Colfer (1949) to follow stimulation of the hypothalamus for four 1 hr periods on each of 2 days. No optimum site in the hypothalamus was found but control stimulation of the thalamus or corpus callosum gave negative results. Somewhat similar results were obtained by Del Conte, Ravello & Stux (1955), who found that diffuse electric shocks applied through the cranium of the guinea-pig resulted in an increase in the TSH concentration in the blood within half an hour of the stimulus. In the experiments described below electrical stimulation was applied for prolonged periods, 24–72 hr, to various regions of the hypothalamus and pituitary gland in rabbits. The rate of release of ^{131}I from the gland was used to detect changes in thyroid activity. Since hypothalamic stimulation is known to evoke release of the adrenocorticotrophic hormone (ACTH) (de Groot & Harris, 1950; and others), and since a rise in concentration of blood adrenal corticoids is known to depress thyroid activity (Brown-Grant, Harris & Reichlin, 1954b), both normal and adrenalectomized animals were studied.

[*Editor's Note:* Material has been omitted at this point.]

DISCUSSION

The technique of remote control stimulation has been modified from that described previously (Harris, 1947; de Groot & Harris, 1950). In earlier studies the coil and electrode system was made as a solid unit and implanted under the scalp, whereas in the work described above the coil was buried under the skin over the lumbar region of the vertebral column and flexible insulated leads ran to electrodes fixed to the cranium. This method had been attempted on previous occasions (G. W. Harris, unpublished) but had failed from fracture of the leads or insulation in the cervical region. The success of the present units depended on the use of many-stranded tinsel wire insulated with two sheaths of polyvinylchloride. The advantages of the method may be summarized as follows. (1) It is possible to implant a larger coil under the skin of the back than under the scalp; this makes it easier to induce the required voltage, and so to economize on the electrical components of the primary circuit. (2) The present method makes it as easy to implant bipolar as unipolar electrodes; it also makes it possible to use X-ray control when implanting the electrodes, a procedure which greatly increases the accuracy of electrode placement. (3) The use of stainless steel screws and dental cement for fixing the electrodes to the bones of the skull has been found eminently satisfactory; no movement of the electrodes has been detected in any of the forty-three animals used in the present series. (4) After obtaining any given response by stimulation, it would be a simple matter to anaesthetize the animal, extract a portion of one lead through a small incision, cut the lead, pass a direct current of a few milliamperes through the unit and thus produce a lesion around the tips of the electrodes, reunite and reinsulate the lead, and repeat the experiment; such a procedure would seem to offer a good internal control for experiments on any one animal. (5) Whilst the animals are being killed with Nembutal the occasion is taken to extract the leads through a small incision in the skin of the neck and to record the voltages on an oscilloscope with the animal in similar positions in the field of the primary coil as were used in the previous experiment. In this way the voltages between the electrodes were measured for the individual rabbits. (6) After killing the animal, the leads are cut near the skull, and the coil and attached parts of the leads removed, cleaned, sterilized and used in further experiments. After formol fixation of the head, the dental cement is dissolved in chloroform and the electrodes and stainless steel screws are recovered for further use.

Rabbits with intact adrenal tissue respond to hypothalamic stimulation in the region of the supraopticohypophysial tract with an increase of thyroid activity. Many workers have reported that lesions in the hypothalamus may interfere with the normal secretion of TSH (Bogdanove & Halmi, 1953; Bogdanove, Spirtos & Halmi, 1955; Greer & Erwin, 1956; Ganong et al. 1955; D'Angelo & Traum, 1956; Reichlin, 1957). Ganong et al. (1955) found that lesions in the anterior part of the median eminence reduced thyroid activity in dogs to the level seen in hypophysectomized animals. Greer (1951), in commenting on the region of the hypothalamus in which lesions result in reduced thyroid function, says: 'The impression gained so far, however, is that the area is anterior to the ventro-median nucleus and lies along or near the ventral surface of the hypothalamus, possibly near the ventral extension of the supraopticohypophysial tract.' The evidence derived from studies of lesions and stimulation are in good agreement. Both indicate that it is the anterior part of the median eminence that is involved in the control of TSH secretion and thyroid activity. Although stimulation in the region of the supraopticohypophysial tracts resulted in increased thyroidal secretion, it is not certain that this result can be ascribed to the supraopticohypophysial tracts themselves. The microanatomy of the hypothalamus is highly complex and there is little knowledge of the detailed pathway of the multitude of unmyelinated fibre tracts in this region. It is likely that other tracts run closely associated with the supraopticohypophysial tract, and this probability should be taken into account before associating the present results with any particular nervous pathway. In the twelve rabbits in which both thyroidal and antidiuretic responses were studied, the association between the two responses in the different animals was suggestive but not entirely uniform. In one case, in which a marked antidiuretic response but no increase in thyroid activity followed stimulation, the electrodes were found to be situated in the pars distalis in a position to stimulate the nerve fibres of the infundibular stem but not those of the median eminence. The data from this animal then cannot be related to the question of which nerve tracts of the hypothalamus are concerned with the regulation of TSH secretion. One other rabbit, however, showed a thyroidal response to stimulation but no antidiuretic response. In this case the electrodes were situated in the anterior tuber cinereum, slightly posterior to the supraopticohypophysial tract (Pl. 4, fig. 11). Since an antidiuretic response forms a very sensitive test of electrical stimulation of the supraopticohypophysial tract, this evidence suggests that stimulation of the tract is not essential in evoking a thyroid response. On the other hand, the findings of Dubreuil & Martini (1956), that the uptake of radioactive iodine by the thyroid gland of male rats is increased by previous administration of vasopressin, is compatible with the view that the supraopticohypophysial tract regulates pituitary secretion of TSH by releasing a vasopressin-like substance into the hypophysial portal vessels.

The evidence that hypothalamic stimulation causes increased thyroid activity through the agency of thyrotrophic hormone may be summarized. First, hypothalamic stimulation is effective in exciting the activity of the transplanted thyroid as well as of the normal gland: the effect is thus humorally mediated. Secondly, the effect of hypothalamic stimulation on thyroid activity may be closely simulated by injection of appropriate doses of TSH (see Text-fig. 8). And thirdly, it may be recalled that von Euler & Holmgren (1956*b*), and Brown-Grant *et al.* (1957) have shown, by different methods, that the central nervous system may influence thyroid activity through the mediation of hypothalamo-hypophysial connexions.

It has been suggested that the hypothalamus may be 'mapped', three-dimensionally, in terms of pituitary hormones (Harris, 1955). In such a map the control of TSH secretion would be localized in the anterior parts of the median eminence and tuber cinereum. It would seem inadvisable to term such an area a 'centre'; it probably represents some neural mechanism akin to a 'final common path' by which the nervous system acting through this area and the pituitary stalk controls the secretion of TSH. This region of the hypothalamus then would give the maximum effects on TSH release when damaged or stimulated. It is likely, however, that many reflex paths from the

[*Editor's Note:* Plate 4 and Text-figure 8 are not reproduced here.]

brain stem, hippocampus, amygdaloid nuclei, thalamus, cerebral cortex and other parts of the central nervous system play upon and influence this final common path. If this is so, then it is to be expected that a more detailed investigation will reveal further hypothalamic areas, through which pass such reflex paths, that may exert an influence on TSH discharge. It is of interest that the anterior part of the median eminence, concerned with thyroid activity, is adjacent to the anterior hypothalamic and preoptic region known to be concerned with the regulation of body temperature (Magoun, Harrison, Brobeck & Ranson, 1938; von Euler, 1952).

Complete adrenalectomy, with maintenance on small and constant doses of cortisone, was performed in thirty-two out of the total of forty-three rabbits studied. The difference in the thyroid response seen after adrenalectomy, as compared with that in the same animal in experiments before adrenalectomy, may be summarized as follows: (*a*) Four animals that showed an increase in thyroid activity to stimulation before complete adrenalectomy, showed a greater increase after. (*b*) Thirteen animals that had shown inhibition, or no change of thyroid activity, previous to complete adrenalectomy, exhibited a clear-cut acceleration of thyroid function afterwards; the increased function of the thyroid was assessed by measurements of the release curve of thyroidal radio-iodine, and by measurements of the blood concentration of $PB^{131}I$; the changes recorded by the two methods were in good agreement. (*c*) Twelve animals that previous to complete adrenalectomy had shown inhibition, or no change of thyroid activity, gave responses of the same two types afterwards but showed a significant decrease in the number of responses of the inhibitory type.

The reason for the differences observed before and after adrenalectomy is not entirely clear. The most likely hypothesis is that some substance is liberated from the adrenal gland during hypothalamic stimulation which in turn inhibits either TSH secretion or the thyroid gland itself. It is known that electrical stimulation of certain areas of the hypothalamus evokes secretion of adrenaline (Magoun, Ranson & Hetherington, 1937) and that adrenaline may inhibit thyroid activity in the rabbit, probably by a vasoconstrictor action on the vessels of the gland (Haigh, Reiss & Reiss, 1954; Brown-Grant *et al.* 1954*a*; Brown-Grant & Gibson, 1956). However, it is unlikely that adrenal medullary secretion is the only factor involved in the present experiments since (*a*) the median eminence is not a particularly effective site for localized electrical stimulation to excite adrenaline secretion (Magoun *et al.* 1937), (*b*) the dose of adrenaline necessary to produce prolonged inhibition of the thyroid gland of the rabbit is high (Brown-Grant *et al.* 1954*a*), (*c*) in the case of one rabbit adrenal denervation did not have the same effect as adrenal removal, and (*d*) rabbits with an adrenal gland intact may show a reversal of the thyroid response to stimulation if under high cortisone administration.

It is likely that adrenal cortical secretion is the major factor involved, since: (i) hypothalamic stimulation is known to evoke release of ACTH (de Groot & Harris, 1950; Hume & Wittenstein, 1950; Hume, 1953; Porter, 1954); (ii) the dose of adrenal steroids necessary to produce prolonged inhibition of the thyroid gland in the rabbit seems to be within the physiological range (Brown-Grant et al. 1954b; Brown-Grant, 1956); and (iii) rabbits which possess an intact adrenal gland may show a reversal of thyroid response, so that hypothalamic stimulation results in thyroidal acceleration, if given large doses of cortisone in an attempt to 'blockade' ACTH secretion. It is possible that the adrenal steroids affect thyroid activity by suppressing the secretion of TSH from the anterior pituitary, since cortisone was found not to influence the response of the thyroid gland of the hypophysectomized rabbit to injection of exogenous TSH (Brown-Grant et al. 1954b).

Hypothalamic stimulation might evoke a rise of adrenal steroid concentration in the blood for a variety of reasons. First, stimulation of hypothalamic nerve fibres may excite release of anterior pituitary ACTH. Secondly, the slight noise and flickering of lights from the thyratron valves during stimulation may evoke some emotional disturbance and so some ACTH secretion; and thirdly, any rise in the blood level of thyroid hormone might in itself stimulate the pituitary-adrenal axis (Wallach & Reineke, 1949; Timiras & Woodbury, 1955). It is likely that the most important of these factors is the first, since the type of response both before and after adrenalectomy was related to the electrode position in the hypothalamus.

Stimulation of the most anterior part of the tuber cinereum resulted in thyroidal acceleration both before and after adrenalectomy, and similarly stimulation of the superior region of the hypothalamus or areas posterior to the median eminence failed to result in thyroidal acceleration either before or after complete adrenalectomy. In the intermediate zone between the above two areas, that is, in the region of the median eminence, stimulation after adrenalectomy in many rabbits evoked increased thyroid activity though stimulation before had given inhibition of, or no change in, thyroidal function. A possible explanation of this finding is that the median eminence is a zone where the ACTH and TSH 'fields' of the hypothalamus overlap. De Groot & Harris (1950) have shown in rabbits that stimulation of the more posterior parts of the tuber cinereum and mammillary region excites secretion of ACTH, whilst in the present study stimulation of the anterior area of the tuber cinereum excited TSH release. Since the evidence is strongly in favour of the view that both neural mechanisms act on the anterior pituitary through the pituitary stalk, it seems likely that in the region of the median eminence there is overlap of the areas in which stimulation might evoke both ACTH and TSH release. In that case it is possible that stimulation at this site would act rapidly to raise the blood level of adrenal steroids, and that this might inhibit any TSH secretion that would otherwise have been elicited. Such a view would at the moment fit the experimental findings.

A point of interest arising from the above results is that eight rabbits died during or shortly after hypothalamic stimulation. Six of these animals were adrenalectomized, and seven had shown thyroid acceleration following the start of stimulation. It is well known that thyrotrophic hormone or thyroid hormone should be administered with caution to patients suffering from Addison's disease. It is possible that, in the present work, the thyroid acceleration resulting from hypothalamic stimulation was responsible for precipitating a state of acute adrenal insufficiency.

The presence or absence of the ovaries was not related to the type of thyroid response following hypothalamic stimulation. Further, the occurrence of ovulation following stimulation could not be correlated with the thyroid responses. The incidental observation, that ovulation had occurred in a proportion of the rabbits following stimulation in the region of the median eminence, confirms the older observations of Harris (1937, 1948), Haterius & Derbyshire (1937) and Markee, Sawyer & Hollinshead (1946).

Animals in which the stimulating tips of the electrodes were situated deeply in the pars distalis of the pituitary gland failed to show any sign of thyroidal activation on stimulation, either before or after complete adrenalectomy. This is again in conformity with previous results that electrical stimulation of the anterior pituitary gland, at a strength that does not produce spread of current to the hypothalamus, fails to excite release of gonadotrophic hormone (Markee *et al.* 1946; Harris, 1948), or adrenocorticotrophic hormone (de Groot & Harris, 1950). This suggests that the stimulus from the hypothalamus which evokes anterior pituitary secretion is not transmitted to the gland cells by nerve fibres. Taken in conjunction with the findings of Brown-Grant *et al.* (1957), who reported the loss of nervous reflex control of TSH release from the adenohypophysis after pituitary stalk section, but the return of such control if regeneration of the hypophysial portal vessels occurred, the evidence would suggest that hypothalamic regulation of TSH discharge occurs through the mediation of the hypophysial portal vessels.

In a preliminary report of this work (Harris & Woods, 1956b), the possible relationships between the present findings and the aetiological factors involved in Graves's disease have been discussed in some detail. The two factors that have been described many times as of importance in the development of exophthalmic goitre, emotional trauma and adrenal cortical deficiency, may be compared with the electrical stimulation of the central nervous system and the bilateral adrenalectomy utilized in the present experiments. Such a comparison might imply that the onset of Graves's disease is associated with an increase in the blood concentration of TSH. This has been reported by several groups of workers (Querido & Lameyer, 1956; Gilliland & Strudwick, 1956).

The results of McCullagh, Clamen & Gardner (1957) are directly related to the hypothesis that central nervous factors and some degree of adrenal cortical insufficiency are connected with Graves's disease. These workers found that the exophthalmos and other features of hyperthyroidism improve or completely disappear on treatment by (a) administration of ACTH and hydrocortisone or (b) operative section of the pituitary stalk. Also pertinent is the observation of Purves (1957) that patients in whom a raised blood concentration of TSH has been demonstrated possess also a raised plasma protein-bound iodine, and that the simultaneous increase in TSH and thyroid hormone in the blood is strong evidence that some pathological condition exists in the 'feed-back mechanism', probably at a hypothalamic or pituitary level.

SUMMARY

1. Various areas in the hypothalamus and pituitary gland have been electrically stimulated for periods of 24–72 hr, using a remote control method, in forty-three conscious rabbits. The effect of such stimulation on thyroid activity has been assessed by measuring the rate of release of ^{131}I-labelled hormone from the gland and by studies of the blood concentration of PB^{131}I.

2. Stimulation in rabbits with intact adrenal tissue results in increased thyroid activity if the electrode tips are situated in the anterior part of the median eminence adjacent to the supraopticohypophysial tract. Stimulation of more posterior and superior areas of the hypothalamus, and different regions of the pituitary gland, did not elicit thyroid activation. That the supraopticohypophysial tract is the neural path involved in the thyroid response is not certain, since concurrent experiments in which both the thyroid and antidiuretic responses were measured in twelve rabbits revealed a discrepancy in the responses in the case of one animal.

3. Stimulation was repeated in thirty-two of the above forty-three animals after complete adrenalectomy and maintenance with small daily doses of cortisone. In four cases in which thyroid activation had occurred before adrenalectomy, a greater thyroidal response was observed after adrenalectomy. In thirteen other animals in which no increased thyroid function was observed before adrenalectomy, constant and marked thyroidal activation in response to stimulation was observed after adrenalectomy. In these latter thirteen rabbits the electrode positions were found to be in the median eminence, but posterior to the supraopticohypophysial tract.

4. The mechanism of the change in thyroidal response after complete adrenalectomy was investigated in animals subjected to adrenal denervation or to adrenal cortical 'blockade' with high doses of cortisone. The evidence indicates that it is removal of the adrenal cortex, rather than the adrenal medulla, which is effective in reversal of the thyroid response after adrenalectomy. Since stimulation of the hypothalamus is known to activate release of

pituitary ACTH, and since adrenal corticoids have been shown to inhibit TSH secretion, it is suggested that the effect of adrenalectomy is to prevent a sudden rise of adrenal steroids in the blood simultaneous with the period of stimulation.

5. In one animal a typical thyroid acceleration was observed in response to hypothalamic stimulation after the thyroid gland had been transplanted to the anterior surface of the infrahyoid muscles.

6. Eight rabbits died during, or shortly after, prolonged or repeated periods of hypothalamic stimulation. An increase in thyroid hormone in the blood tends to a state of adrenal cortical insufficiency.

7. It was observed incidentally that twenty rabbits had ovulated after periods of stimulation. In these cases the electrodes were situated in the anterior or middle tuber cinereum. These observations confirm previous reports.

Our thanks are due to Mr W. F. Piper for his skilled assistance in building the apparatus; to Messrs S. A. Renner and S. A. Williams who assisted in the operative and histological work and Mr F. A. Smith for photography; to the United States Air Force for support of this work (Contract No: AF61(514)-953), and to the Research Fund of the Maudsley Hospital. Thyrotrophic hormone was obtained through the kindness of Armour and Co., Chicago. This work was carried out, in part, during the tenure of a fellowship (by J. W. W.) from the American Cancer Society.

REFERENCES

BOGDANOVE, E. M. & HALMI, N. S. (1953). Effects of hypothalamic lesions and subsequent propylthiouracil treatment on pituitary structure and function in the rat. *Endocrinology*, **53**, 274–292.

BOGDANOVE, E. M., SPIRTOS, B. N. & HALMI, N. S. (1955). Further observations on pituitary structure and function in rats bearing hypothalamic lesions. *Endocrinology*, **57**, 302–315.

BROWN-GRANT, K. (1956). The effect of ACTH and adrenal steroids on thyroid activity, with observations on the adrenal–thyroid relationship. *J. Physiol.* **131**, 58–69.

BROWN-GRANT, K. & GIBSON, J. G. (1956). The effect of exogenous and endogenous adrenaline on the uptake of radio-iodine by the thyroid gland of the rabbit. *J. Physiol.* **131**, 85–101.

BROWN-GRANT, K. HARRIS, G. W. & REICHLIN, S. (1954a). The effect of emotional and physical stress on thyroid activity in the rabbit. *J. Physiol.* **126**, 29–40.

BROWN-GRANT, K., HARRIS, G. W. & REICHLIN, S. (1954b). The influence of the adrenal cortex on thyroid activity in the rabbit. *J. Physiol.* **126**, 41–51.

BROWN-GRANT, K., HARRIS, G. W. & REICHLIN, S. (1957). The effect of pituitary stalk section on thyroid function in the rabbit. *J. Physiol.* **136**, 364–379.

COLFER, H. F. (1949). Thyroid response to hypothalamic stimulation. *Trans. Amer. Goiter Ass.* pp. 376–378.

D'ANGELO, S. A. & TRAUM, R. E. (1956). Pituitary-thyroid function in rats with hypothalamic lesions. *Endocrinology*, **59**, 593–595.

DE GROOT, J. & HARRIS, G. W. (1950). Hypothalamic control of the anterior pituitary gland and blood lymphocytes. *J. Physiol.* **111**, 335–346.

Del Conte, E., Ravello, J. J. & Stux, M. (1955). The increase of circulating thyrotrophin and the activation of the thyroid by means of electroshock in guinea pigs. *Acta endocr. Copenhagen*, **18**, 8–14.

Dubreuil, R. & Martini, L. (1956). Possible mechanism of the hypothalamic control of thyrotrophic hormone secretion. *Abstr. XX int. physiol. Congr., Brussels*, p. 257.

Ganong, W. F., Frederickson, D. S. & Hume, D. M. (1955). The effect of hypothalamic lesions on thyroid function in the dog. *Endocrinology*, **57**, 355–362.

Gilliland, I. C. & Strudwick, J. I. (1956). Clinical application of an assay of thyroid-stimulating hormone in relation to exophthalamos. *Brit. med. J.* i, 378–381.

Greer, M. A. (1951). Evidence of hypothalamic control of the pituitary release of thyrotrophin. *Proc. Soc. exp. Biol. N.Y.*, **77**, 603–608.

Greer, M. A. (1952). The role of the hypothalamus in the control of thyroid function. *J. clin. Endocrin.* **12**, 1259–1268.

Greer, M. A. & Erwin, H. L. (1956). Evidence of separate hypothalamic centers controlling corticotropin and thyrotropin secretion by the pituitary. *Endocrinology*, **58**, 665–670.

Haigh, C. P., Reiss, M. & Reiss, J. M. (1954). Measurements of absolute radioiodine uptake in the assessment of human thyroid activity. *J. Endocrin.* **10**, 273–283.

Harris, G. W. (1937). The induction of ovulation in the rabbit by electrical stimulation of the hypothalamo-hypophysial mechanism. *Proc. Roy. Soc.* B, **122**, 374–394.

Harris, G. W. (1947). The innervation and actions of the neurophypophysis; an investigation using the method of remote control stimulation. *Phil. Trans.* B, **232**, 385–441.

Harris, G. W. (1948). Electrical stimulation of the hypothalamus and the mechanism of neural control of the adenohypophysis. *J. Physiol.* **107**, 418–429.

Harris, G. W. (1955). The function of the pituitary stalk. *Johns Hopk. Hosp. Bull.* **97**, 358–375.

Harris, G. W. & Woods, J. W. (1956b). Aetiology of Graves's Disease in relation to recent experimental findings. *Brit. med. J.* ii, 737–739.

Haterius, H. O. & Derbyshire, A. J., Jr. (1937). Ovulation in the rabbit following upon stimulation of the hypothalamus. *Amer. J. Physiol.* **119**, 329–330.

Hume, D. M. (1953). The neuro-endocrine response to injury; present status of the problem. *Ann. Surg.* **138**, 548–557.

Hume, D. M. & Wittenstein, G. J. (1950). The relationship of the hypothalamus to pituitary-adrenocortical function. *Proc. 1st clin. ACTH Conf.* Ed. J. R. Mote, pp. 134–146. Philadelphia: Blakiston and Co.

Magoun, H. W., Harrison, F., Brobeck, J. R. & Ranson, S. W. (1938). Activation of heat loss mechanisms by local heating of the brain. *J. Neurophysiol.* **1**, 101–114.

Magoun, H. W. Ranson, S. W. & Hetherington, A. (1937). The liberation of adrenin and sympathin induced by stimulation of the hypothalamus. *Amer. J. Physiol.* **119**, 615–622.

Markee, J. E., Sawyer, C. H. & Hollinshead, W. H. (1946). Activation of the anterior hypophysis by electrical stimulation in the rabbit. *Endocrinology*, **38**, 345–357.

McCullagh, E. P., Clamen, M. & Gardner, W. J. (1957). Clinical progress in the treatment of exophthalmos of Graves' disease; with particular reference to the effect of pituitary surgery. *J. clin. Endocrin.* **17**, 1277–1292.

Porter, R. W. (1954). The central nervous system and stress-induced eosinopenia. *Recent Progr. Hormone Res.* **10**, 1–18.

Purves, H. D. (1957). In discussion, *Ciba Foundation Colloquia on Endocrinology*, **10**, 17–18.

Querido, A. & Lameyer, L. D. F. (1956). Thyrotrophic hormone content of human sera in normals and patients with thyroid disease. *Proc. R. Soc. Med.* **49**, 209–212.

Reichlin, S. (1957). The effect of hypothalamic lesions upon the thyroid response to partial thyroidectomy. *Endocrinology*, **60**, 567–569.

Timiras, P. S. & Woodbury, D. M. (1955). Adrenocortical function after administration of thyroxine and triiodothyronine in rats. *J. Pharmacol.* **115**, 144–153.

von Euler, C. (1952). Slow 'temperature potentials' in the hypothalamus. *J. cell. comp. Physiol.* **36**, 333–350.

von Euler, C. & Holmgren, B. (1956a). The thyroxine 'receptor' of the thyroid-pituitary system. *J. Physiol.* **131**, 125–136.

von Euler, C. & Holmgren, B. (1956b). The role of hypothalamo-hypophysial connexions in thyroid secretion. *J. Physiol.* **131**, 137–146.

Wallach, D. P. & Reineke, E. P. (1949). The effect of varying levels of thyroidal stimulation on the ascorbic acid content of the adrenal cortex. *Endocrinology*, **45**, 75–81.

15

Copyright © 1962 by The Journal of Endocrinology
Reprinted from pages 147 and 151-153 of *J. Endocrinol.* 25:147-154 (1962)

HYPOPHYSIOTROPHIC AREA IN THE HYPOTHALAMUS

B. HALÁSZ, L. PUPP AND S. UHLARIK

Department of Anatomy, University Medical School of Pécs, Hungary

(*Received* 31 *January* 1962)

SUMMARY

Anterior pituitary tissue was implanted into the hypothalamus, other parts of the brain and beneath the renal capsule of rats. Grafts in the ventral hypothalamus could retain a normal histological appearance despite a lack of any contact with the capillary loop system of the median eminence.

By observing the location of basophils in the grafts a 'hypophysiotrophic' area has been defined. In other sites the histological structure of the grafts was not maintained.

In animals with grafts in the hypophysiotrophic area the target organs might be well preserved, though sometimes the gonads were preserved and other target organs atrophied. Grafts in other sites always led to atrophy of the target organs.

It is concluded that the material from the hypothalamus essential for the maintenance of anterior pituitary structure and function is not simply a synaptic mediator discharged by nerve terminals into the portal circulation, but a true neurosecretory substance produced by and available from small neurones in the hypothalamus.

INTRODUCTION

Transplantation experiments (Greep, 1936; Harris & Jacobsohn, 1952; Nikitovitch-Winer & Everett, 1958, 1959; Smith, 1961) have shown that direct vascular contact with the characteristic capillary loops of the median eminence is essential for the maintenance of normal function and histological structure of anterior lobe tissue. These studies, however, have not shown whether the substances conveyed by the portal veins to the anterior lobe are produced in the walls of the capillary loops of the median eminence, or are already present in an active form elsewhere and, if so, in what part of the hypothalamus.

This paper reports the results of intrahypothalamic grafts of anterior pituitary tissue. Histological and functional evidence has been obtained which defines what may be called the 'hypophysiotrophic' region of the hypothalamus.

[*Editor's Note:* Material has been omitted at this point.]

[*Editor's Note:* Text-figure 1, Plate 1, and Table 1 are not reproduced here.]

DISCUSSION

The results substantiate those of other workers (Nikitovitch-Winer & Everett, 1958, 1959; Smith, 1961) who grafted the anterior pituitary into heterotopic sites and then replanted it in the natural position below the median eminence. Further conclusions can also be drawn. It seems that direct contact of the graft with the characteristic capillary system of the median eminence is not essential for the maintenance of anterior pituitary structure and function. Therefore, the material which normally is carried by the portal circulation from the hypothalamus to the pituitary is not of necessity a synaptic mediator produced in and discharged by nerve endings solely into the capillary tufts of the median eminence. The material must be available already in an active form in a well circumscribed region of the hypothalamus (Text-fig. 1) which may be called the hypophysiotrophic area. Without any portal circulation, contact with this area preserves the function and histological appearances of anterior pituitary tissue if the size and vascularization of the graft is adequate. As it cannot be supposed that there are any specific nerve terminals in the grafts, the hypophysiotrophic material presumably produced in nerve cell bodies can, under our experimental conditions, pass directly to the graft. The sharp lateral boundaries of the hypophysiotrophic area suggest that the neurosecretory substance in question has little tendency to diffuse through the hypothalamic tissue. Many grafts outside the hypophysiotrophic area were bulging into the third ventricle and in contact with the cerebrospinal fluid (CSF). They were not preserved, showing that the material is not contained in adequate amounts in the CSF.

The shape of the hypophysiotrophic area suggests that it might coincide with the course of the paraventriculo–hypophysial tract. This is disproved, however, by the graft shown in Pl. 1, figs. 5 and 6, which contained no basophils in spite of being in direct contact with the magnocellular part of the paraventricular nucleus. The hypophysiotrophic area includes the whole of the arcuate nucleus, the ventral part of the anterior periventricular nucleus and the parvocellular region in the retrochiasmatic area. This corresponds fairly well with the regions from which the fine calibered tubero–hypophyseal tract originates (Spatz, 1951; Nowakowski, 1951). We shall present later (Szentágothai et al., 1962) histological evidence of a parvicellular neurone system in the hypophysiotrophic area, the axons of which can be traced to the characteristic capillary loops of the median eminence and particularly to the surface of the proximal part of the pituitary stalk. It seems probable that the neurosecretory hypophysiotrophic material is synthesized in the small neurones of the arcuate, anterior periventricular and retro-chiasmatic region and carried by the fine fibre system of Spatz and Nowakowski to the zone in contact with the pituitary circulation.

An alternative explanation is suggested by the approximate correspondence of the hypophysiotrophic area to the region of the ventral hypothalamus which contains a peculiar type of ependymal glia. Löfgren (1961) suggested that these glial elements might carry the neurosecretory material to the capillary loops of the median eminence. This seems unlikely because hypertrophy of the ependymal glial tissues, which often occurs around intrahypothalamic pituitary grafts, has an adverse effect, presumably by preventing contact between the graft and nervous tissue, rather than helping to preserve the structure and function of the implant.

In this study the preservation of function of the pituitary grafts can be estimated only from the weights and histological structure of the target organs. Group *a* (Table 1) shows that intrahypothalamic pituitary grafts may completely (or almost completely) take over the functions of the hypophysis of the host.

With other grafts, however, the preservation of target organs was often dissociated. It has been shown by partial hypophysectomy (Ganong & Hume, 1956) that the gonads are the most and the adrenal glands the least sensitive to the loss of anterior pituitary tissue. The results after partial lesions of the pituitary stalk are essentially the same (Halász, Pupp & Uhlarik, 1962). On the other hand, the preservation of target organs after intrahypothalamic grafts of pituitary tissue in completely hypophysectomized animals is exactly the reverse. Similar dissociation, with better preservation of the male gonads, has been described following pituitary grafts into the anterior chamber of the eye and beneath the renal capsule (Goldberg & Knobil, 1957; Hertz, 1959).

In the present study, dissociated preservation of the target organs was never seen with grafts in non-hypothalamic parts of the brain or beneath the renal capsule. No explanation is offered for the different effects on the target organs of progressive pituitary ablation and intrahypothalamic grafting.

It is tempting to relate the degree of preservation of the different target glands to the exact location of the graft within the hypophysiotrophic area. The positions of the grafts in groups *a* and *b* are not significantly different except that those in group *b* are perhaps further away from the median eminence. Group *c* might be helpful by suggesting that the stimulators of thyrotrophin and adrenocorticotrophin production are produced in more anterior regions than the gonadotrophin stimulators, but this group contains only a single animal. Further experiments are needed before any definite conclusions can be drawn. Finally, it would be of interest to know whether the material essential for the maintenance of normal pituitary structure is the same as one or other of the trophic hormone 'releasing factors' which have been shown to exist in the median eminence by investigation into the effect of hypothalamic extracts (Guillemin & Rosenberg, 1955; McCann, Taleisnik & Friedman, 1960; Royce & Sayers, 1960; Schally, Andersen, Lipscomb, Long & Guillemin, 1960; Campbell, Feuer, Garcia & Harris, 1961). It was not possible to obtain evidence concerning this interesting question from the present study.

REFERENCES

Campbell, H. J., Feuer, G., Garcia, J. & Harris, G. W. (1961). The infusion of brain extracts into the anterior pituitary gland and the secretion of gonadotrophic hormone. *J. Physiol.* **157**, 30P.

Flerkó, B. & Szentágothai, J. (1957). Oestrogen sensitive nervous structures in the hypothalamus. *Acta endocr., Copenhagen*, **26**, 121.

Ganong, W. F. & Hume, D. M. (1956). The effect of graded hypophysectomy on thyroid, gonadal and adrenocortical function in the dog. *Endocrinology*, **59**, 292.

Goldberg, R. C. & Knobil, E. (1957). Structure and function of intraocular hypophyseal grafts in the hypophysectomized male rat. *Endocrinology*, **61**, 742.

Greep, R. O. (1936). Functional pituitary grafts in rats. *Proc. Soc. exp. Biol., N.Y.*, **34**, 754.

Guillemin, R. & Rosenberg, B. (1955). Humoral hypothalamic control of anterior pituitary: a study with combined tissue cultures. *Endocrinology*, **57**, 599.

Halász, B., Pupp, L. & Uhlarik, S. (1962). Pituitary-target gland system after pituitary-stalk lesion. *Acta Morph. Hung.* (in the Press).

Harris, G. W. & Jacobsohn, D. (1952). Functional grafts of the anterior pituitary gland. *Proc. roy. Soc. B*, **139**, 263.

Hertz, R. (1959). Growth in the hypophysectomized rat sustained by pituitary grafts. *Endocrinology*, **65**, 926.

Löfgren, F. (1961). The glial-vascular apparatus in the floor of the infundibular cavity. *Lunds Universitets Årsskrift*, N.F., Avd. 2. 57/2, 1. Lund Gleerup.

McCann, S. M., Taleisnik, S. & Friedman, H. M. (1960). LH-releasing activity in hypothalamic extracts. *Proc. Soc. exp. Biol., N.Y.*, **104**, 432.

Nikitovitch-Winer, M. & Everett, J. W. (1958). Functional restitution of pituitary grafts re-transplanted from kidney to median eminence. *Endocrinology*, **63**, 916.

Nikitovitch-Winer, M. & Everett, J. W. (1959). Histologic changes in grafts of rat pituitary on the kidney and upon retransplantation under the diencephalon. *Endocrinology*, **65**, 357.

Nowakowski, H. (1951). Infundibulum und Tuber cinereum der Katze. *Dtsch. Z. Nervenheilk.* **156**, 261.

Royce, P. C. & Sayers, G. (1960). Purification of hypothalamic corticotropin releasing factor. *Proc. Soc. exp. Biol., N.Y.*, **103**, 447.

Schally, A. V., Andersen, R. N., Lipscomb, H. S., Long, J. M. & Guillemin, R. (1960). Evidence for the existence of two corticotrophin-releasing factors, α and β. *Nature, Lond.*, **188**, 1192.

Smith, P. E. (1961). Postponed homotransplants of the hypophysis into the region of the median eminence in hypophysectomized male rats. *Endocrinology*, **68**, 130.

Spatz, H. (1951). Neues über die Verknüpfung von Hypophyse und Hypothalamus. *Acta neuroveg., Wien*, **3**, 1.

Szentágothai, J., Flerkó, B., Mess, B. & Halász, B. (1962). Hypothalamic control of the anterior pituitary gland. *Akadémiai Kiadó, Budapest.* (In the Press.)

Editor's Comments on Papers 16 and 17

16 BOWERS et al.
Excerpts from *Effect of Thyrotropin-Releasing Factor in Man*

17 FOLKERS et al.
Discovery of Modification of the Synthetic Tripeptide-Sequence of the Thyrotropin Releasing Hormone Having Activity

The isolation of the thyrotropin-releasing factor (TRF) in a state of "near purity" from porcine hypothalami achieved in Schally's laboratory enabled Bowers et al. (Paper 16) to conduct the first clinical studies with TRH. They demonstrated that highly purified natural porcine TRH stimulated TSH release in humans, as measured by both bioassay and radioimmunoassay determinations of TSH levels. The rises were found to occur quickly (by six minutes) in all subjects studied. Maximal rises in TSH were seen at six to thirty minutes, followed by a gradual decline of TSH levels over the next forty-five minutes to basal levels. This pattern of TSH response to TRH has been recurrently demonstrated in subsequent human studies. The results of this study demonstrated that TRF is not species specific since porcine TRF was active in mouse and rat TSH bioassays, as well as human studies.

In 1969 the thyrotropin-releasing hormone (TRH) was characterized and synthesized by Folkers et al. (Paper 17), based on much laborious effort in Schally's laboratory in which 100,000 porcine hypothalami were processed and three amino acids—histidine, glutamic acid, and proline—were identified upon acid hydrolysis of the purified porcine hypothalami. Schally's group characterized TRH as being a tripeptide pyroglutamyl-histidylprolinamide and then synthesized it using amino acid sequencing, mass spectrophotometry of natural and synthetic preparations, gel filtration and sephadex chromatography. Folkers et al., using this type of methodology, were able to modify both the amino and carboxyl groups of the tripeptide Glu-His-Pro, yielding a ninhydrin-negative and Pauly-positive tripeptide (pyro) Glu-His-Pro (NH_2), which displayed biological TSH-releasing activity in the mouse bioassay system and in-vitro hypophysial preparations. They demonstrated that, like natural porcine TRH, the TSH response to the synthetic preparation was inhibited by triiodothyronine and that incubation for fifteen minutes in human plasma inactivated the synthetic preparation. This synthetic preparation was also found to elevate plasma levels of TSH in rats at two minutes after intravenous injection, with levels peaking at ten to fifteen minutes and remaining elevated for sixty minutes, similar to the temporal TSH response to natural TRH. At approximately the same time in Guillemin's laboratory, Burgus et al., using high-resolution mass spectrometry, characterized ovine TRH as the tripeptide (pyro) Glu-His-Pro NH_2 and prepared a synthetic preparation that displayed physiochemical and biological characteristics quantitatively and qualitatively indistinguishable from a highly purified preparation of hypothalamic ovine origin. These elegant studies in which TRH was characterized and synthesized led to a Nobel prize shared by Schally and Guillemin.

Effect of Thyrotropin-Releasing Factor in Man

C. Y. BOWERS, A. V. SCHALLY, W. D. HAWLEY, CARLOS GUAL, AND ALBERT PARLOW

Tulane University School of Medicine, Department of Medicine, and Endocrine and Polypeptide Laboratories, Veterans Administration Hospital, New Orleans, Louisiana, Instituto Nacional de la Nutricion, Mexico, D. F., and University of California School of Medicine, Department of Obstetrics and Gynecology, Los Angeles, California

A SERIES of beautiful and specific studies was performed within the last 20 years which indicated that thyrotropin (TSH) released from the anterior pituitary gland (APG) was dependent on the hypothalamus (1, 2). To increase the release of TSH with electrodes placed into the hypothalamus, it was necessary to stimulate the preoptic area. To decrease the release of TSH it was found that either the removal of the pituitary gland and its transplantation away from its normal anatomical site, the severing of the anatomical connection between the hypothalamus and pituitary gland, or the localized destruction of specific areas in the hypothalamus was effective in each instance. It was concluded from these studies that the hypothalamus and anterior pituitary gland functioned as a unit to regulate TSH release. Since it had been established that a vascular link in which blood flowed from the hypothalamus to the APG was the only connection between these two organs, it was also concluded that a humoral substance had been formed in the hypothalamus and secreted into the vascular link to stimulate TSH release. Investigators who attempted to find this TSH neuroregulator were indeed successful (3–5). This chemical or hormone was designated as the thyrotrophin-releasing factor (TRF) or thyrotrophin-releasing hormone (TRH) (6) and was found in the hypothalamus of the sheep, ox, pig, rat and human (4, 7–9). Earlier studies indicated that TRF was a peptide (10, 11); however, more recently this was disproven (12, 13). Although some of the chemical properties of ovine and porcine TRF were previously described, at the present time the chemical structure of the compound is still unknown (12, 13).

Since TRF purified from the hypothalamus of the ox, sheep and pig released TSH from the APG of rats and mice, a certain lack of species specificity exists, and therefore it was of special interest to determine its effect in man. This study reports the changes of plasma TSH levels which occurred when a highly purified preparation of porcine TRF was given to man. The *in vivo* conditions used to obtain a response to TRF were previously determined in mice and rats. These same conditions were used for the study of the effects of TRF in man.

Received November 27, 1967; accepted March 5, 1968.

[*Editor's Note:* Material has been omitted at this point.]

Discussion

By definition, TRF should stimulate release of TSH by acting directly on the APG without the intervention of hypothalamo-hypophysial connections. This perhaps is best demonstrated *in vitro* by the "isolated" pituitary method described by Saffran and Schally (4, 7, 17). The magnitude of the TRF-TSH release response in mice depends not only on the amount of TRF given but also on the amount of T_3 and T_4 present (16). This relationship between the thyroid hormones and TRF is considered to be one of the important *in vivo* criteria by which to characterize a substance as TRF. The highly purified preparation of TRF, obtained from hypothalami of pigs and used in these studies, when given to animals has produced the above-described biological changes. It also has been found to elevate TSH levels in rats, to decrease pituitary TSH content in mice, and to be inactive in hypophysectomized mice. For these reasons this preparation has been designated TRF.

Prior to these TRF studies in humans, the effect of TRF on plasma TSH levels of thyroidectomized rats was determined. Three hours after giving these rats a small amount of T_3, TRF was given as a single quick iv injection and a rise in the plasma TSH level occurred within two minutes (18) and was higher 15 minutes after the injection. Thus, the sudden release of TSH following the injection of TRF is another important *in vivo* criterion by which to characterize a substance as TRF. TRF was also active when given sc and ip but not when given im (19). As the dose of TRF was increased the response increased. When TRF was given as a two to four hour infusion into the femoral vein of the rat, plasma TSH levels increased (unpublished). The disadvantages of the latter method of administration are that it requires more TRF and, if given to an intact animal, the TSH released stimulates the release of T_4 and T_3, which then block the TRF effect. Of course, when the test subject does not have a thyroid gland, this does not need to be considered. A final point is that serum or plasma from rats and man rapidly inactivates TRF (19). Therefore, it is unlikely that TRF recirculates through the APG even if it is not retained, inactivated, or destroyed there.

Some conditions considered to be important for testing the activity of TRF in man were: inhibition of endogenous TSH release before injecting TRF, maintenance or increase in the content of TSH in the APG, maintenance or increase of the sensitivity of the APG to TRF, and the demonstration of the TRF response by measuring a change in TSH levels of the plasma. Athyrotic cretins, on no T_4 or T_3 for at least six months, were chosen for this study and thought to be ideal subjects to establish whether porcine TRF was active in man. Levels of TSH had been found to be elevated in the APG of untreated cretins. In these patients the TSH blood levels were measurable by bioassay and in two patients by both bioassay and radioimmunoassay. Since release of TSH was high in these untreated patients, a single small 25 µg dose of T_3 was given orally to the patients 12 to 24 hours before the studies were performed to decrease this release. By the use of a single small dose of T_3, the plasma TSH levels were decreased but could still be measured, the pituitary TSH content was thought to be maintained or increased, and the sensitivity of the APG to TRF was considered to be optimal.

Although the TSH blood levels of the cretins did not significantly change six minutes after the iv injection of saline, they were significantly elevated six minutes after the iv injection of TRF. Even at three minutes there was a significant rise. The greatest rise was from six to 30 minutes and was followed by a gradual decline of the TSH level over the next 45 minutes. The plasma TSH levels were still elevated 60 minutes after the TRF was injected. When the plasma level of TSH was measured in one of the patients 120 minutes after injecting TRF, it had returned to the base line level. Because of the limited supply, it was not possible to determine if the above were the optimal conditions for detecting the TRF response in man.

It is probable that only limited studies will be performed in man with this hypothalamic pituitary neuroregulator until the structure of this compound is determined and it has been synthesized. Only 2.7 mg of pure TRF has been obtained from the hypothalami of 100,000 pigs (13). Since the recovery of TRF has been high with the purification procedures used, it indicates that domestic animals are an impractical source of this regulator for clinical studies. These and other findings also suggest that very small amounts of TRF are stored in the hypothalamus and that the hypothalamus may continuously synthesize and secrete it. Comparison of the results of our animal studies using pure porcine TRF and those obtained in these studies indicate that it would be necessary to give 20 µg of pure TRF to these cretins to elicit comparable responses. These findings only help to support the importance of the vascular link which joins the hypothalamus and APG. There is little dilutional change, only a brief contact with the plasma, and no intervening organs to change the concentration of the hypothalamic regulators in their short transit to the APG.

TRF can be appropriately thought of as a regulator since it specifically controls TSH secretion, acts quickly and is rapidly destroyed. Recent studies indicate that T_3 or T_4 and TRF do not directly interact or compete for the same chemical site in the APG (20, 21) and that an intact thyrotropin cell may be necessary for the action of TRF (22, 23) to release TSH.

These present results in man indicate a certain lack of species specificity since TRF prepared from the hypothalami of pigs is active in the mouse and rat as well as man. It is of interest, however, that TRF has not been found to be active in the tadpole (19).

Acknowledgments

The authors wish to thank Dr. José A. Bermudez, Dr. Ofelia Gonzales and Fr. Augusto Diaz Infante from the Department of Endocrinology, Instituto Nacional de la Nutricion, Mexico, D. F., for their expert clinical assistance in performing these studies, Miss George-Ann Reynolds for performing the bioassay, and Dr. William Locke for help in preparing this manuscript.

References

1. Harris, G. W., Neural Control of the Pituitary Gland, E. Arnold, London, 1955.
2. D'Angelo, S. A., In Nalbandov, A. V. (ed.), Advances in Neuroendocrinology, University of Illinois Press, Urbana, 1963, p. 158.
3. Schreiber, V., A. Echertova, Z. Franz, J. Koei, M. Rybak, and V. Kimentova, Experientia 17: 264, 1961.
4. Guillemin, R., E. Yamazaki, D. A., Gard, M. Jurioz, and E. Sakiz, Endocrinology 73: 564, 1963.
5. Reichlin, S., In Cameron, M. P. (ed.), Brain Thyroid Relationship, Little, Brown and Co., Boston, 1964, p. 17.
6. Schally, A. V., A. Arimura, C. Y. Bowers, A. J. Kastin, S. Sawano, and T. W. Redding, Recent Progr Hormone Res (in press).
7. Bowers, C. Y., T. W. Redding, and A. V. Schally, Endocrinology 77: 609, 1965.
8. Shina, D., and J. Meites, Neuroendocrinology 1: 4, 1966.
9. Schally, A. V., E. E. Muller, A. Arimura, C. Y. Bowers, T. Saito, T. W. Redding, S. Sawano, and P. Pizzolato, J Clin Endocr 27: 755, 1967.
10. Guillemin, R., Proc. Int. Cong. Physiol., Tokyo, Excerpta Med. Int. Congress Series No. 87, 1965, p. 284.
11. Schally, A. V., C. Y. Bowers, and T. W. Redding, Endocrinology 78: 726, 1966.
12. Guillemin, R., R. Burgus, E. Sakiz, and D. N. Ward, C R Acad Sci (Paris) 262: 2278, 1966.
13. Schally, A. V., C. Y. Bowers, T. W. Redding, and J. F. Barrett, Biochem Biophys Res Commun 25: 165, 1966.
14. Redding, T. W., C. Y. Bowers, and A. V. Schally, Endocrinology 79: 229, 1966.
15. Schally, A. V., C. Y. Bowers, and T. W. Redding, Proc Soc Exp Biol Med 121: 718, 1966.
16. Bowers, C. Y., A. V. Schally, G. A. Reynolds, and W. D. Hawley, Endocrinology 81: 741, 1967.
17. Saffran, M., and A. V. Schally, Canad J Biochem 33: 408, 1955.
18. Bowers, C. Y., T. W. Redding, and A. V. Schally, Clin Res 14: 97, 1966.
19. Bowers, C. Y., T. W. Redding, and W. D. Hawley, Endocrine Society Abstracts, 48th Meeting, 1966, p. 48.
20. Bowers, C. Y., K. L. Lee, and A. V. Schally, Endocrinology 82: 75, 1968.
21. ———, Ibid., p. 303.
22. Bowers, C. Y., and K. L. Lee, Endocrine Society Abstracts, 49th Meeting, 1967, p. 89.
23. Bowers, C. Y., K. L. Lee, and A. V. Schally, Clin Res 16: 1, 1968.

17

Copyright © 1969 by Academic Press, Inc.

Reprinted from *Biochem. Biophys. Res. Commun.* 37:123-126 (1969)

DISCOVERY OF MODIFICATION OF THE SYNTHETIC TRIPEPTIDE-SEQUENCE OF THE
THYROTROPIN RELEASING HORMONE HAVING ACTIVITY.

by K. Folkers, F. Enzmann, and J. Bøler
The University of Texas at Austin, Texas

C. Y. Bowers, and A. V. Schally
Tulane University School of Medicine and Veteran Administration
Hospital, New Orleans, Louisiana

The isolation of the thyrotropin releasing factor or hormone (TRF or TRH) in a state of "near-purity" from porcine hypothalami was achieved by Schally et al., in 1966. Since only 2.8 mg. of TRH was obtained from the hypothalami of 100,000 pigs, the investment of this amount in further work to "absolute-purity" or in structure determination became one of stepwise decision. Most notably, this TRH was subjected to acid hydrolysis and three amino acids were obtained; they were histidine, glutamic acid and proline. These three amino acids were present in essentially equimolar amounts and accounted for about 30% of the particular sample which was hydrolyzed. This evidence indicated that His, Glu and Pro are moieties in TRH. It was advantageous that TRH showed only one Pauly-positive spot (the histidine moiety) on chromatograms.

Extension of the isolation process to 165,000 hypothalami has recently been described in detail, and the TRH appeared to be homogeneous by TLC, electrophoresis and paper chromatography (Schally et al., 1969). Such isolated TRH released thyrotropin (TSH) from the pituitary glands of mice in doses of about one nanogram. In vitro, about ten picograms of such TRH stimulated the secretion of TSH. Again, only three amino acids, histidine, glutamic acid and proline, were obtained in equimolar ratio by hydrolysis. The structural sequence of the three amino acids was determined by the Edman procedure to be Glu-His-Pro.

The knowledge of the presence of the three amino acids was the first basis for organic syntheses on this problem. Dr. Frederick W. Holly of the Merck, Sharp and Dohme Research Laboratories had kindly provided in 1966 gift-samples of the following sequences of the three amino acids and Gln modifications of Glu: Pro-Glu-His; Glu-Pro-His; His-Glu-Pro; Glu-His-Pro;

His-Pro-Glu; Pro-His-Glu; His-Pro-Gln; Pro-His-Gln. Although these samples included Glu-His-Pro, none of them showed the hormonal activity of TRH, either in vitro or in vivo at relatively high dose levels (Schally et al., 1968).

The lack of activity of the unsubstituted tripeptide, Glu-His-Pro, is not particularly surprising since TRH does not appear to have a free amino or carboxyl group; TRH appears to be a substituted or modified form of Glu-His-Pro. Taking into account the known structural characteristics of TRH, including the knowledge of the sequence, synthetic experiments were carried out on Glu-His-Pro to modify both the amino and carboxyl groups. This tripeptide was treated with anhydrous methanol containing hydrogen chloride to form a dimethyl ester. The dimethyl ester was dissolved in anhydrous methanol saturated with ammonia at -5° and allowed to stand for 24 hours at room temperature to yield preparation A. The conditions used to give preparation A may be expected (Coleman, 1951; Beecham, 1954, Shiba et al., 1958) to give predominately, but not exclusively, (pyro)Glu-His-Pro(NH$_2$) (I). Preparation A was not specially purified partly because the tripeptide used as starting material was estimated to be not over 80% pure, and the reactions were carried out on a milligram-basis. Preparation A was ninhydrin-negative and Pauly-positive.

Samples of preparation A were subjected directly to biological tests for hormonal activity by the T$_3$-TRH method in mice (Bowers et al., 1965, '67, '69). The response is determined by the increase of I^{125} in the blood as Δ cpm two hours after the i.v. injection of TRH and the synthetic preparations. The increase is proportional to the amount of TSH released from the pituitary. Since the doses of the synthetic preparations represent the weights of the starting material, they are the "relative" rather than the actual amounts of the products given; although products were visualized chromatographically, the yields are unknown. Nevertheless, levels of "6 - 54" nanograms of preparation A in the mouse increased I^{125} in the range of Δ cpm 670 - 8000 and in comparison with Δcpm 140 - 170 for acid-saline controls. Levels of 2 - 6 - 18 nanograms of porcine TRH increased I^{125} in the range of Δ cpm 2000 - 6000. It is significant that preparation A is extremely active in comparison with porcine TRH although a precise comparison of activities is not yet known. Graded responses were obtained when the doses of preparation A was increased, and two of the important biological characteristics of natural TRH were observed: (a) the degree of the response depended upon the amount of T_3 injected; (b) incubation for fifteen minutes at 37°C in normal human plasma inactivated the synthetic preparation.

The synthetic preparation was also active _in vitro_ by the method of Bowers et al. (1965). The amount of TSH released from the pituitary into the medium was estimated by the release of I^{125} from the thyroid gland of mice. Activity is measured as I^{125} in Δ cpm and is proportional to the amount of TSH present in the medium. More TSH (Δ cpm, 2300 - 3100) was released when "50" nanograms of the preparation A was added to the medium than in the control (Δ cpm 275). It appeared that T_3 added, _in vitro_, or given, _in vivo_, partially or completely inhibited the activity.

A comparison was made of the changes in blood levels of I^{125} in mice at various time-intervals after the i.v. injection of acid-saline, the synthetic preparations, porcine and bovine TSH. The time-response curves of the active compounds are essentially the same. There was a definite rise at 60 minutes; the levels were higher at 90 minutes and remained elevated at 120 and 180 minutes.

Preparation A elevated the plasma levels of TSH in rats (Bowers et al., 1965), and produced an increase within two minutes in plasma levels of TSH, after its i.v. injection in mice (Bowers et al., 1967, 1969). The plasma levels of TSH were highest at 10 and 15 minutes, and remained elevated for 60 minutes, and started to fall at 120 minutes. Preparation A was active in mice when given i.v., i.p., but not i.m. or orally.

Similar synthetic reactions were carried out upon Glu-Pro-His; Pro-His-Gln; Pro-His-Glu, but none of the resulting preparations showed the hormonal activity of TRH under comparable conditions. To this limited extent, the sequence of Glu-His-Pro shows organic structural specificity for hormonal activity.

While these structural and synthetic studies have been on TRH isolated from porcine hypothalami, Guillemin and his group have similarly investigated TRH which they isolated from ovine hypothalami. Burgus et al., 1969, found TRH-activity at microgram levels for acetylation products of Glu-His-Pro and observed that TRH is active at 1×10^{-3} of the level of these particular synthetic preparations.

These mutually independent synthetic studies on porcine and ovine TRH show at this stage of structural elucidation that the hormone from the two mammalian species may be chemically identical.

ACKNOWLEDGMENT. - Gratitude is expressed to Dr. Sheldon J. Segal and The Population Council for their interest and support which have contributed to this research.

REFERENCES

Beecham, A. F., J. Am. Chem. Soc., 76, 4615 (1954).

Bowers, C. Y., Redding, T. W., and Schally, A. V., Endocrinology, 77, 609, (1965).

Bowers, C. Y., Schally, A. V., Reynolds, G. A., and Hawley, W. D., Endocrinology, 81, 741 (1967).

Bowers, C. Y., and Schally, A. V., (J. Meites, ed.) Proceedings of NIH Conference on Hypothalamic Hypophysiotropic Hormones, Tuscon, Arizona (1969) in press.

Burgus, R., Dunn, T. F., Ward, D. N., Vale, W., Amoss, M., and Guillemin, R., C. R. Acad. Sc. Paris, 268, 2116 (1969).

Coleman, D., J. Chem. Soc., 2294 (1951).

Schally, A. V., Bowers, C. Y., Redding, T. W., and Barrett, J. F., Biochem. Biophys. Res. Commun., 25, 165 (1966).

Schally, A. V., Arimura, A., Bowers, C. Y., Kastin, A. J., Sawano, S., and Redding, T. W., Recent Progress in Hormone Research, 24, 497 (1968).

Schally, A. V., Redding, T. W., Bowers, C. Y., and Barrett, J. F., J. Biol. Chem., April 10, (1969).

Shiba, T., Imai, S., Kameko, Bull. Chem. Soc., Japan, 31, 244 (1958).

Editor's Comments on Papers 18 and 19

18   MARTIN and REICHLIN
     Thyrotropin Secretion in Rats after Hypothalamic Electrical Stimulation or Injection of Synthetic TSH-Releasing Factor

19   BROWNSTEIN et al.
     Thyrotropin-Releasing Hormone in Specific Nuclei of Rat Brain

Martin and Reichlin (Paper 18) demonstrated that electrical stimulation of sites in the medial-basal and paraventricular areas of the hypothalamus resulted in a rapid increase in circulating levels of TSH as measured by a specific radioimmunoassay (RIA). The ability to measure TSH in small samples of blood using the RIA allowed them to perform time-course studies of TSH release after hypothalamic stimulation. TSH rose within five minutes and was maximally elevated at ten to twenty-five minutes following stimulation. Intravenous synthetic TRH induced a maximal rise in five minutes. The results of this study indicate that there are neuronal elements within the medial-basal hypothalamus (MBH) that release TRH. The rapid responses of TSH release following stimulation of the MBH suggested that there was release of previously synthesized TRH from these cells.

Brownstein et al. (Paper 19) made use of a sensitive and highly specific RIA, which they developed to measure TRH, and a new method, which allowed discreet brain nuclei to be isolated by stereomicroscopically controlled techniques to study TRH distribution in rat brain nuclei. The highest concentrations of TRH were found in the hypothalamus, with relatively large amounts of TRH being found in the preoptic and septal areas; lesser amounts were also found in the mammary body, the cerebral cortex, and the brain stem. The highest concentration of TRH within the hypothalamus was in the region of the median eminence (ME). The highest concentration outside the ME was found in the ventromedial hypothalamus; there was a concentration gradient with lesser quantities of TRH peripheral to the portion of the hypothalamus adjacent to the third ventricle. The results of this study suggest that TRH is produced in several hypothalamic nuclei and by axonal transport reaches the ME, where it is stored and can be discharged into the portal system to act on the adenohypophysis to release TSH. The authors suggested that TRH might act as a neurotransmitter in other areas of the brain. The anatomical area of distribution of TRH demonstrated in this study corresponds to the hypophysiotrophic area of the hypothalamus that was described by Halász in 1962. The role of TRH as a neurotransmitter has been further suggested by the localization of TRH in the gut, pancreas, and placenta in the laboratories of Hershman and Wilber, as well as those of others.

Thyrotropin Secretion in Rats after Hypothalamic Electrical Stimulation or Injection of Synthetic TSH-Releasing Factor

Joseph B. Martin and Seymour Reichlin

A number of authors have claimed that electrical stimulation of the hypothalamus causes an increase in pituitary thyroid-stimulating hormone (TSH) secretion. Most of these studies have measured changes in thyroid function as an index of TSH release (1). Certain of these experiments suffer from the criticism that non-TSH changes such as vasopressin release (in the rabbit), epinephrine release (in the dog), or other unknown factors such as vascular changes due to sympathetic stimulation might have accounted for the observed results. Increases in plasma TSH as measured by bioassay have been reported in the rat and the rabbit following hypothalamic stimulation (2, 3). The studies in the rat used repeated daily stimulations. Elevation of plasma TSH was found several hours after the last stimulation, but no increases could be detected 1 to 2 hours after a single stimulation of 20 minutes' duration (2). In the experiments performed in the rabbit, plasma TSH levels were shown to be increased within 15 minutes after the onset of stimulation, with peak responses occurring in some animals between 15 and 45 minutes. This is the only report of the time course of plasma TSH response after hypothalamic stimulation.

The development of a sensitive and specific radioimmunoassay for TSH in the rat (4) has provided the methodology for determination of TSH in small samples of plasma, permitting repeated sampling from the same animal. With this method we have made detailed time-course studies of the effect of electrical stimulation of the hypothalamus. Since it has been hypothesized that the regulation of TSH release is dependent upon the secretion of a hypothalamic "releasing factor" (thyrotropin-releasing factor, TRF), changes in plasma TSH following electrical stimulation were compared with those obtained following the intravenous administration of "synthetic" TRF. Recently two laboratories have reported that a tripeptide amide, pyroglutamyl-histidyl-proline-amide, has thyrotropin-releasing activity identical with that of TRF isolated from hypothalamic extracts and is virtually indistinguishable chemically from the isolated native material (5, 6).

Male Sprague-Dawley rats weighing 250 to 450 g were used. Plasma samples were obtained under pentobarbital (50 mg/kg) or ether anesthesia either by puncture of the external jugular vein or from indwelling jugular cannulas. For electrical stimulation, bipolar .032 gauge Nichrome electrodes, insulated with Insl-X except at the tip, were placed stereotactically into various areas of the medial-basal hypothalamus. The electrodes were soldered to a connector which was affixed to the skull with screws and dental cement. Electrical stimulations were performed 10 to 14 days later. Biphasic square waves from a constant-current stimulator were delivered for 5 or 10 minutes in trains of 4 seconds on and 4 to 10 seconds off, with current of 0.5 to 1.0 ma, frequency of 60 cycle/second, and pulse duration of 1 to 2 msec.

Two separate experiments were undertaken. In the first, electrodes were placed in various regions of the basal hypothalamus extending from the anterior hypothalamus to the posterior ventromedial nucleus. Plasma samples were taken prior to and at several intervals for a period of 1 to 2 hours after stimulation. In the second experiment, electrodes were implanted in the median eminence [de Groot coordinate (7): anterior (+)5.6, lateral 0.5, depth (−)3.0], and samples were taken at 0, 5, 10, 15, and 25 minutes.

Two kinds of controls were used. Five sham-stimulated animals with electrodes in place were anesthetized, and blood samples were withdrawn

Table 1. Plasma thyrotropin response to electrical stimulation or "synthetic" TRF administration. Values are milliunits of plasma TSH per 100 milliliters, ± standard error.

Experiment	Time (min)				
	0	5	10	15	25
Hypothalamic stimulation	8.6 ± 3.2	14.9 ± 3.2	20.6 ± 3.8	23.3 ± 8.9	20.9 ± 9.4
Cortex stimulation	11.3 ± 2.0	10.5 ± 2.1	9.3 ± 2.7	6.8 ± 1.0	10.6 ± 3.7
100 ng TRF intravenously	9.5 ± 2.0	97.0 ± 13.3	74.5 ± 15.1	59.4 ± 11.7	
0.9 percent NaCl intravenously	10.6 ± 3.2	12.0 ± 4.0	5.4 ± 0.4	6.6 ± 1.6	

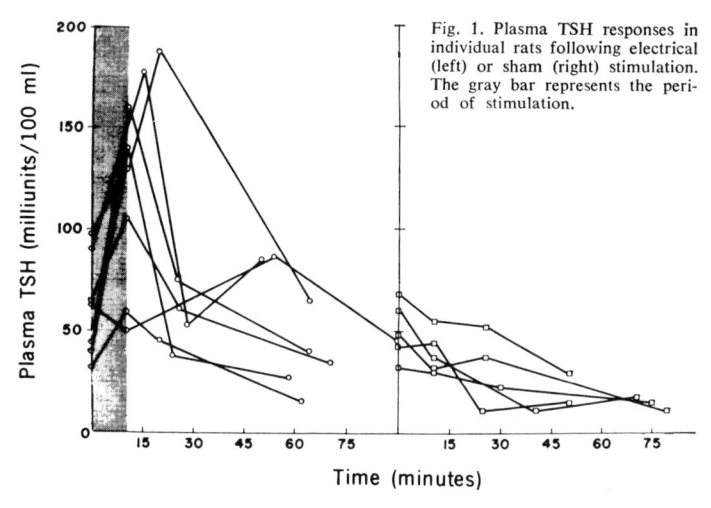

Fig. 1. Plasma TSH responses in individual rats following electrical (left) or sham (right) stimulation. The gray bar represents the period of stimulation.

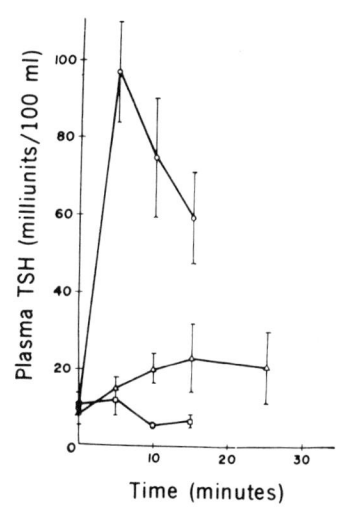

Fig. 2. Comparison of the plasma TSH response following electrical stimulation with that following intravenous administration of "synthetic" TRF. Each point represents the mean of five animals in the experimental groups and four animals in the control group. Circles, "synthetic" TRF; triangles, electrical stimulation; squares, controls; vertical bars, standard errors of the means.

without application of current. Five other animals were stimulated with identical currents through electrodes placed 1 mm below the surface of the parietal cortex. Histological verification of electrode sites was obtained by serial sections of paraffin-embedded brains stained with Luxol fast blue and cresyl violet. There was no evidence of lesions at the site of stimulation. Further proof that the effects were not due to tissue damage was the finding that repeated stimulations at intervals of 2 to 4 weeks in the same animal gave comparable TSH responses.

The amide of the synthetic tripeptide pyroglutamyl-histidyl-proline-acetate (furnished through the courtesy of Hoffman-LaRoche Laboratories) was prepared in our laboratory according to the method described by Burgus et al. (5). Proof that the product obtained was similar to the material synthesized by Bøler and co-workers (6) was shown by thin-layer chromatography of the reaction products in three different solvent systems. One hundred nanograms of the amide were injected into the jugular vein and blood samples were taken for TSH assay at 5-, 10-, and 15-minute intervals. Control rats received normal saline which was used as the diluent for the amide.

Electrical stimulation of a number of sites in the medial-basal hypothalamus resulted in rapid, marked increases in plasma TSH levels, which reached a peak at 10 to 25 minutes after the onset of stimulation (Fig. 1). Positive responses were obtained in seven of eight animals. The electrode placements were all within 1 mm of the midline and no more than 1.5 mm from the base of the hypothalamus; locations extended from the posterior portion of the anterior hypothalamic region to the posterior arcuate nucleus. In the animal in which no response occurred (not shown in the figure), the electrode was located slightly dorsolateral to the ventromedial nucleus, a location which did give a positive response in another animal. One animal showed a later response than the others, a result which may have been in part due to the sampling sequence, since the peak response may have been missed. In the sham-stimulated animals plasma TSH continued to fall during the period of anesthesia, an effect on plasma TSH which has been consistently found in our laboratory with pentobarbital or ether anesthesia.

Since consistent responses appeared to occur with median eminence placements, the time course of TSH release was determined by frequent sampling in animals with electrodes in this region. Stimulation was applied for 5 minutes. The results are shown in Table 1 and Fig. 2. An increase in plasma TSH occurred in all of the five animals stimulated, but the increases were much less than that following the 10-minute stimulations used in the first experiment. An increase in plasma TSH was evident at 5 minutes, but the increase was not significant until 10 minutes ($P < .05$, Student's t-test). The peak response appeared to occur at 15 minutes. Stimulation of the cerebral cortex had no effect on plasma TSH levels.

The administration of 100 ng of "synthetic" TRF produced a much more rapid and dramatic response similar in magnitude to the response following 10 minutes of electrical stimulation in the first experiment (Table 1 and Fig. 2). The response was already maximal in the samples taken at 5 minutes and reached levels comparable to those obtained in our laboratory following thyroidectomy. The time course of this response is similar to that which is observed following administration of hypothalamic extracts with TSH-releasing activity (unpublished results).

Control injections of 0.9 percent NaCl, crude extracts of porcine cerebral cortex (equivalent in weight to five stalk median eminences), synthetic mast cell releaser 48/80 (0.03 to 0.5 mg), histamine phosphate (0.25 mg), and Pitressin (0.5 unit) were all without effect on plasma TSH levels.

These experiments demonstrate for the first time the time course of TSH release in the rat following hypothalamic electrical stimulation. The increases in plasma TSH levels were rapid and corresponded closely to those reported for growth hormone following stimulation of the ventromedial hypothalamic nucleus in the rat (8). Since peripheral blood was sampled in these experiments, the quantity of TSH secreted must be considerable in order to elevate blood levels two- to fivefold. It is hypothesized that release of TSH from the pituitary is dependent upon a thyrotropin-releasing factor synthesized in the neurons of the basal hypothalamus. The rapid responses which occur following electrical excitation of this region are suggestive of release of preformed TRF from these cells. The administration of "synthetic" TRF in the present experiments produced a more rapid increase in plasma TSH levels, which reached thyroidectomy levels (perhaps a maximal response) within 5 minutes. It is probable that the earlier response following a single injection of TRF reflects the difference between a sudden stimulus and a more sustained release of smaller quantities of TRF during the period of hypothalamic stimulation.

References and Notes

1. G. W. Harris and J. W. Woods, *J. Physiol. (London)* **143**, 246 (1958); H. J. Campbell, R. George, G. W. Harris, *ibid.* **152**, 527 (1960); K. Shizume, K. Matsuda, M. Irie, S. Iino, J. Ishii, S. Nagataki, F. Matsuzaki, S. Okinaka, *Endocrinology* **70**, 298 (1962); W. C. Boop and J. Story, *Neurology* **16**, 1167 (1966); M. Vertes, Z. Vertes, S. Kovacs, *Acta Physiol. Acad. Sci. Hung.* **27**, 229 (1965); R. L. W. Averill and T. H. Kennedy, *N.Z. Med. J.* **65** 398 (1966).
2. S. A. D'Angelo and J. Snyder, *Endocrinology* **73**, 75 (1963).
3. ——— and J. M. Grodin, *ibid.* **75**, 417 (1964); R. L. W. Averill and D. F. Salaman, *ibid.* **81**, 173 (1967).
4. S. Reichlin, J. B. Martin, R. L. Boshans, D. S. Schalch, J. G. Pierce, J. Bollinger, in preparation.
5. R. Burgus, T. F. Dunn, D. Desiderio, W. Vale, R. Guillemin, *C. R. Hebd. Seances Acad. Sci. Paris* **269**, 226 (1969).
6. J. Bøler, F. Enzmann, K. Folkers, C. Y. Bowers, A. V. Schally, *Biochem. Biophys. Res. Commun.* **37**, 705 (1969).
7. J. de Groot, *J. Comp. Neurol.* **113**, 389 (1959).
8. L. A. Frohman, L. L. Bernardis, K. J. Kant, *Science* **162**, 580 (1968).
9. We thank Drs. Roger Guillemin and Andrew V. Schally who have allowed us to read their manuscripts in advance of publication. Supported by PHS grant AM 13695-01.

Thyrotropin-Releasing Hormone in Specific Nuclei of Rat Brain

Michael J. Brownstein, Miklos Palkovits, Juan M. Saavedra, Rabim M. Bassiri, and Robert D. Utiger

In 1947 Green and Harris (*1*) proposed that neurons located in the hypothalamus might secrete into the portal circulation certain substances which are essential for the normal function of the pituitary (*2*). In the late 1950's and early 1960's hypothalamic extracts were prepared which could stimulate thyrotropin secretion (*3*). The active principle in such extracts, which is called thyrotropin-releasing hormone (TRH), was ultimately isolated, and its structure was determined to be pyroglutamyl-histidyl-prolineamide (*4*) Synthetic TRH has been produced, and a highly sensitive and specific radioimmunoassay has been developed using the synthetic hormone (*5*).

Recently a technique has been described which allows discrete nuclei to be dissected from the brain of the rat (*6*). This technique involves punching small pellets of tissue from frozen sections of the brain under stereomicroscopic control. The method has been used to study the distribution of several putative transmitters among the hypothalamic nuclei of the rat (*7–10*). We report here the localization of TRH in hypothalamic and extrahypothalamic brain nuclei.

Female rats (Osborne-Mendel, NIH strain) (average weight, 150 g) were used. The animals, which were housed in diurnal lighting conditions (light 6 a.m. to 6 p.m., dark 6 p.m. to 6 a.m.) with free access to food and water, were killed by decapitation at 9:00 a.m. Their brains were removed quickly, frozen on a block of Dry Ice, and sectioned with a cryostat-microtome. Sections 300 μm thick were cut through the brain in the frontal plane. In initial experiments relatively large regions of the brain (for example, septum, amygdala, and mammillary body) were cut or punched from the sections. The tissues obtained from two rats were pooled and homogenized in 200 μl of 2.0N acetic acid; 5 μl of each homogenate was removed for protein determination according to the method of Lowry et al. (*11*). Bovine serum albumin (BSA) served as the standard. The homogenates were centrifuged and the supernatants were lyophilized. Subsequently, the samples were dissolved in a solution consisting of 0.25 percent BSA, 0.01M phosphate, and 0.15M NaCl (pH 7.5), and their TRH contents were determined by radioimmunoassay (*5*). Results were expressed as nanograms of TRH per milligram of protein. Of exogenous TRH (1 ng) added to brain homogenates and carried through the entire assay procedures, 96.2 ± 5.6 percent (mean ± standard error of the mean) was recovered.

In the preliminary experiments described above, the protein content of each sample was in the range 0.2 to 1 mg. No TRH was detected in samples from the following regions (*12*): pineal gland, habenula, central gray, reticular formation, tegmentum, cerebellar cortex, amygdala, hippocampus, cingulate cortex, parietal cortex, olfactory tubercle, caudate nucleus, and anterior pituitary. When larger samples than those used in this study were assayed, TRH was found in the thalamus, brain-

Table 1. Distribution of TRH in the hypothalamus, preoptic area, and septum. The abbreviations are as used in Fig. 1; *N*, number of samples assayed; ng/mg, nanograms per milligram of protein (mean ± standard error of the mean).

Brain region	Abbreviation	N	TRH content ng/mg	Nanograms per nucleus
Hypothalamus			1.3*	
Nucleus periventricularis†	NPE	4	4.25 ± 0.69	0.22
Nucleus suprachiasmaticus	NSC	4	1.79 ± 0.18	0.05
Nucleus supraopticus	NSO	4	0.85 ± 0.17	0.02
Nucleus anterior	NHA	4	0.82 ± 0.28	0.15
Nucleus hypothalamicus lateralis anterior	MFB	4	0.70 ± 0.23	
Nucleus paraventricularis	NPV	4	2.60 ± 0.74	0.15
Nucleus arcuatus	NA	6	3.92 ± 0.90	0.41
Nucleus ventromedialis pars medialis	NVMm	4	9.02 ± 3.3	0.80
Nucleus ventromedialis pars lateralis	NVMl	4	2.95 ± 0.59	0.16
Nucleus dorsomedialis	NDM	4	3.95 ± 0.75	0.29
Nucleus perifornicalis	NPF	4	2.03 ± 0.71	0.06
Area hypothalamica lateralis posterior	MFB	4	1.15 ± 0.49	
Nucleus posterior	NHP	4	1.79 ± 0.20	0.10
Nucleus premammillaris dorsalis	NPMD	4	1.48 ± 0.16	0.03
Nucleus premammillaris ventralis	NPMV	4	1.34 ± 0.27	0.02
Median eminence	ME	4	38.38 ± 8.27	0.89
Mammillary body	MB	6	< 0.32‡	
Preoptic area		6	1.09 ± 0.08	
Nucleus preopticus medialis	NPOm	4	1.95 ± 0.13	0.20
Septum		6	0.72 ± 0.09	
Nucleus medialis	Sm	3	0.35 ± 0.07	
Nucleus dorsalis	Sd	3	1.86 ± 0.38	
Nucleus dorsalis pars intermedia	Si	3	0.47 ± 0.11	
Nucleus fimbrialis		3	0.62 ± 0.24	
Nucleus triangularis		3	0.51 ± 0.04	
Nucleus lateralis	Sl	3	2.97 ± 0.34	

* This is based on the data of Winokur and Utiger (*13*), who found 0.129 ± 0.007 ng of TRH per milligram of tissue (wet weight) (*N* = 30) in hypothalamic fragments with an average weight of 32.6 mg.   † The periventricular nucleus was removed from brain sections with a small knife. The nucleus consists of a fine line of cells and was contaminated by tissue lying lateral to it in our samples. Therefore the concentration of TRH in the periventricular nucleus may be greater than reported.   ‡ TRH could be measured in only three of the six samples assayed. The mean TRH concentration in these samples was 0.32 ng/mg.

stem, and cerebral cortex (see *13, 14*).

As expected, TRH was found in high concentrations in the hypothalamus (Table 1). There were also relatively large amounts of TRH in the preoptic and septal areas, and a small amount was found in the mammillary body (Table 1). Therefore, the distribution of TRH among discrete nuclei of the hypothalamus, septum, and preoptic area was studied. Sixteen hypothalamic nuclei, the median eminence, the medial preoptic nucleus, and six septal nuclei could be dissected from the brain of each rat (*7*). These nuclei were removed from frozen brain sections 300 μm thick with small punches (*6*). The inner diameter of the punch was 300 or 500 μm and never exceeded the smallest cross-sectional diameter of the nucleus that was being removed. For each nucleus two to four pellets of tissue were removed from each brain. Nuclei from five rats were pooled and homogenized in 200 μl of 2.0N acetic acid in microhomogenizers (Micrometric Instrument Co.). The homogenates were extracted and assayed as described above.

The concentrations of TRH in isolated nuclei of rat brain are listed in Table 1. Since the volumes of the hypothalamic nuclei (except for the lateral anterior and lateral posterior nuclei), the medial preoptic nucleus, and the median eminence were known (*15*) the amount of TRH in these regions could be calculated. These amounts also appear in Table 1.

The median eminence contained 1.04 ng of TRH; this is about 25 percent of the TRH found in a 30-mg fragment of hypothalamus (*13, 14*). The concentration of TRH in the median eminence was four times greater than that in the medial part of the ventromedial nucleus, the nucleus with the highest TRH concentration. Of the TRH located within the hypothalamic nuclei, approximately 32 percent was found in the medial part of the ventromedial nucleus, 12 percent in the dorsomedial nucleus, 16 percent in the arcuate nucleus, 7 percent in the lateral part of the ventromedial nucleus, 9 percent in the periventricular nucleus, and 23 percent in the eleven remaining nuclei (*16*). The three subdivisions of the medial part of the ventromedial nucleus were separated and assayed for TRH. The amount of TRH per subdivision and the contribution of each subdivision to the total TRH in the medial part of the ventromedial nucleus were determined. The medial posterior subdivision contributed 51 percent to the total, the medial anterior subdivision 46 percent, and the ventromedial anterior nucleus 3 percent.

The medial preoptic nucleus, which comprises one-half of the preoptic area, contained most of the TRH in that area (Table 1). The dorsal and lateral septal nuclei had much higher concentrations of the peptide than did the other four septal nuclei (Table 1).

These results show that TRH is scattered among several hypothalamic nuclei and that it is present in extrahypothalamic sites. Figure 1 shows the distribution of TRH. It was found in highest concentrations adjacent to the third ventricle in the hypothalamus and adjacent to the lateral ventricles in the septum.

In all likelihood, the TRH found in the median eminence is present in axons and nerve endings which terminate on or near the portal vessels. It is not clear, however, whether the TRH measured elsewhere is present in cell bodies, axons, or nerve terminals. Cell bodies that produce TRH may reside solely in one, two, or three nuclei which send their axons to the median eminence and to other areas of the brain. Thus, the peptide might act as a releasing hormone at the anterior pituitary and as a transmitter in other regions. The development of an immunohistochemical technique for visualizing TRH in nervous tissue should help to resolve these questions.

A variety of techniques have been used to study the neural control of thyrotropin secretion. The earliest studies involved examination of the effect of brain lesions on the function of the thyroid (*17*). Greer (*18*) used this technique to delineate a "thyrotrophic area" of the brain. This area is found in the midline between the paraventricular nuclei and the median eminence. Elec-

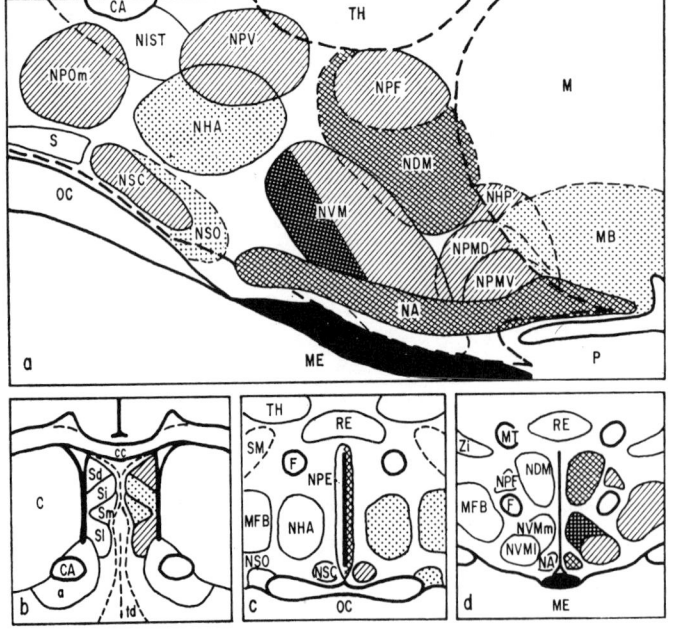

Fig. 1. Localization of TRH in the hypothalamus, septum, and preoptic area. Drawing (a) is of a parasagittal section through the rat hypothalamus and (b) to (d) are of frontal sections. Drawing (b) depicts the septal region, (c) the anterior hypothalamus, and (d) the tuberal region. Abbreviations: *C*, nucleus caudatus; *CA*, comissura anterior; *CC*, corpus callosum; *F*, fornix; *M*, mesencephalon; *MT*, tractus mammillothalamicus; *NIST*, nucleus interstitialis striae terminalis; *OC*, chiasma opticum; *P*, pituitary; *RE*, nucleus reuniens thalami; *S*, nucleus preopticus suprachiasmaticus; *SM*, stria medullaris; *TH*, thalamus; *Zi*, zona incerta; *q*, nucleus accumbens; and *td*, nucleus tractus diagonalis. The remainder of the abbreviations appear in Table 1. Key: nanograms of TRH per milligram of protein.

■ 38
▨ 9
▦ 3.5–4.5
▥ 1–3
⋯ <1

trical stimulation of this region of the hypothalamus produced an increase in plasma thyrotropin concentration (*19*), and pituitary implants in this area show thyrotrope differentiation and stimulate thyroid function (*20*). Measurements of TRH remaining in the hypothalamus after lesions were also compatible with its being localized in the thyrotrophic area (*21*). In our study TRH was found in highest concentrations within nuclei of the thyrotrophic area, but was found outside this area as well.

The distribution of TRH differs from that of the luteinizing hormone releasing hormone, which is found almost exclusively in the arcuate nucleus and median eminence (*22*). The fact that TRH is distributed among several nuclei suggests that more detailed anatomical, physiological, and pharmacological studies of these nuclei are needed to ascertain their individual roles in generating the neuroendocrine (*4, 23*) and behavioral (*24*) effects that have been attributed to TRH. In addition, it has recently proved possible to measure norepinephrine (*7*), dopamine (*7*), serotonin (*8*), histamine (*9*), and choline acetyltransferase (*10*) in isolated hypothalamic nuclei. It is hoped that the part played by one or more of the biogenic amines in the control of TRH release can be established.

References and Notes

1. J. D. Green and G. W. Harris, *J. Endocrinol.* **5**, 136 (1947).
2. G. W. Harris, *J. Anat.* **81**, 343 (1947); *J. Physiol. (Lond.)* **107**, 418 (1948).
3. K. Shibusawa, S. Saito, K. Nishi, T. Yamamoto, C. Abe, T. Kawai, *Endocrinol. (Jap.)* **3**, 151 (1956); K. Shibusawa, S. Saito, K. Nishi, T. Yamamoto, K. Tomizawa, C. Abe, *ibid.*, p. 116; K. Shibusawa, T. Yamamoto, K. Nishi, C. Abe, S. Tomie, K. Shirota, *ibid.* **6**, 149 (1959); V. Schreiber *et al.*, *Experientia (Basel)* **17**, 264 (1961); R. Guillemin, E. Yamazaki, M. Jutisz, E. Sakiz, *C. R. Hebd. Seances Acad. Sci.* **255**, 1018 (1962).
4. J. Boler, F. Enzmann, K. Folkers, C. Y. Bowers, A. V. Schally, *Biochem. Biophys. Res. Commun.* **37**, 705 (1969); R. Burgus, T. F. Dunn, D. Desiderio, R. Guillemin, *C. R. Hebd. Seances Acad. Sci.* **269**, 1870 (1969).
5. R. M. Bassiri and R. D. Utiger, *Endocrinology* **90**, 722 (1972).
6. M. Palkovits, *Brain Res.* **59**, 449 (1973).
7. ———, M. Brownstein, J. M. Saavedra, J. Axelrod, *ibid.*, in press.
8. J. M. Saavedra, M. Palkovits, M. Brownstein, J. Axelrod, *ibid.*, in press.
9. M. Brownstein, J. M. Saavedra, M. Palkovits, J. Axelrod, *ibid.*, in press.
10. M. Brownstein, R. Kobayashi, M. Palkovits, J. M. Saavedra, *J. Neurochem.*, in press.
11. O. H. Lowry, N. J. Rosebrough, A. L. Farr, R. J. Randall, *J. Biol. Chem.* **193**, 265 (1951).
12. The concentration of TRH in these regions is less than 0.3 ng per milligram of protein.
13. A. Winokur and R. D. Utiger, *Science* **185**, 265 (1974).
14. I. M. D. Jackson and S. Reichlin, personal communication; J. C. Porter, *Endocrinology*, in press.
15. M. Palkovits, in preparation.
16. These estimates were obtained by summing the TRH nanograms per nucleus values in Table 1 and dividing the value for each area by the total. Since the contributions of the lateral anterior and lateral posterior nuclei to this total could not be taken into account, our estimates may be somewhat high. It is of note that the sum of the values (3.35 ng) is roughly equal to the amount of TRH measured in 30-mg hypothalamic fragments by Winokur and Utiger (*13*).
17. A. B. Houssay, A. Biasotti, R. San Martino, *C. R. Seances Soc. Biol. Fil.* **120**, 725 (1935); M. Cahane and T. Cahane, *Acta Med. Scand.* **94**, 320 (1938); *Rev. Fr. Endocrinol.* **14**, 472 (1936).
18. M. A. Greer, *Recent Prog. Horm. Res.* **13**, 67 (1959).
19. S. A. D'Angelo, J. Snyder, J. M. Grodin, *Endocrinology* **75**, 417 (1964); J. B. Martin and S. Reichlin, *Science* **168**, 1366 (1970).
20. B. Halasz, L. Pupp, S. Uhlarik, *Endocrinology* **25**, 147 (1962); J. Flament-Durand and L. Desclin, *J. Endocrinol.* **41**, 531 (1968).
21. B. Mess, in *Hypothalamic Control of the Anterior Pituitary*, J. Szentagothai, B. Flerko, B. Mess, B. Halasz, Eds. (Akademiai, Kiado, Budapest, 1968), p. 250.
22. M. Palkovits, A. Arimura, M. Brownstein, A. V. Schally, J. M. Saavedra, *Endocrinology*, in press.
23. C. Y. Bowers, H. G. Friesen, P. Hwang, H. J. Guyda, K. Folkers, *Biochem. Biophys. Res. Commun.* **45**, 1033 (1971); L. Jacobs, P. Snyder, R. Utiger, W. Daughaday, *J. Clin. Endocrinol. Metab.* **33**, 996 (1971); D. S. Schalch, D. Gonzales-Barcena, A. J. Kastin, A. V. Schally, L. A. Lee, *ibid.* **35**, 609 (1972); M. Irie and T. Tsushima, *ibid.*, p. 97.
24. N. P. Plotnikoff, A. J. Prange, Jr., G. R. Breese, M. S. Anderson, I. C. Wilson, *Science* **178**, 417 (1972); A. J. Kastin, R. H. Ehrensing, D. S. Schalch, M. S. Anderson, *Lancet* **1972-I**, 740 (1972); A. J. Prange, Jr., I. C. Wilson, P. P. Lara, L. B. Allsop, G. R. Breese, *Lancet*, *ibid.*, p. 999; I. C. Wilson, A. J. Prange, Jr., P. P. Lara, L. B. Allsop, R. A. Stikeleather, M. A. Lipton, *Arch. Gen. Psychol.* **29**, 15 (1973).
25. We are grateful to Dr. Julius Axelrod for his encouragement and advice and to Ms. Kathleen Kelley for technical assistance. R.M.B. and R.D.U. are supported by grants 5 RO1 AM 14039 and 5 TO 1 AM 05649 from the U.S. Public Health Service.

Part IV
THE HYPOTHALAMIC-HYPOPHYSIAL-GONADAL AXIS

Editor's Comments
on Papers 20 Through 24

20 HARRIS
Excerpts from *The Induction of Ovulation in the Rabbit, by Electrical Stimulation of the Hypothalamo-hypophysial Mechanism*

21 SAWYER, MARKEE, and HOLLINSHEAD
Excerpts from *Inhibition of Ovulation in the Rabbit by the Adrenergic-Blocking Agent Dibenamine*

22 BARRACLOUGH and SAWYER
Excerpts from *Induction of Pseudopregnancy in the Rat by Reserpine and Chlorpromazine*

23 BARRACLOUGH and GORSKI
Excerpts from *Evidence That the Hypothalamus Is Responsible for Androgen-Induced Sterility in the Female Rat*

24 SAWYER and MARKEE
Excerpts from *Estrogen-Facilitation of Release of Pituitary Ovulating Hormone in the Rabbit in Response to Vaginal Stimulation*

Harris (Paper 20) performed studies in the rabbit, a reflex ovulator, which played an important role in the development of hypothalamo-hypophyseal hypothesis of neurovascular adenohypophysial secretion. Previous studies by Westman had demonstrated that intact vascular connections between the hypophysis and the hypothalamus were essential for the release of a so-called ovulating hormone upon copulation. Harris showed that localized electrical stimulation of the median eminence and preoptic-suprachiasmatic regions of the hypothalamus in rabbits evoked ovulation, presumably by causing release of gonadotropins from the adenohypophysis. Harris thus concluded that the hypothalamus is an integral part of a reflex pathway that results in stimulation of the hypophysis with gonadotropin release after sexual excitement and that the functional link between the hypothalamus and the adenohypophysis is the hypophysial stalk. He speculated that the hypothalamus not only controlled gonadotropic hormone secretion but that there also existed similar hypothalamic control of thyrotropic, adrenotropic, lactogenic, and growth hormone release from the adenohypophysis, all of which was documented in the next several decades of research in neuroendocrinology. Markee et al. (1946), using carefully controlled degrees of intensity of electrical stimulation, were able to induce ovulation by directly stimulating the hypothalamus with currents so low as to be ineffective when applied to the hypothalamus. These findings were interpreted as indicating that ovulation was enhanced by activation of nerve tracts present in the hypothalamus but absent from the hypophysis. These results confirmed Harris's earlier studies and suggested that hypothalamic control involved a hormonal pathway between the hypothalamus and hypophysis.

Sawyer, Markee, and Hollingshead (Paper 21) studied the role of adrenergic mechanisms in the copulation-induced neurogenic release of LH by employing Dibenamine, an adrenergic blocking agent. Dibenamine given intravenously within one minute after copulation prevented ovulation in sixteen of nineteen rabbits but was ineffective if administration was delayed for three minutes or more following coitus. This study led to the hypothesis that copulation-induced ovulation in rabbits dependent upon a humoral pathway of an adrenergic nature and that stimulation of the adenohypophysis is completed rapidly following copulation. Thus it was suggested that during the first minute after mating, an adrenergically induced releasing factor was liberated near the emergence of the hypophysial stalk from the median eminence of the hypothalamus and passed along the portal system to the adenohypophysis, resulting in activation of gonadotropin release. The role of nor-adrenergic neurotransmitters in the regulation of gonadotropin secretion was further demonstrated by Barraclough and Sawyer (Paper 22), who showed that reserpine, a catecholamine-depleting agent, blocked ovulation in rats and rabbits. Subsequent studies documented that norepinephrine stimulates hypophysial LH release by increasing hypothalamic release of luteinizing hormone–releasing hormone (LH-RH). Immunohistochemical studies have demonstrated that impinging on hypothalamic LH-RH–containing peptidergic neurons are nor-adrenergic fibers arising from the locus ceruleus of the midbrain, which is connected to the limbic system. Thus, the LH-RH peptidergic neurons have been demonstrated to be regulated by a central aminergic system, which links gonadotropin regulation to the remainder of the brain.

On the basis of physiological studies, Barraclough and Sawyer (Paper 22) proposed a dual hypothalamic control of LH-RH secretion, mediated by two separate anatomical areas of the hypothalamus. Barra-

Editor's Comments on Papers 20 Through 24

clough and Gorski (Paper 23) conducted studies that demonstrated convincingly the existence of a dual hypothalamic control mechanism involving two anatomically distinct regions of the hypothalamus: a region responsible for the tonic discharge of gonadotropins in sufficient quantity to cause secretion but not ovulation and one responsible for activating the cyclic discharge of gonadotropins responsible for ovulation. The arcuate-ventromedial complex of the median eminence was the region associated with basal tonic secretion of gonadotropins and the anterior preoptic (suprachiasmatic) area of the hypothalamus with cyclic gonadotropin discharge. These investigators also presented evidence that prepubertal androgen treatment causes sterility in female rats by interfering with the function of the ovulation-controlling preoptic region of the hypothalamus. They proposed that the anterior preoptic area of the prepubertal female rat is undifferentiated at birth with regard to control of gonadotropin secretion and, when allowed to differentiate normally, regulated the cyclic release of gonadotropins. However, they showed that during a critical period of development, this area, when exposed to androgen, becomes refractory to both intrinsic and extrinsic activation, and the tonic type of male gonadotropin secretion occurs.

Sawyer and Markee (Paper 24) demonstrated that priming the estrus rabbit with estrogen for two days or the anestrus rabbit for longer periods set the stage for release of hypophysial ovulating hormone in response to artificial stimulation of the vagina. The ovarian follicles, ruptured in this response, became functional corpus lutea as evidenced by the decidual reaction to uterine trauma. This was the first evidence of the facilitating role of rising estrogen levels exerted at the hypothalamic level in the gonadotropic surge in reflexogenic ovulation or in midcycle ovulation.

REFERENCE

Markee, J. E., C. H. Sawyer, and W. H. Hollinshead. 1946. Activation of the Anterior Hypophysis by Electrical Stimulation in the Rabbit. *Endocrinology* 38:345.

The Induction of Ovulation in the Rabbit, by Electrical Stimulation of the Hypothalamo-hypophysial Mechanism

By G. W. Harris, *Department of Anatomy, Cambridge*

In two recent papers, by Marshall and Verney (1936), and by Harris (1936), the mechanism concerned with ovulation in the rabbit has been fully discussed. In view of this, only a brief summary of the present position will be given here.

Ovulation in the rabbit occurs normally only after some form of sexual excitement. There is much evidence to show that the factors involved are: first, a nervous stimulation from the genital region and perhaps from the cortex, acting on the anterior lobe of the pituitary gland; and secondly, a hormonal factor, the pituitary gland secreting a gonadotropic hormone which affects the ovaries.

The nervous pathway by which the pituitary gland is stimulated has not yet been fully determined. Cajal (1894) was the first to show that the posterior lobe of this gland is in direct nervous connexion with the hypothalamus. More recently, Greving (1925, 1926) and Pines (1925) have shown that the supra-optic and paraventricular nuclei supply the posterior lobe with fine non-medullated nerve fibres passing through the infundibulum. The only known nerve supply of the anterior lobe is from the superior cervical ganglion, through the carotid plexus (Dandy 1913). No fibres have been traced from the pars nervosa to the pars anterior.

The three main hypotheses which have been put forward concerning the pathways of nervous impulses to the anterior lobe of the pituitary are as follows:

(1) That the impulses pass along sympathetic fibres in the superior cervical ganglion and the carotid plexus. These are the only nerves which have been found entering this lobe of the gland. That this is not the only path has been shown by Vogt (1931, 1933), Hinsey and Markee (1933),

and Brooks (1935), who have all found that rabbits ovulate in a perfectly normal manner after extirpation of the superior cervical ganglia. On the other hand, Haterius (1933) showed that sympathectomized rats failed to become pseudo-pregnant following artificial stimulation, whilst Friedgood and Pincus (1935) managed to obtain ovulation in rabbits after electrical stimulation of the superior cervical ganglia, a result that Haterius (1934) had previously failed to obtain.

There is therefore evidence that the cervical sympathetic system plays some part in this mechanism, but presumably not a very large part.

(2) That there are sympathetic fibres from the central nervous system which supply the pituitary gland, other than those passing through the superior cervical ganglion. Thus Hinsey and Markee (1933) suggest that stimuli may pass to the anterior lobe, via the greater superficial petrosal nerve and the carotid plexus, that is, along paths described by Cobb and Finesinger (1932) and by Chocobski and Penfield (1932).

There appears to have been no experimental evidence put forward for or against this theory.

(3) The third possibility is that there occurs a humoral or nervous transmission of stimuli from the posterior to the anterior lobe of the pituitary, the posterior lobe itself being affected by nerve fibres from the hypothalamus. The evidence for this has been mainly of a negative character, concerning the effect of hypothalamic and pituitary-stalk lesions, on the sex cycles of various animals. Camus and Roussy (1920) showed that, in dogs, damage of the hypothalamus performed with a hot needle led to genital atrophy, though the pituitary gland was left intact by the operation. Bailey and Bremer (1921) found that genital atrophy in dogs followed lesions to the tuber cinereum performed by the temporal route so that there was no danger of concurrent damage to the pituitary gland. Smith (1926) found that lesions of the tuber cinereum in rats produced, amongst other effects, genital atrophy. Cushing (1932a), in discussing Smith's results, says that "in all probability this gonadal effect is merely another instance of interference with hypophysial blood supply or of interrupted nerve supply". Richter (1934) cut the stalk, also in rats, and obtained great prolongation of the oestrous cycle.

This evidence certainly seems to suggest that the hypothalamus and stalk of the pituitary gland are concerned with sexual activity, probably as a functional unit, together with the anterior lobe.

The purpose of the present work was to discover whether the hypothalamus and stalk of the pituitary gland played any part in the mechanism underlying ovulation in the rabbit. Three types of experiments were performed to find the effects on the ovaries of; first, lesions of the stalk; secondly, electrical stimulation of the pituitary gland directly; and thirdly, electrical stimulation of the hypothalamus.

[*Editor's Note:* Material has been omitted at this point.]

Discussion

Previous workers have noted various effects on stimulation of the pituitary gland. Cyon (1898, 1899, 1900) obtained slowing of the heart with increased amplitude of the beat on stimulation by pressure or electrical excitation. Weed, Cushing and Jacobson (1913) showed stimulation of the exposed pituitary in dogs gave variation in the blood sugar. This they put down to stimulation of the posterior lobe. Keeton and Becht (1915) also found that stimulation in dogs produced glycosuria, but not if the splanchnic nerves had been previously cut. It is possible, therefore, that this effect is not due to action of the pituitary gland.

The experiments described above have shown that ovulation in the rabbit can be obtained by electrical stimulation of the pituitary and the hypothalamus. There is evidence that the effects originate definitely in the gland, or through the intermediation of the gland, for the effects upon the ovary are very similar to those obtained by the injection of extracts, either of the pituitary or of pregnancy urine. These effects, besides those of normal ovulation, include the production of cystic follicles,* of cystic follicles becoming haemorrhagic and of large haemorrhagic follicles (figs. 12, 13, 14, Plate 17).

One difference between stimulation and injection of extracts is that the injection of extracts will produce ovulation, formation of luteal tissue, and haemorrhagic follicles in the immature and anoestrous rabbit; but so far as has been observed, to obtain any result by electrical excitation the rabbit must be well on heat. It is possible that after a more delicate technique for stimulating this gland has been obtained, prolonged stimulation over many days might produce different results.

As regards the conclusions to be drawn from the results of the hypothalamic stimulation, one difficulty arises. It is just possible that the positive results obtained were due to general spread of the stimulating current to the pituitary gland, and not due to stimulation of nerve fibres running through the hypothalamus.

At first sight the obvious experiment to perform is stimulation of this region after preliminary transection of the stalk. This is technically extremely difficult, for, as shown previously, after section of this structure, the animals enter into a state of anoestrous. Therefore, unless the stimulation was carried out immediately following the preliminary operation, the experiment would be useless. If the two operations were performed together, the time of the whole experiment and the damage committed would be so great that almost certainly no results of value would be obtained.

Another possible way of deciding the question would be to try to define more accurately the exact regions in the hypothalamus from which the reactions could be obtained and to follow the probable nervous pathway through the mid-brain, so increasing the distance between the stimulating electrode and the pituitary gland. This would require a more delicate stereotaxic instrument than was available in the present research, and further that rabbits of the same breed and nearly uniform in size should be used, thus ensuring more accurate localization when inserting the electrode.

Concerning this question, the evidence at present available is:

(1) That during hypothalamic stimulation, no changes in pupil size were observed, although the eyeballs, eyelids and nictitating membrane were

---

* One observation may be of agricultural interest. In one animal (rabbit 60), cystic and haemorrhagic follicles were obtained following pituitary stimulation (fig. 12, Plate 17). Fifty hours after stimulation and just before being killed, this rabbit was put with a buck. The experimental animal showed intense sexual excitement, manifested by continuous "jumping" on to the male rabbit. The condition produced by this stimulation is thus very suggestive of the pathological condition, nymphomania.

[Editor's Note: Plate 17 is not reproduced here.]

seen to flicker. The conclusion drawn is that the spread of current to the oculomotor nerves was sufficient to stimulate the somatic fibres, but insufficient to stimulate the autonomic fibres which have a higher threshold of excitability. Now in the rabbit oculomotor nerves lie in closer anatomical relationship to the tuber cinereum than does the pituitary gland, so that it would be justifiable to assume that if the current spread did not excite the autonomic fibres in the third nerve it would not excite fibres of a presumably similar nature in the gland.

(2) The results show that the threshold current needed to produce ovulation was the same whether the electrode was in the hypothalamus or in the pituitary. This would indicate that spread of current during hypothalamic stimulation would be insufficient to account for the results obtained.

(3) In rabbit 17, stimulated in the posterior hypothalamus (see fig. 15, Plate 17), the tip of the electrode was 4–5 mm. distant from the nearest point of the pituitary gland. This animal ovulated about 35 hr. post-stimulation. After taking into consideration the fact that, in a case of intended pituitary gland stimulation with the same voltage in which the electrode was found on post-mortem to be lying outside the gland but directly adjacent to it, no ovulation was obtained, it seems safe to conclude again that the results were not due to spread of current.

Therefore, the evidence at present indicates strongly, though not certainly, that ovulation in the rabbit may be induced by stimulation of nerve fibres in the hypothalamus as well as by pituitary stimulation.

If this view be accepted, it would follow that the hypothalamus forms part of a reflex path used in stimulating the pituitary gland after sexual excitement. It therefore becomes of considerable interest to discuss the pathway in detail.

It seems highly probable that the stimulation of the pituitary directly is acting on non-medullated nerve fibres in the anterior lobe and that these fibres have a very high threshold of excitability. The functional links between the hypothalamus and the anterior lobe of the pituitary that have been suggested are, the cervical sympathetic nerves, the greater superficial petrosal nerves and the pituitary stalk. Of these, it cannot be the cervical sympathetic nerves alone, for, as previously stated, ovulation can be obtained in a normal fashion after extirpation of these nerves. It may be the greater superficial petrosal nerves, but on this point there is little evidence. It appears more probable that the functional link is the pituitary stalk. The main evidence for this is that genital atrophy follows lesions of the tuber cinereum and pituitary stalk which has been noted by several previous workers and confirmed in the rabbit in this present account.

The hypothesis that the hypothalamus influences the anterior lobe via nervous impulses passing down the stalk is open to one obvious objection: that is, the fact that nerve fibres have never been seen passing from the posterior to the anterior lobe. By the use of the de Castro technique of staining, nerve fibres may be seen passing from the pars nervosa to the pars intermedia (Cushing 1932b). Serial sections through several rabbit pituitaries have been obtained, demonstrating this fact. It is difficult to trace these fibres to their termination owing to their extremely fine character. It may be mentioned in passing that although the pars nervosa and intermedia may take the stain perfectly, the pars anterior takes it poorly. In order to surmount the above objection, it is necessary to suppose either that the nerve fibres seen to enter the pars intermedia eventually pass round the cleft into the anterior lobe, or else that the posterior or intermediate lobe can influence the anterior lobe hormonally. The former supposition is felt to be the more probable of the two.

This suggested pathway (hypothalamus, stalk, posterior lobe, anterior lobe) may possibly be active in several phenomena which have previously been difficult to explain. It is well known that in some birds and in the ferret, the sex cycle may be influenced by extra radiation. It is probable that the radiation, at least in the ferret, acts on the anterior lobe of the pituitary through the intermediation of the eyes (Bissonnette 1936). Collin (1935) has brought forward evidence that there is a nervous connexion passing from the optic tract through the hypothalamus to the stalk of the pituitary. On correlation, these two facts fit in well with the above theory.

Again, it is highly probable that the uterus may affect the anterior lobe of the pituitary gland by nervous reflex paths, for it has been shown that hysterectomy in the pseudo-pregnant rabbit, or guinea-pig, will prolong the life of corpora lutea in the ovaries (Loeb 1923, 1927; Loeb and Smith 1936; Asdell and Hammond 1933). Selye (1934) showed in rats that Caesarian section initiates lactation and the recurrence of oestrous cycles, though this does not occur if the uterus is distended with wax after removal of the foeti.

From the work of Selye and McKeown (1934), it appears that mechanical stimulation of the nipples is the cause of lactation dioestrus in rats and mice.

Thus there is evidence that the anterior lobe may be influenced by nervous effects from the eyes, uterus and mammary glands, as well as from the vaginal region. Also, Haterius (1933) produced evidence that a psychic factor normally plays a part in the induction of pseudo-pregnancy in rats, whilst Theobald (1936), who has collected clinical evidence for a diencephalic centre governing the menstrual cycle in women, states that psychic factors such as fear of pregnancy and hypnosis may affect this cycle through the supposed centre.

It might be theorized that the hypothalamus controls the secretion of hormones, other than the gonadrotropic hormone, from the anterior lobe. In a recent review on the relationship between the hypothalamus and the pituitary, Dodds and Noble (1936) draw attention to the well-known facts that hypothalamic damage may cause glycosuria, adiposity, and genital atrophy, which are possibly all anterior lobe effects. Here then is evidence that the hypothalamus controls the secretion of the hormones influencing sugar and fat metabolism. There is no reason to doubt that the thyrotropic, adrenotropic, lactogenic, parathyrotropic and growth hormones are not similarly controlled.

Finally, much evidence has accumulated in the past few years indicating that the hypothalamus contains centres controlling the autonomic nervous system. If it is further shown that the pituitary gland and, through the intermediation of the structure, the thyroid, parathyroids, adrenals and gonads are likewise influenced by this important region of the brain, then it would be possible to say that a very large part of both the nervous and chemical links which unite one part of the body functionally with another part are controlled by this region of the diencephalon.

I wish to express my sincerest thanks to Professor H. A. Harris and Professor E. D. Adrian for their ever willing advice. In particular, my deepest gratitude is due to Dr F. H. A. Marshall, first, for suggesting this work to me, and secondly for his constant aid and encouragement. Also I should like to thank Mr E. Powell for the care he bestowed on the animals.

The expenses of this research were in part defrayed by a grant from the Medical Research Council.

Summary

Lesions in the stalk of the pituitary gland have been shown to cause genital atrophy in male and female rabbits.

Direct stimulation of the pituitary gland in female rabbits induced ovulation 15–40 hr. later and sometimes the formation of cystic and haemorrhagic follicles.

Stimulation of the hypothalamus gave results similar to the above.

Evidence is adduced that this is an effect on nerve fibres in the hypothalamus rather than due to spread to the pituitary gland.

The control of the anterior lobe of the pituitary by the hypothalamus is discussed, with particular reference to the nervous pathway involved.

References

Asdell, S. A. and Hammond, J. 1933 *Amer. J. Physiol.* **103**, 600.
Bailey, P. and Bremer, F. 1921 *Arch. Intern. Med.* **28**, 773.
Bissonnette, T. H. 1936 *J. Hered.* **27**, 171.
Brooks, C. McC. 1935 *Amer. J. Physiol.* **113**, 18.
Cajal, R. y 1894 *An. Soc. esp. Hist. nat.* **2**, 214.
Camus, J. and Roussy, G. 1920 *Endocrinology*, **4**, 507.
Chocobski, J. and Penfield, W. 1932 *Arch. Neurol. Psychiat., Chicago*, **28**, 1257.
Cobb, S. and Finesinger, J. E. 1932 *Arch. Neurol. Psychiat., Chicago*, **28**, 1243.
Collin, R. 1935 *C.R. Soc. Biol., Paris*, **118**, 1560.
Cushing, H. 1932*a* "Papers relating to the Pituitary Body, Hypothalamus, and Para-sympathetic Nervous System," p. 42. Baltimore: Thomas.
— 1932*b* "Papers relating to the Pituitary Body, Hypothalamus, and Para-sympathetic Nervous System," p. 22. Baltimore: Thomas.
Cyon, A. von 1898, 1899, 1900 A series of papers in *Pflug. Arch. ges. Physiol.*
Dandy, W. E. 1913 *Amer. J. Anat.* **15**, 333.
Dodds, E. C. and Noble, R. L. 1936 *Brit. Med. J.* No. 3956, p. 878.
Friedgood, H. B. and Pincus, G. 1935 *Endocrinology*, **19**, 710.
Greving, R. 1925 *Klin. Wschr.* **4**, 2181.
— 1926 *Dtsch. Z. Nervenheilk.* **89**, 179.
Harris, G. W. 1936 *J. Physiol.* **88**, 361.
Haterius, H. O. 1933 *Amer. J. Physiol.* **103**, 97.
— 1934 *Proc. Soc. Exp. Biol., N.Y.*, **31**, 1112.
Hinsey, J. C. and Markee, J. E. 1933 *Proc. Soc. Exp. Biol., N.Y.*, **31**, 270.
Keeton, R. W. and Becht, F. C. 1915 *Amer. J. Physiol.* **39**, 109.
Loeb, L. 1923 *Proc. Soc. Exp. Biol., N.Y.*, **20**, 441.
— 1927 *Amer. J. Physiol.* **83**, 202.
Loeb, L. and Smith, M. G. 1936 *Amer. J. Anat.* **58**, 1.
Marshall, F. H. A. and Verney, E. B. 1936 *J. Physiol.* **86**, 327.
Pines, I. 1925 *Z. ges. Neurol. Psychiat.* **100**, 123.
Richter, C. P. 1934 *Amer. J. Physiol.* **106**, 80.
Selye, H. 1934 *Proc. Soc. Exp. Biol., N.Y.*, **31**, 488.
Selye, H. and McKeown, T. 1934 *Surg. Gynec. Obstet.* **59**, 886.
Smith, P. E. 1926 *Anat. Rec.* **32**, 221.
Theobald, G. W. 1936 *Brit. Med. J.* No. 3933, p. 1038.
Vogt, M. 1931 *Arch. Exp. Path. Pharmak.* **162**, 197.
— 1933 *Arch. Exp. Path. Pharmak.* **170**, 72.
Weed, L. H., Cushing, H. and Jacobson, C. 1913 *Johns Hopk. Hosp. Bull.* **24**, 40.

INHIBITION OF OVULATION IN THE RABBIT BY THE ADRENERGIC-BLOCKING AGENT DIBENAMINE

C. H. SAWYER, J. E. MARKEE AND W. HENRY HOLLINSHEAD

From the Department of Anatomy, Duke University School of Medicine
DURHAM, NORTH CAROLINA

INTRODUCTION

IN PREVIOUS papers (Markee, Sawyer and Hollinshead, 1946, 1947 a, b) we have reported the results of investigations of the mechanism by which the central nervous system exerts its control over the release of luteinizing hormone in the rabbit. Using unipolar and bipolar electrical stimulation of known voltage and current we found that direct stimulation of the hypophysis by a unipolar electrode was effective in producing ovulation in the rabbit only with relatively strong currents, which gave signs of considerable spread to the central nervous system. On the other hand, localized bipolar stimulation of the hypothalamic region with a current which was ineffective when applied by the same electrode directly to the hypophysis, produced ovulation in three out of four animals. From these results we concluded that the pathway of excitation from the hypothalamus to the anterior lobe of the hypophysis was probably not through the hypothalamico-hypophyseal nerve tract, even though its fibers have been described as ending in the anterior lobe (Brooks and Gersh, 1941; Truscott, 1944) as well as in the posterior. Rather, we believed our evidence was in favor of the existence of a humoral link in the pathway between hypothalamus and anterior lobe—a humoral link considerably longer than that usually involved between nerve endings and effector organs.

Subsequently, we attempted to determine if either of the known neurohumoral agents, acetylcholine or adrenaline, might be effective in producing ovulation in estrus rabbits if applied directly to the anterior pituitary gland. While Taubenhaus and Soskin (1941) have reported that the application of acetylcholine to the hypophysis of the rat results in the production of pseudopregnancy—i.e. in the release of luteotrophic substance (lactogenic hormone) from the anterior hypophysis—we found instillation of acetylcholine into the anterior hypophysis of the rabbit to have no patent effect in inducing release of luteinizing hormone, upon which ovulation in this species depends. However, the introduction of adrenaline into the hypophysis was followed by ovulation in a significant number of cases (with the most favorable dilution, 1/1000 five out of ten animals receiving it ovulated). Since adrenaline so applied was found to be effective in producing ovulation, this finding was interpreted as indicating that an adrenergic mechanism is involved in the anterior lobe stimulation produced by coitus, or by other forms of sexual stimulation.

In the present paper we have attempted to secure additional evidence as to the adrenergic nature of the proposed humoral link, in so far as the release of luteinizing hormone is concerned, by the use of Dibenamine (N, N-dibenzyl-B-chloroethylamine) which Nickerson and Goodman (1947) have shown to be one of the more effective of the new adrenergic blocking agents, and by the use of Priscol (benzylimedazoline hydrochloride) which also has certain adrenolytic and sympatholytic actions (Chess and Yonkman, 1946), but is ineffective in counteracting several effects of adrenaline (Ahlquist et al., 1947). Since our results indicate that the ovulation normally following coitus in the rabbit can be prevented by the prompt injection of Dibenamine, we have also attempted to estimate the time which must elapse following coitus, in order that hypophyseal stimulation may be effective. Fee and Parkes (1929) have shown that the hypophysis must remain *in situ* for approximately an hour, in order that sufficient luteinizing hormone to produce ovulation may be released; our results with Dibenamine indicate that the actual stimultion of the hypophysis is effective within about one minute after the termination of coitus.

[*Editor's Note:* Material has been omitted at this point.]

DISCUSSION

That the animals used were in estrus and capable of ovulating is indicated both by their willingness to accept the male and by the fact that ovulation invariably followed copulation when lower or delayed doses of Dibenamine were administered or, with the single exception noted above, when Priscol or nembutal were given. In viewing these observations, the preponderant percentage of cases in which the administration of higher doess of dibenamine within a minute after coitus was followed by failure of the animal to ovulate cannot be attributed to chance. The failure of these animals to ovulate seems indubitably the result of the Dibenamine injection.

The adrenolytic and other pharmacological properties of Dibenamine have been investigated by Nickerson and Goodman (op. cit.), who report that it has a high specificity of action and that the adrenergic block which it produces is unusually complete and prolonged. Its toxic effects are reported to be primarily local tissue damage and central excitation. In the present experiments, the sympatholytic effect was obvious in the pronounced pupillary constriction. Since, however, it is possible that the blocking of ovulation produced by Dibenamine in these experiments might be due, at least in part, to the deleterious action of large doses administered quickly, this possibility must be examined.

Although the excitation and prostration induced by Dibenamine varied somewhat in detail from that produced by Priscol, it was not apparently more severe. Indeed, it was our impression that of the two drugs Priscol, in the dosages given, exerted the more profound effect upon the activity of the animal, certainly in the first few minutes following the injection. Moreover, only a very slight delay in giving the Dibenamine was sufficient to allow ovulation to proceed apparently normally, in spite of the fact that the release of luteinizing hormone from the hypophysis requires approximately an hour to be effected, and that reaction of the ovary to this hormone requires some ten to eighteen hours or more to reach its culmination. As is indicated also by the few experiments with nembutal, there seems to be no correlation between the degree of prostration or other toxic symptoms produced, and the occurrence or prevention of ovulation. It seems proper to conclude, therefore, that the action of Dibenamine in preventing ovulation from following coitus in the rabbit is due to its specific adrenolytic properties, and not to a general effect upon the animal as a whole.

Since our previous experiments indicated that ovulation could be artificially induced in the rabbit by the intrahypophyseal instillation of adrenaline, and the present ones apparently demonstrate that the ovulation normally following coitus may be prevented by the adrenolytic action of Dibenamine, the evidence seems strong that there is a humoral link involved in the hypothalamico-hypophyseal ovulatory mechanism of the rabbit, and that this humoral link is of an adrenergic nature.

Our experiments on electrical stimulation of the hypothalamus and hypophysis suggest that the link is a relatively long one, arising outside of the anterior lobe of the hypophysis. There is as yet no definite evidence as to the locus of origin of the humoral adrenergic mediator whose action we believe we have demonstrated. The adrenal medulla can apparently be excluded from consideration in this regard; in our experiments, neither intravenous nor intracarotid injections of adrenaline were effective in producing ovulation and there is a considerable body of evidence to indicate that ovulation cannot depend upon the output of adrenaline from the adrenal. According to Nickerson and Goodman (op. cit.) Dibenamine probably acts directly upon the effector cells, and, therefore, the present experiments contribute no information upon this point. Green (1946) has pointed out that the portal system of veins of the hypophyseal stalk is admirably adapted for serving in the transmission of a neurohumoral agent from median eminence to the anterior lobe of the hypophysis. This is certainly the pathway by which one would expect specific humoral agents destined for the hypophysis to reach the gland; perhaps therefore the source of the adrenergic substance should be sought in the median eminence, rather than in the hypothalamus itself.[1] Green has also (1947) described nerve endings, of presumable hypothalamico-hypophyseal tract origin, in intimate association with the capillary loops of the median eminence, and imbedded in the sheaths of the portal veins. Whether these endings are cholinergic or adrenergic is not known, but Green has suggested that some of them may be secretory. If the nerve endings actually liberate an adrenergic substance into the portal circulation, they may be the site of the formation of an adrenergic agent arising outside of the anterior lobe which our theory postulates.

While a humoral control over the hypophysis by way of the portal circulation has been frequently suggested as a possibility, our experiments with the instillation of adrenaline into the hypophysis, and the present ones concerning the blocking of ovulation with Dibenamine, constitute, so far as we know, the first definite evidence as to the existence and nature of this control in the ovulatory mechanism of the rabbit. Eskin (1944) had previously concluded that adrenaline inhibited the secretion of luteinizing hormone in rat and rabbit. In so far as the rabbit is concerned, at least, his experiments and their interpretation are open to serious question. The dose of adrenaline which

---

[1] Most or all of the median eminence is regarded by Weaver and Bucy (1940) and Rioch, Wislocki and O'leary (1940) as being actually a part of the posterior lobe, rather than of the hypothalamus proper.

he administered was close to the lethal dose for a rabbit of average size; it is somewhat surprising that even four out of eleven animals receiving this dose would mate within the following 15 minutes, and the lack of ovulation in these four (although three were said to have hemorrhagic follicles, probably an indication of some hypophyseal stimulation) can hardly in this case be attributed to specific inhibitory action of adrenaline upon the hypophysis.

In regard to the non-effect of Priscol in blocking ovulation, it should be pointed out that this drug possesses many different pharmacological actions, including both sympathomimetic and sympatholytic qualities (Ahlquist et al., 1947). As judged by our results with Dibenamine, the action of Priscol upon the anterior pituitary gland is not predominantly adrenolytic. The one case in which ovulation failed to occur following the administration of Priscol is presumably due to the condition of the ovaries rather than to the action of this drug.

While it has been impossible to establish physiologically exact times within our experiments, they give evidence as to the approximate time during which stimulation of the hypophysis is necessary in order to produce a liberation of luteinizing hormone adequate for the production of ovulation. While Fee and Parkes (op. cit.), and others have shown that the liberation of the luteinizing hormone from the anterior hypophysis requires approximately an hour, our experiments indicate that the stimulation necessary to produce this liberation is of the order of no more than one to three minutes. Dibenamine in adequate doses given within a minute after the end of coitus rather effectively blocked ovulation, while it was ineffective when its administration was delayed for 3 minutes or more.

The results presented here, therefore, reenforce our belief that an adrenergic humoral agent is normally concerned in the liberation of luteinizing hormone from the hypophysis of the rabbit following coitus, and indicate that this humoral agent produces its full effect upon the hypophysis within a very few minutes. The delay in the release of luteinizing hormone is apparently due to the necessary adjustments within the glandular cells, and not to the necessity of repeated or very prolonged stimulation of these cells.

Certain other events in the ovulatory mechanism may be given time values. Claesson and Hillarp (1947) have found that within 3 to 5 hours after mating most of the sterol granules are mobilized from the interstitial gland of the rabbit ovary. Markee (1933) reported that enough estrogen had reached the endometrium to induce vasodilatation in intraocular transplants within about 7 hours of mating. The events in the ovulatory mechanism, in the rabbit, proceed at about the following speed: stimulation of the hypophyseal cells requires about one to three minutes; an adequate amount of L. H. is discharged in about an hour; the cholesterol like sterols are mobilized from the interstitial gland of the ovary within 3 to 5 hours; estrogen sufficient to induce dilatation of endometrial vessels is secreted in about 7 hours; and, the follicles rupture about 10 to 14 hours after mating.

SUMMARY

In previous experiments, we found that ovulation can be induced in the rabbit by the instillation of adrenaline into the hypophysis, and advanced the theory that the ovulatory mechanism includes an adrenergic humoral link between hypothalamus and anterior hypophysis. As a test of this hypothesis, we have, in the present experiments, tried to determine whether the ovulation normally following coitus in the rabbit can be blocked by some of the available sympatholytic and adrenolytic drugs.

Twenty-five to thirty-two mg./kg. of Dibenamine, given intravenously within 1 minute after the end of copulation, prevented ovulation in sixteen of nineteen animals. The same doses of Dibenamine were ineffective if injection was delayed for three minutes or more following coitus. These experiments support the hypothesis that ovulation in the rabbit is dependent upon a humoral pathway of an adrenergic nature, and indicate that the necessary stimulation of the hypophysis is completed within little more than one minute following copulation.

Priscol was found to be ineffective in preventing ovulation following coitus.

ACKNOWLEDGMENTS

The authors wish to express their appreciation to Drs. Arnold Lehman and Keith Grimson for samples of Dibenamine and Priscol with which preliminary experiments were performed, and to Dr. William Gump of Givaudan-Delawanna Chemical Works and Drs. F. L. Mohr and Ernst Oppenheimer of Ciba Pharmaceutical Products, Inc., for generous quantities of Dibenamine and Priscol respectively.

REFERENCES

AHLQUIST, R. P., R. A. HUGGINS AND R. A. WOODBURY: *J. Pharmacol. & Exper. Therap.* 89: 271. 1947.
BROOKS, C. M., AND I. GERSH: *Endocrinology* 28: 1. 1941.
CHESS, D., AND F. F. YONKMAN: *Proc. Soc. Exper. Biol. & Med.* 61: 127. 1946.
CLAESSON, L., AND N. A. HILLARP: *Acta physiol. Scandinav.* 13: 115. 1947.
ESKIN, I. A.: *Byull. eksper. biol. i. med.* 18: 68. 1944.
FEE, A. R., AND A. S. PARKES: *J. Physiol.* 67: 383. 1929.
GREEN, J. D.: *Alexander Blain Hospital Bulletin* 5: 186. 1946.
GREEN, J. D.: *Anat. Rec.* 97: 338. 1947.
MARKEE, J. E.: *Surg., Gynec. & Obstet.* 56: 51. 1933.
MARKEE, J. E., C. H. SAWYER AND W. H. HOLLINSHEAD: *Endocrinology* 38: 345. 1946.
MARKEE, J. E., C. H. SAWYER AND W. H. HOLLINSHEAD: *Anat. Rec.* 97: 398. 1947 (a).
MARKEE, J. E., C. H. SAWYER AND W. H. HOLLINSHEAD: Laurentian Conferences. In press. 1947 (b).
NICKERSON, M., AND L. S. GOODMAN: *J. Pharmacol. & Exper. Therap.* 89: 167. 1947.
RIOCH, D. McK., G. B. WISLOCKI AND J. L. O'LEARY: *Research Publ., Nerv. Ment. Dis.* 20: 3. 1940.
TAUBENHAUS, M., AND S. SOSKIN: *Endocrinology* 29: 958. 1941.
TRUSCOTT, B. L.: *J. Comp. Neurol.* 80: 235. 1944.
WEAVER, T. A., JR., AND P. C. BUCY: *Endocrinology* 27: 227. 1940.

22

Copyright © 1959 by J. B. Lippincott Company

Reprinted from pages 563–564, 568, and 570–571 of *Endocrinology*
65:563–571 (1959)

INDUCTION OF PSEUDOPREGNANCY IN THE RAT BY RESERPINE AND CHLORPROMAZINE[1]

CHARLES A. BARRACLOUGH AND CHARLES H. SAWYER

Department of Anatomy, School of Medicine, University of California at Los Angeles, Los Angeles, California and Research Division, Veterans Administration Hospital, Sepulveda, California

ABSTRACT

Treatment of female rats with reserpine or chlorpromazine interrupts normal estrous cycles. To establish whether this effect is related to the discharge of luteotropin from the adenohypophysis or to the previously demonstrated inhibition of the ovulatory release of pituitary gonadotropin (LH), the pseudopregnancy response in the normal 5-day cyclic rat was tested. When single subcutaneous injections of reserpine (1 mg./kg.) or chlorpromazine (50 mg./kg.) were given to animals during the proestrous or estrous phase of the cycle, 50–60% of the animals became pseudopregnant as indicated by deciduoma formation following uterine traumatization. In contrast, 100% of the rats treated on the first day of diestrus became pseudopregnant and gave maximal decidual responses. Prolongation of the diestrus phase also occurred in cyclic animals treated on day 2 or 3 of diestrus, but decidual formation, in response to uterine traumatization, was minimal or absent. Nembutal (35 mg./kg.) administered under similar conditions failed to alter the estrous cycle of a third group of rats. Chronic treatment of female rats on alternate days with reserpine produced and maintained deciduomata for 15- but not for 20-day periods. These results indicate that the prolonged interruption of normal estrous cycles in rats treated with reserpine or chlorpromazine is due to the release of luteotropin from the adenohypophysis.

ONE of the more consistent alterations in the reproductive performance of animals treated with reserpine or chlorpromazine is the interruption of normal estrous and menstrual cycles (1–6). In addition, galactorrhea frequently occurs in female mammals and patients receiving these drugs (7–11). In rats, prolongation of the diestrus phase of the estrous cycle has been noted to resemble superficially that observed earlier with chronic morphine sulfate treatment (12). Seemingly, the morphine-induced irregularity of estrous cycle and the acyclic behavior which ensues following "tranquilization" are due to different imbalances in pituitary gonadotropic hormone secretion. The ovaries of morphine addicted rats lack corpora lutea, suggesting a blockade of the ovulatory release of luteinizing hormone from the adenohypophysis (12). In contrast, the ovaries of rats subjected to chronic reserpine treatment contain numerous large corpora

[1] This work was supported by a grant, NSF-G2226, from the National Science Foundation.

lutea similar in size and appearance to those observed during pregnancy. Nevertheless, in spite of these differences and the fact that they are pharmacologically unrelated, morphine, reserpine and chlorpromazine are all equally effective in inhibiting the neurogenically-controlled release of ovulating hormone (LH) when administered before the "critical period" on the day of proestrus (12, 13).

In the current study we have attempted to establish whether the prolongation of diestrus and the related ovarian histology of the tranquilized rat is correlated with the secretion of a third gonadotropin, luteotropic hormone (LTH). It has long been recognized that the release of LTH in the rat normally depends upon the reflex activation of the hypothalamus at coitus or by artifical stimulation of the vaginal cervix. However, in an interesting series of experiments, Desclin (14) and Everett (15) found that the rat adenohypophysis, when isolated from the diencephalon and autotransplanted to the kidney capsule, selectively secreted LTH. From these observations, Everett suggests that the hypothalamus may ordinarily exert a "tonic" inhibitory control over the secretion of this gonadotropin during the estrous cycle. If this is so then the secretion of luteotropic hormone from the adenohypophysis might also be fostered by factors which depress hypothalamic activity. Thus an evaluation of the ability of two tranquilizers, a barbiturate and an alkaloid to induce pseudopregnancy in the cyclic rat, is of considerable interest, especially since these drugs have been shown to inhibit one phase of the hypothalamic control of gonadotropin secretion in blocking ovulation. The results of these experiments have been reported previously in abstract form (16).

[*Editor's Note:* Material has been omitted at this point.]

DISCUSSION

These results clearly indicate that the acyclic condition of the "tranquilized" rat is produced by an atypical release of luteotropic hormone from the adenohypophysis. Velardo (7) has observed that pseudopregnancy can likewise be induced by Trilifon, a tranquilizer with properties somewhat different from the drugs used in these experiments. In other species reserpine treatment induces lactation in the rabbit (8, 9, 10) and suppresses menstruation and ovulation in the rhesus monkey (6). Whitelaw (11) observed that clinical use of chlorpromazine would delay ovulation in the female patient, and there are several reports that it also induces galactorrhea (12, 18).

It is difficult to reconcile the findings of the present experiments with those of other investigators who report involution of the corpus luteum in the cyclic or pregnant rat after treatment with reserpine or chlorpromazine (3, 5, 19, 20). Not only is it apparent that the corpus luteum becomes functional after treatment of the rat with these drugs, but also that it remains functional beyond the normal period of pseudopregnancy (12–14 days). Furthermore, DeFeo (28) has shown that reserpine will not interrupt uterine deciduoma formation during a pseudopregnancy which results from stimulation of the vaginal cervix in the rat. It is more probable that the abortions which occur in the tranquilized rat are due to a general debilitation of the mother or to a deleterious drug action at the placenta or directly on the embryo.

The mechanism or mechanisms by which reserpine and chlorpromazine induce, or at least permit, the secretion of LTH in the absence of coitus is speculative. Everett (16) has shown that autotransplantation of the adenohypophysis to the kidney capsule results in a gland which selectively secretes luteotropic hormone at the expense of the other tropic hormones. He suggests from these experiments that in the normal cyclic rat the hypothalamus by way of its neurovascular linkage to the pars distalis partially inhibits LTH secretion and that the inhibitory agents may be the same as those which induce the secretion of the other gonadotropins. In a somewhat different series of experiments, Rothchild (21) found that unilateral ovariectomy during normal pseudopregnancy was not followed by hypertrophy of the remaining ovary as would be the case in the cyclic rat. He proposed that factors which suppressed the secretion of FSH-LH also fostered the secretion of LTH. The present results are not inconsistent with either hypothesis. Reserpine and chlorpromazine will block ovulation when administered prior to the 2–4 P.M. "critical period" on the day of proestrus. Furthermore, both compounds induce pseudopregnancy even when given as single injections. Although morphine and Nembutal similarly block ovulation in the rat, they are ineffective in inducing pseudopregnancy when given as single injections. It should be remembered, however, that these latter compounds have a relatively short central nervous action as compared with the 24 to 48 hour effect of reserpine. Thus it may be that it is necessary not only for hypothalamic function to be depressed, but that such function be depressed for a somewhat extended period of time in order for LTH to be released.

Assuming that reserpine and chlorpromazine induce pseudopregnancy by blocking hypothalamic function, and thus permit LTH to be released, the differential effectiveness of the agents during the various phases of the estrous cycle still needs to be explained. One might invoke cyclic changes in thresholds of hypothalamic function in response to different levels of circulating ovarian steroids. Recent experiments have shown that steroids can act directly on the brain (22, 23, 24, 25), and Kawakami and Sawyer have found that systemic administration of ovarian steroids can alter functional thresholds in the brain (26). An explanation of the present problem based on this type of evidence would simply imply that the tranquilizers release more LTH during day 1 (V^1) of diestrus than during the other days of the cycle.

It seems more likely, in view of the recent experiments of Nikitovitch-Winer and Everett (27) that a decreasing responsiveness of the corpora lutea toward the end of the 5-day cycle may explain the differential effects. These authors found that pseudopregnancy was not induced by a pituitary transplanted on the day of proestrus due to luteolysis of the corpora. When a new generation of corpora lutea was induced artificially the same pituitary graft supported deciduoma formation. In the present experiments the somewhat better "score" at proestrus is possible because the tranquilizer was purposely administered too late to block ovulation and, the new generation of corpora was the group stimulated in the pseudopregnancy cases. Such an explanation of the variations in terms of differential responsiveness of the target organs is consistent with the results of reserpine-induced lactogenesis in rabbits. In this animal, the condition of the mammary gland is more important than the level of ovarian steroids or the retention or release of pituitary LH. If the mammary gland were in a responsive condition lactogenesis (as an indicator of the release of lactogenic hormone-LTH) occurred whether or not the reserpine blocked ovulation (9).

Acknowledgments

We wish to express our appreciation to Dr. R. Gaunt of Ciba Pharmaceutical Company for the Serpasil and to Dr. A. E. Heming of Smith, Kline and French Laboratories for the Thorazine.

REFERENCES

1. Gaunt, R., A. A. Renzi, N. Antanehak, G. T. Miller and M. Gilman: *Ann. N. Y. Acad. Sci.* **59:** 22. 1954.
2. Dasgupta, S. R.: *Bull. Calcutta School Trop. Med.* **3:** 1. 1955.
3. Tuchmann-Duplessis, H. and L. Mercier-Parot: *C. R. Acad. Sci. Paris* **242:** 1233. 1956.
4. Mercier-Parot, L. and H. Tuchmann-Duplessis: *C. R. Acad. Sci. Paris* **240:** 1935. 1955.
5. Tuchmann-Duplessis, H.: *Pr. Med.* **64:** 2189. 1956.
6. DeFeo, V. J. and S. R. M. Reynolds: *Science* **124:** 726. 1956.
7. Velardo, J. T.: *Fertility and Sterility* **9:** 60. 1958.
8. Kehl, R., A. Audibert, C. Gage and J. Amarger: *C. R. Soc. de Biol. Paris* **150:** 981. 1956.
9. Sawyer, C. H.: *Anat. Rec.* **127:** 362. 1957.
10. Meites, J.: *Proc. Soc. Exper. Biol. and Med.* **96:** 728. 1957.
11. Whitelaw, J. M.: *J. Clin. Endoc. and Metab.* **16:** 972. 292.
12. Polishuk, W. Z. and S. Kulcsar: *J. Clin. Endoc. and Metab.* **16:** 292. 1956.
13. Barraclough, C. A. and C. H. Sawyer: *Endocrinology* **57:** 32. 1955.
14. Barraclough, C. A. and C. H. Sawyer: *Endocrinology* **61:** 341. 1957.
15. Desclin, L.: *Ann. d'Endocrinol.* **11:** 656. 1950.
16. Everett, J.: *Endocrinology* **54:** 685. 1954.
17. Barraclough, C. A.: *Anat. Rec.* **127:** 262. 1957.
18. Sulman, F. G. and H. Z. Winnik: *Nature* **178:** 365. 1956.
19. Tuchmann-Duplessis, H., R. Gershon and L. Mercier-Parot: *J. de Physiol.* **49:** 1007. 1957.
20. Chambon, Y.: *Ann. d'Endocrinol.* **18:** 80. 1957.
21. Rothchild, I.: Unpublished Work.
22. Flerkó, B.: *Acta Morph. Hung.* **4:** 475. 1954.
23. Flerkó, B. and J. Szentagothai: *Acta Endocrinol.* **26:** 121. 1957.
24. Kent, G. C. and M. J. Liberman: *Endocrinology* **45:** 29. 1949.
25. Michael, R. P.: *Nature* **181:** 567. 1958.
26. Kawakami, M. and C. H. Sawyer: *The Physiologist* **1:** 48. 1957.
27. Nikitovitch-Winer, I. M. and J. W. Everett: *Endocrinology* **62:** 522 1958.
28. DeFeo, V. J.: *Anat. Rec.* **127:** 409. 1957.

EVIDENCE THAT THE HYPOTHALAMUS IS RESPONSIBLE FOR ANDROGEN-INDUCED STERILITY IN THE FEMALE RAT[1]

CHARLES A. BARRACLOUGH AND ROGER A. GORSKI

Department of Anatomy, School of Medicine, University of California at Los Angeles, and Research Division, Veterans Administration Hospital, Sepulveda, California

ABSTRACT

The data presented in the current study suggest that the sterility which ensues from androgen treatment of prepubertal female rats is not the result of malfunction of the adenohypophysis. Rather, the pituitaries of such animals will respond to electrical stimulation of the hypothalamus by discharging sufficient gonadotropin to cause ovulation. It is further suggested from these experiments that there are two regions within the hypothalamus which control adenohypophyseal gonadotropin secretion: (a) a region responsible for activating the cyclic discharge of ovulating hormone: the anterior preoptic (suprachiasmatic) area of the hypothalamus, and (b) a region independently responsible for the tonic discharge of luteinizing hormone in a sufficient quantity to cause estrogen secretion but not ovulation: the arcuate-ventromedial nuclei complex of the median eminence. Evidence is presented which suggests that prepubertal androgen treatment deleteriously alters the function of the "ovulation controlling" preoptic region of the hypothalamus.

INTRODUCTION

PREVIOUS studies have demonstrated a period of steroid sensitivity in the female rat between birth and the tenth day of age during which a single injection of androgen will result in permanent infertility (1). It was originally proposed by Pfeiffer that such sterility was the consequence of a deleterious effect of androgen on the adenohypophysis, resulting in a gland that secreted only follicle stimulating hormone (2). Since the time of these early observations it has become apparent that the pituitary of the androgen-sterilized rat elaborates both follicle stimulating and luteinizing hormone. Not only are vesicular follicles present in the sterile rat ovary but estrogen is secreted as evidenced by the persistence of a cornified vaginal mucosa, cystic enlargement of the uterine endometrial glands and hypertrophy of the ovarian interstitial tissue (1, 3). Seemingly, the particular adenohypophyseal malfunction is a failure to release sufficient gonadotropin to cause ovulation, a phenomenon generally held to be regulated by the hypothalamus. This suggests either that the pituitary of the androgen-sterilized rat is refractory to hypothalamic activation or, more likely, that the malfunction in the ovulatory mechanism is inherent

---

[1] Supported by grant RG-5496 from the United States Public Health Service.

within the hypothalamus itself. Some support for the latter hypothesis is offered by the observations of Harris and Jacobsohn (4) and Martinez and Bittner (5) that male hypophyses transplanted beneath the median eminence of hypophysectomized female rats would restore normal estrous cycles. Apparently, the sex difference in gonadotropin secretion is not resident within the adenohypophysis as such, but a higher neural level.

The current studies were designed to answer two questions: (a) will the pituitary of the anovulatory female rat respond to stimulation of the hypothalamus by the release of sufficient gonadotropin to cause ovulation and (b) if so, can a specific region of the hypothalamus be implicated as the site of the deleterious androgen action? The results of these experiments have been presented previously in abstract form (6).

[*Editor's Note:* Material has been omitted at this point.]

DISCUSSION

These results suggest that the adenohypophysis of the androgen-sterilized rat can function normally, provided: (a) proper gonadotropin storage is permitted and (b) an impetus for its release is supplied by the hypothalamus. We have interpreted the failure of the persistent-estrous rat to ovulate on artificial hypothalamic stimulation as due to insufficient pituitary gonadotropin stores. When such animals are primed with progesterone they readily ovulate in response to such hypothalamic stimulation. Presumably progesterone permits sufficient gonadotropin to be accumulated in the adenohypophysis to cause ovulation when released. Segal has reported that the pituitary gonadotropin content of the androgen-sterilized rat is comparable to that of the normal male rat (9). However, his assays are based on glands of 60-day-old rats which have exhibited only

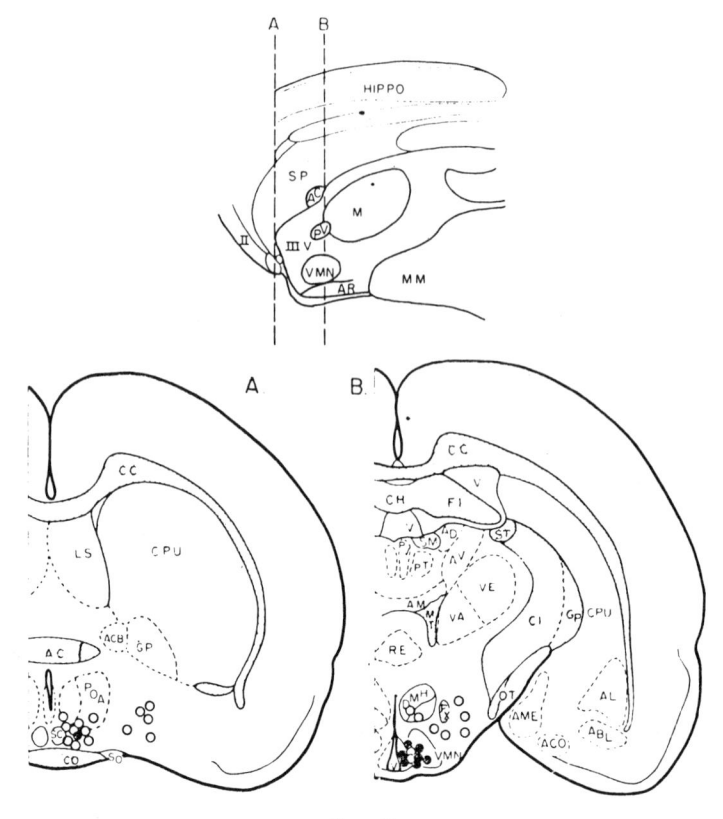

FIG. 5.

2–3 weeks of persistent vaginal cornification, whereas the animals employed in these studies have undergone an additional 60–120 days of persistent estrus (120–180 days of age). It is probable that the pituitary, when subjected to prolonged estrogen stimulation would be depleted of its stored gonadotropin. Preliminary assay data of the pituitary LH content of progesterone-primed persistent estrous rats suggest a twofold increase in content (unpublished observations).

A second mode of progesterone action also deserves consideration. Everett (10) has shown that progesterone will advance ovulation 24 hours in the normal cyclic rat provided this steroid is administered on the last day of diestrus. Furthermore, Kawakami and Sawyer (11) have observed that progesterone, in facilitating ovulation in the rabbit, also lowers various central nervous thresholds to electrical stimulation. There is thus the possibility that treatment of the androgen-sterilized female rat with progesterone may facilitate the electrical stimulus to result in ovulation rather than having a direct effect on pituitary gonadotropin content. Regardless of its site of action, progesterone priming is necessary, prior to hypothalamic stimulation, for ovulation to occur.

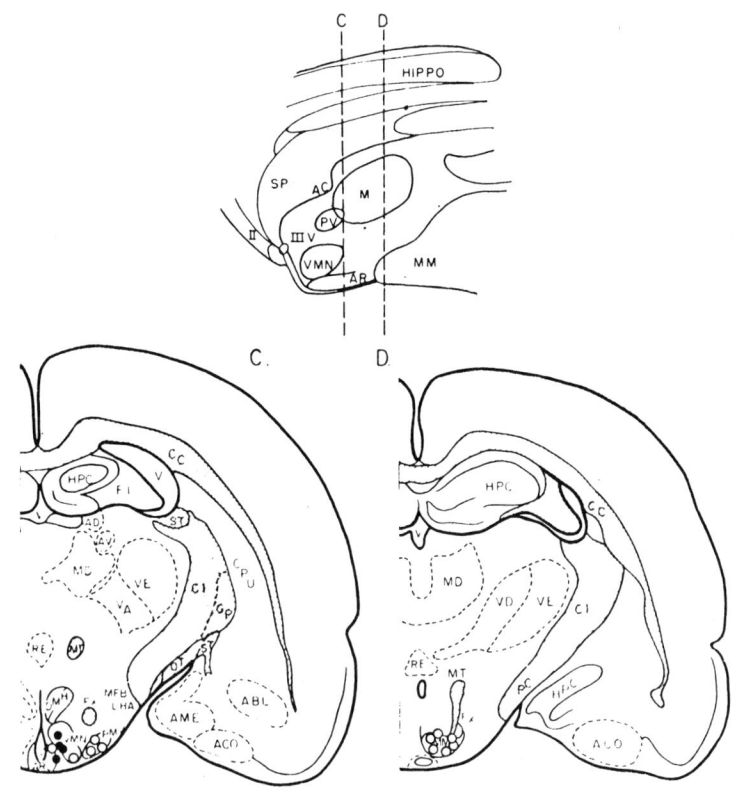

FIG. 6.

FIGS. 5, 6. Midsagittal and coronal sections of rat hypothalamus indicating points of stimulation. Diagrams from DeGroot's "The rat forebrain in stereotaxic coordinates" (15). *Closed circles* indicate hypothalamic sites in which stimulation induced ovulation. *Open circles* represent areas in which stimulation failed to induce ovulation. Abbreviations used in this and subsequent figures: AC, anterior commissure; ACB, area parolfactoria lateralis; AR, arcuate nucleus; CC, corpus callosum; CPU, nucleus caudatus/putamen; CO, optic chiasm; DMH, dorsal medial nucleus; MN, medial mamillary nucleus; MT, mamillothalamic tract; POA, preoptic area; VMN, ventral medial nucleus.

What is the mechanism by which androgen induces sterility? Apparently prepubertal androgen treatment so alters normal hypothalamic function as to render it incapable of activating the cyclic ovulatory discharge of gonadotropin (presumably LH). In contrast, such treatment fails to cause complete cessation of LH secretion. This is evidenced by the syndrome which ensues following prepubertal treatment: persistent vaginal cornification and ovarian interstitial cell, adrenal and pituitary hypertrophy which are either directly or indirectly (through estrogen secretion), the consequence of a tonic discharge of adenohypophyseal LH.

To establish a hypothalamic locus which is deleteriously affected by

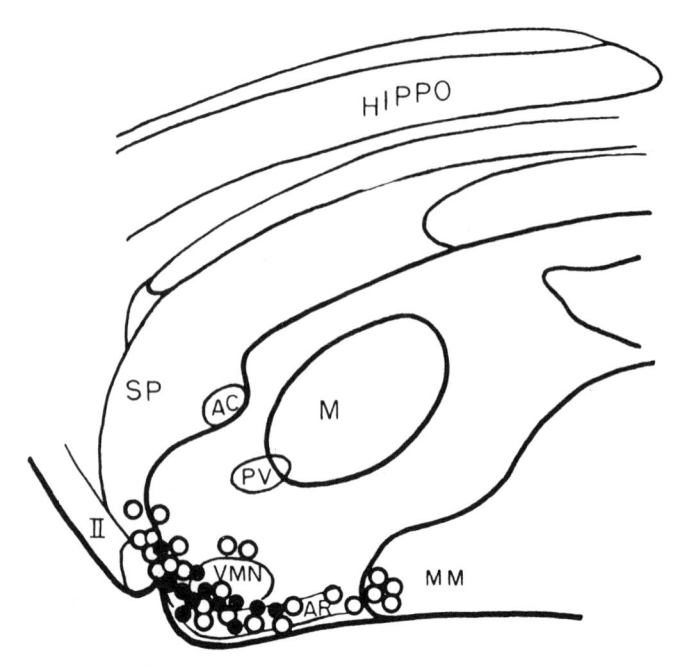

FIG. 7. Midsagittal reconstruction of rat hypothalamus indicating extent of area in which stimulation resulted in ovulation. Abbreviations: hippo, hippocampus; M, massa intermedia; PV, paraventricular nucleus; SP, septum; II, optic nerve.

androgen requires an evaluation of the specific hypothalamic areas proposed to be responsible for the control of ovulation in the normal rat. Critchlow initially demonstrated that electrical stimulation of hypothalamic regions extending from the basal area, from the optic chiasm to the infundibular stalk, consistently induced ovulation in Nembutal-blocked rats (7). The more recent studies of Everett have extended these observations to include the preoptic area rostral to the suprachiasmatic nucleus (8). Furthermore, when small, specific lesions are made in the suprachiasmatic nucleus, reproductive behavior is so affected so as to result in anovulatory-persistent-estrous animals similar in every respect to the androgen-sterilized rat (12).

The hypothalamic locus thus implicated as the site of deleterious androgen action is the midline suprachiasmatic-preoptic area. Lesions of this region result in an imbalance in gonadotropin secretion which imitates that observed in the sterilized rat (12) and ovulation can readily be induced by stimulation of this region in normal but not in androgen-sterilized animals.

The observations of these and previous investigations suggest a dual hypothalamic control of adenohypophyseal gonadotropin secretion in the female rat. The first level of hypothalamic control involves the tonic discharge of gonadotropin in sufficient quantity to maintain estrogen production but cannot independently initiate the ovulatory surge of gonadotropin.

This control is apparently resident in the arcuate-ventromedial nuclei region of the median eminence. Evidence for this primary control and localization is based on the observations that estrogen is secreted in the anovulatory-persistent estrous rat and that electrical stimulation of these structures in the sterile rat will induce LH secretion. Furthermore, destruction of these areas results in the cessation of estrogen production, ovarian atrophy and anestrus (12).

Of fundamental importance is the second and higher control which results in the cyclic discharge of gonadotropin to cause ovulation. The specific region responsible for such control may, most likely, be placed in the preoptic area of the hypothalamus. Furthermore, this region of "ovulation control" is dependent for its activation on exteroceptive (light, etc.) (13), and interoceptive (steroid [14], higher neural control) influences.

Thus it may be that the hypothalamic events which occur during the normal cycle in the female rat are these: the preoptic (suprachiasmatic) area responds under proper environmental and hormonal circumstances,

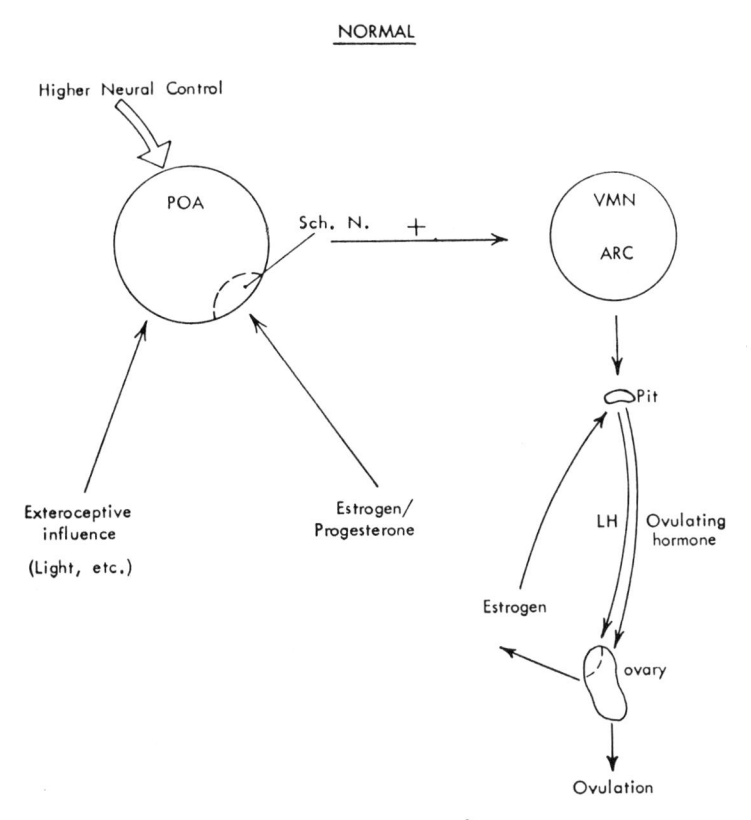

FIG. 8. Diagrammatic representation of hypothalamic events which regulate the discharge of gonadotropin to cause ovulation (ovulating hormone) and/or the tonic release of ovarian estrogen. Abbreviations: POA, preoptic area; Sch. N., suprachiasmatic nucleus; VMN, ventral medial nucleus; ARC, arcuate nucleus.

ANDROGEN-STERILE OR LESION

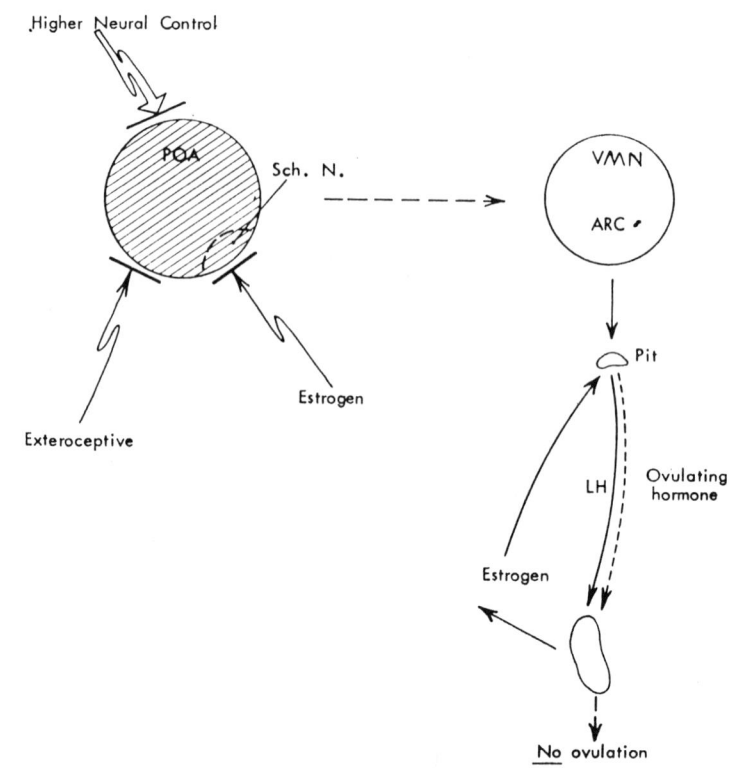

FIG. 9. Hypothalamic events which occur on prepubertal treatment of female rats with androgen or destruction of the anterior preoptic area.

(which are fulfilled on the day of proestrus) by an activation of the more terminal infundibular regions to cause an ovulatory discharge of gonadotropin from the adenohypophysis (Fig. 8). In the absence of this higher control, the terminal structures (arcuate-ventromedial nuclei) still function normally to stimulate LH secretion, but the ovulatory surge of gonadotropin is absent and sterility ensues (Fig. 9).

Seemingly, the anterior preoptic area of the prepubertal female rat is undifferentiated at birth with regard to its subsequent control of gonadotropin secretion. When allowed to differentiate normally it regulates the release of ovulating hormone. However, if differentiated in the presence of androgen, this area becomes refractory to both intrinsic and extrinsic activation and the more tonic type of male gonadotropin secretion is observed.

Acknowledgments

The authors wish to express their appreciation for the technical assistance rendered by Miss Theresa Mangold and Mr. Leroy Brown during this study.

REFERENCES

1. BARRACLOUGH, C. A.: *Endocrinology*. This issue.
2. PFEIFFER, C. A.: *Amer. J. Anat.* **58**: 195. 1936.
3. FEVOLD, H. L.: *Endocrinology* **28**: 33. 1941.
4. HARRIS, G. W. AND D. JACOBSOHN: *J. Physiol.* **113**: 35. 1951.
5. MARTINEZ, C. AND J. J. BITTNER: *Proc. Soc. Exper. Biol. & Med.* **91**: 506. 1956.
6. BARRACLOUGH, C. A.: *Anat. Rec.* **133**: 248. 1959.
7. CRITCHLOW, V.: *Amer. J. Physiol.* **195**: 171. 1958.
8. EVERETT, J.: Harvard Conference on Control of Ovulation, Pergamon Press (in press).
9. SEGAL, S. J. AND D. C. JOHNSON: *Arch. D'Anat. Micro. Morph. Exper.* **48**: 261. 1959.
10. EVERETT, J.: *Endocrinology* **43**: 389. 1948.
11. KAWAKAMI, M. AND C. H. SAWYER: *Endocrinology* **65**: 631. 1959.
12. FLERKÓ, B. AND V. BARDOS: *Acta Neuroveg.* **20**: 248. 1959.
13. CRITCHLOW, V. AND J. DEGROOT: *Anat. Rec.* **136**: 179. 1960.
14. FLERKÓ, B. AND J. SZENTAGOTHAI: *Acta Endoc.* **26**: 121. 1957.
15. DEGROOT, J.: *Trans. Roy. Neth. Acad. Sci.* **52**: 1. 1959.

24

Copyright © 1959 by J. B. Lippincott Company

Reprinted from pages 614–615 and 618–621 of *Endocrinology*
65:614–621 (1959)

ESTROGEN FACILITATION OF RELEASE OF PITUITARY OVULATING HORMONE IN THE RABBIT IN RESPONSE TO VAGINAL STIMULATION[1]

CHARLES H. SAWYER[2] AND J. E. MARKEE

Departments of Anatomy, University of California at Los Angeles and Duke University, Durham, North Carolina, and Veterans Administration Hospital, Long Beach, California

ABSTRACT

Although naturally estrous rabbits ordinarily ovulate following coital stimulation, very few respond in this manner to simple mechanical stimulation of the vagina. In this regard, among others, they differ from the estrous cat which which readily ovulates in response to glass-rod stimulation of the vagina. The present study reveals that priming the estrous rabbit with moderate dosages of estrogen for two days or the anestrous rabbit for a longer period sets the stage for release of pituitary ovulating hormone in response to artificial stimulation of the vagina in 40–45% of the cases. The ovarian follicles, ruptured in this response, become functional corpora lutea as evidenced by the decidual reaction to uterine trauma. The ovulatory response could not be evoked in pseudopregnant rabbits by these means. The response was blocked in estrous estrogen-treated rabbits by pentobarbital, atropine, dibenamine and reserpine. The report emphasizes the facilitatory function of estrogen in reflexogenous ovulation and discusses its possible sites of action rather than supporting a very important role for vaginal stimulation among the afferent mechanisms triggered at coitus.

INTRODUCTION

AMONG the best known of the species which ordinarily require a coital stimulus to induce ovulation are the rabbit and the cat. In these forms there is strong evidence that sensory or psychic stimulation accompanying copulation activates the adenohypophysis via the hypothalamus to release an ovulatory surge of gonadotropin (here designated ovulatory hormone). In the estrous cat afferent stimuli from the cervix, following introduction of a glass rod into the vagina, are adequate to initiate the ovulatory reflex (1). Although there have been isolated reports of partial success with such stimulation in the rabbit (2, 3), most attempts to induce ovulation in the estrous rabbit by simple vaginal stimulation have led to negative results (4, 5; Markee, unpublished). On the other hand, ovulation following sexual excitement without vaginal penetration is common among estrous female rabbits following mounting or on being mounted by other estrous females. Furthermore, copulation induces ovulation in spite of

---

[1] Supported in part by a grant (B-1162) from the National Institutes of Health.
[2] Fellow of the Commonwealth Fund, 1958–1959.

vaginal anesthesia (6) or denervation (7, 8). These experiments have led to the conclusion that in the rabbit reflexogenous ovulation must ordinarily be triggered by afferent stimuli from sources other than the vagina. A few cases of spontaneous ovulation have been reported in the rabbit (9, 10), but they are apparently quite rare occurrences.

In both reflexly and spontaneously ovulating forms, profound effects on the release of pituitary ovulating hormone are exerted by estrogen. Employing the steroid in short-term experiments, several authors have reported facilitation of the release of pituitary gonadotropin in the rat (11–15). Estrogen will induce ovulation in the pregnant rat (14) and will advance the time of cyclic ovulation if injection is appropriately timed (15). The stimulatory or facilitatory effects have been blocked by drugs whose primary actions are considered to be at the level of the central nervous system, implying that estrogen may exert its ovulatory effects directly or indirectly at this level of organization (16, 17). In the rabbit, while low dosages of estrogen did not lead to spontaneous ovulation (18, 19), they have been shown to facilitate ovulation in response to copper salts (19) and in response to the coital stimulus during pregnancy and pseudopregnancy (20). When injected for several days at high dosage (1 mg./day), estrogen, far from facilitating, actually blocked electrically stimulated ovulation (21). In view of these effects, it became of interest to ascertain whether brief treatment with low dosages of estrogen might set the stage for ovulation in response to vaginal stimulation or, under optimal conditions, even for spontaneous ovulation. The latter phenomenon is considered briefly in the present study, and it will be discussed more completely in a separate communication (22).

The present study reveals that estrogen does indeed facilitate ovulation in response to vaginal stimulation and that such ovulation is followed by formation of functional corpora lutea as evidenced by deciduoma formation. The stimulus is blocked by "anti-neural" drugs, and it is ineffective during pregnancy or pseudopregnancy in spite of estrogen treatment. Most of the experiments were performed at Duke University more than 10 years ago, and they were reported in abstract form at that time (23).

[*Editor's Note:* Material has been omitted at this point.]

DISCUSSION

The result of the present study should be interpreted not as representing support for a major role played by afferent stimuli from the vagina in the copulation-ovulation reflex but rather as providing further evidence for the facilitatory role of estrogen in pituitary activation. The vagina is only one of many sources of afferent impulses at mating, and in the rabbit its stimulation appears to be of only minor importance.

The female rabbit's natural breeding habits include a very prolonged condition of moderate estrus during which copulation, with its stimulation of multiple afferent pathways, will activate the release of pituitary ovulating hormone. In contrast, the female cat has brief periods of intense estrus, probably indicative of a temporary high level of endogenous estrogen, during which a single prodding of the vagina with a glass rod may evoke a behavioral afterreaction (1, 27) and induce ovulation. The cat's ovarian follicles remain ovulable for only a short time, and the acute estrous state is attuned to insuring copulation during this brief period. Behavioral estrus can be induced in the anestrous cat with estrogen alone, but preparation for reflexogenous ovulation also necessitates priming the ovary with a subovulatory dose of exogenous gonadotropin, PMS (28). Exogenous estrogen brings the already moderately estrous rabbit to a condition approaching, but not attaining, the intense heat of the naturally estrous cat.

Vaginal stimulation induces a condition of pseudopregnancy in the rat and, similarly, coitus is a more potent stimulus in this analogous neuroendocrine reflex. Ball (29) suggested that the advantage of coitus over artificial stimulation lay merely in the quantity of vaginal stimulation received. Haterius (30) had contended that qualitative differences including the psychic state of sexual excitement attending coitus made it the more potent activator of the hypophysis. The present results on induction of ovulation in the rabbit may be interpreted consistently in terms of Haterius' proposal; certainly the experimental rabbits received quantitatively more vaginal stimulation than ordinarily occurs at coitus, yet the latter remained a much more uniformly effective stimulus of ovulation. Although it is impossible to assess orgasm as an objective phenomenon in experimental animals, it seems not unlikely that coital stimulation is more successful in activating the pituitary because it induces orgasm in more rabbits than does simple vaginal stimulation.

By processes of elimination the critical sites of estrogen action in facilitating the reflex induction of ovulation have been narrowed to the hypothalamus-hypophysial region. For example, although estrogen is known to act directly upon the ovary (31, 32), the ovary is already sensitive to gonadotropin during periods such as pregnancy when exogenous estrogen must be administered to facilitate reflex ovulation (33). The dramatic effects of estrogen on the uterus and vagina cannot be crucial since the coital stimulus is effective after anesthesia or denervation of these organs (6, 8). The numerous reports of depletion of pituitary gonadotropin by estrogen (11, 12, 13) might suggest that the key reaction site is the adenohypophysis itself. However, estrogen-induced ovulation and even spontaneous ovulation have a neurogenous component (16, 17). Moreover, the ability of estrogen to facilitiate even to the extent of rendering "spontaneous," such sequences as reflex induction of ovulation in the rabbit and pseudopregnancy in the rat (34)—processes which, though utilizing analogous nervous mechanisms, involve different pituitary hormones—suggests the central nervous system as the critical site of estrogen action in these sequences. Flerko and Szentágothai (35) have made pituitary-inhibiting transplants of ovarian tissue to the rat hypothalamus, implying that the inhibitory effects of estrogen are exerted via the nervous system. The induction of sexual behavior patterns by instilling sex steroids directly into the brain (36, 37, 38) supports this hypothesis. The localizing value of such injections has limitations, and the procedure must be combined with discrete electrical stimulating, lesioning and recording technics to localize more sharply the important sites within the brain.

Studies involving stimulating and lesioning methods, of which preliminary reports have appeared (39, 40) have localized two centers in the rabbit hypothalamus. One, located in the basal tuberal region, responds to electrical stimulation by inducing ovulation in the estrogen-treated rabbit, and discrete lesions in this area block copulation-induced ovulation. Rabbits with lesions in this region will, however, mate if given exogenous estrogen. The other center, in the mammillary region, appears to control mating behavior: stimulation does not cause ovulation; lesions do not cause ovarian atrophy; and ovulation can be induced with copper acetate; yet the rabbits will not permit copulation even if supplied with exogenous estrogen. It would seem that estrogen must normally be exerting effects at both of these sites wherever else it may be acting.

In the present studies, the drugs which blocked ovulation in response to vaginal stimulation also forced the rabbits out of behavioral estrus in spite of estrogen treatment. This was probably a non-specific effect, but perhaps a change in neural thresholds at the "sex behavioral center" may contribute to blockade of reflexogenous ovulation. Atropine and pentobarbital, which had earlier been shown to raise reticular formation arousal thresholds (41), were found to block pituitary activation in response to electrical stimulation of the "gonadotropic center" unless the electrode reached the median eminence itself (40). It seems probable that these pharmacological agents affect many regions or components in the nervous system simultaneously rather than exerting isolated effects on discrete centers. The same is true of the sex steroids, and evidence for this observation will be presented in subsequent studies involving electrical recording technics (42).

Acknowledgments

The authors wish to thank the Schering Corporation for supplying estradiol benzoate, Smith, Kline and French Laboratories for dibenamine, and Ciba Pharmaceutical Products, Inc., for reserpine.

REFERENCES

1. Greulich, W. W.: *Anat. Rec.* **58**: 217. 1934.
2. Hammond, J. and S. A. Asdell: *Brit. J Exper. Biol.* **4**: 155. 1926.
3. Bishop, P. M. F.: *Guys Hospital Reports* **83**: 308. 1933.
4. Heape, W.: *Proc. Roy. Soc. B* **76**: 260. 1905.
5. Asdell, S. A.: *Patterns of Mammalian Reproduction.* Comstock Publishing Company, Inc. Ithaca, N. Y. 1946.
6. Fee, A. R. and A. S. Parkes: *J. Physiol. Lond.* **70**: 385. 1930.
7. Friedman, M. H.: *Am. J. Physiol.* **89**: 438. 1929.
8. Brooks, C. M.: *Am. J. Physiol.* **120**: 544. 1937.
9. Walton, A. and J. Hammond: *Brit. J. Exper. Biol.* **6**: 190. 1928–9.
10. Pincus, G.: *Recent Prog. Hormone Research* **2**: 129. 1948.
11. Bradbury, J. T.: *Endocrinology* **41**: 501. 1947.
12. Hisaw, F. L.: *Physiol. Rev.* **27**: 95. 1947.
13. Greep, R. O and I. C. Jones: *Recent Prog. Hormone Research* **5**: 197. 1950.
14. Everett, J. W.: *Endocrinology* **41**: 364. 1947.
15. Everett, J. W.: *Endocrinology* **43**: 389. 1948.
16. Sawyer, C. H., J. W. Everett and J. E. Markee: *Endocrinology* **44**: 218. 1949.
17. Everett, J. W., C. H. Sawyer and J. E. Markee: *Endocrinology* **44**: 234. 1949.
18. Bachman, C.: *Proc. Soc. Exper. Biol. & Med.* **33**: 551. 1936.
19. Dury, A. and J. T. Bradbury: *Am. J. Physiol.* **139**: 135. 1943.
20. Mayer, G. and M. Klein: *C. R. Soc. Biol. Paris* **140**: 1011. 1946.
21. Zondek, B. and J. Sklow: *Endocrinology* **28**: 923. 1941.
22. Sawyer, C. H.: *Endocrinology* **65**: 523. 1959.
23. Sawyer, C. H.: *Anat. Rec.* **103**: 502. 1949.
24. Sawyer, C. H., J. E. Markee and B. F. Townsend: *Endocrinology* **44**: 18. 1949.
25. Sawyer, C. H., J. E. Markee and J. W. Everett: *J. Exper. Zool.* **113**: 659. 1950.
26. Barraclough, C. A. and C. H. Sawyer: *Endocrinology* **61**: 341. 1957.
27. Bard, P.: *Res. Publ. Ass. Nerv. Ment. Dis.* **20**: 551. 1940.
28. Sawyer, C. H. and J. W. Everett: *Proc. Soc. Exper. Biol. & Med.* **83**: 820. 1953.
29. Ball, J.: *J. Comp. Psych.* **18**: 419. 1934.
30. Haterius, H. O.: *Am. J. Physiol.* **103**: 97. 1933.
31. Pencharz, R. I.: *Science* **91**: 554. 1940.
32. Williams, P. C.: *Nature* **145**: 388. 1940.
33. Weinstein, G. L. and A. W. Makepeace: *Am. J. Physiol.* **119**: 508. 1937.
34. Merckel, C. and W. O. Nelson: *Anat. Rec.* **76**: 391. 1940.
35. Flerko, B. and J. Szentagothai: *Acta Endocrinol.* **26**: 121. 1957.
36. Kent, G. C. and M. J. Liberman: *Endocrinology* **45**: 29. 1949.
37. Fisher, A. E.: *Science* **124**: 228. 1956.
38. Harris, G. W., R. P. Michael and P. P. Scott: Ciba Foundation Symposium on *Neurological Basis of Behavior*, 236–251, London, J. & A. Churchill, Ltd. 1958.
39. Sawyer, C. H.: *Anat. Rec.* **124**: 358. 1956.
40. Saul, G. D. and C. H. Sawyer: *Fed. Proc.* **16**: 112. 1957.
41. Sawyer, C. H., B. V. Critchlow and C. A. Barraclough: *Endocrinology* **57**: 345. 1955.
42. Kawakami, M. and C. H. Sawyer: *Endocrinology.* **65**: 652. 1959.

Editor's Comments
on Papers 25 Through 29

25   McCANN, TALEISNIK, and FRIEDMAN
     LH-Releasing Activity in Hypothalamic Extracts

26   CAMPBELL, FEUER, and HARRIS
     Excerpts from *The Effect of Intrapituitary Infusion of Median Eminence and Other Brain Extracts on Anterior Pituitary Gonadotrophic Secretion*

27   RAMIREZ and SAWYER
     Excerpts from *Fluctuations in Hypothalamic LH-RF (Luteinizing Hormone-Releasing Factor) During the Rat Estrous Cycle*

28   IGARASHI and McCANN
     Excerpts from *A Hypothalamic Follicle Stimulating Hormone-Releasing Factor*

29   HALÁSZ and GORSKI
     Excerpts from *Gonadotrophic Hormone Secretion in Female Rats after Partial or Total Interruption of Neural Afferents to the Medial Basal Hypothalamus*

McCann et al. (Paper 25) were the first investigators to demonstrate the presence of an LH-releasing factor in rat hypothalamic extracts by demonstrating that injection of crude acid extracts of the stalk median eminence (SME) resulted in ovarian ascorbic acid depletion from luteinized ovaries of suitably prepared immature rats—the most sensitive and specific assay for LH release available at that time. They termed the substance responsible for LH-releasing activity in those extracts the *LH-releasing factor*. They concluded that this material differs from histamine, serotonin, substance P, epinephrine, and vasopressin or oxytocin.

Campbell et al. (Paper 26) demonstrated that crude extracts of rabbit, cattle, and monkey median eminence tissue could cause ovulation in the estrus rabbit when infused directly via a small cannula implanted in the adenohypophysis. These studies paralleled those of Nikitovitch-

Winer in the same laboratory who showed that direct infusion of rat SME extracts in the adenohypophysis could induce ovulation in the Nembutal-blocked proestrus rat. These studies gave further proof of the existence of a luteinizing hormone-releasing factor in crude extracts of SME of hypothalami. The studies of Campbell et al. further suggested that this releasing factor was the same substance existing in the SME of several different mammals.

Ramirez and Sawyer (Paper 27) established that the hypothalamic content of LH-releasing factor changes during the estrus cycle of the rat; there is a decrease before estrus, suggesting that the release of LH-releasing factor is involved in the discharge of an amount of LH sufficient to cause ovulation. They used a biological assay in which the ovarian ascorbic acid depletion induced by acid extracts of rat SME during the proestrus and early estrus was significantly lower than at other times during the estrus cycle. Thus the study gave proof of an LH-releasing factor that undergoes physiological changes in intact animals related to the function of cyclic release of LH and the mechanisms related to ovulation in the rat.

Igarashi and McCann (Paper 28) were the first investigators to demonstrate direct evidence of the existence of a follicle-stimulating, hormone-releasing factor (FSH-RF) in the hypothalamic SME by using a sensitive bioassay method devised by them in ovariectomized, estrogen-progesterone-blocked rats. They also demonstrated that SME lesions were effective in blocking FSH secretion. They further showed that lesions of the medial basal hypothalamus resulted in anovulation associated with permanent anestrus, indicating reduced hypophysial gonadotropin release.

Halász and Gorski (Paper 29) first demonstrated conclusively that the medial basal hypothalamus (MBH) cannot by itself release LH-RF in amounts necessary for ovulation but that neural afferent tracts from other parts of the CNS reaching the MBH via connections from the anterior hypothalamus are necessary for ovulation. They showed this by making small frontal cuts just posterior to the anterior hypothalamus with the resulting deafferentiation of the MBH preventing ovulation. They presented additional evidence that the MBH is the area necessary for normal basal tonic gonadotropin release by demonstrating that complete deafferentiation of the MBH-median eminence region does not prevent postgonadectomy castration cell formation, which is due to interruption of direct negative feedback to the MBH, exclusive of any other central nervous system input. They concluded that two levels exist in the hypothalamic-hypophyseal-gonadal axis: that represented by the MBH-median eminence region and associated with tonic gonadotropin release, and the second level of control being localized in the anterior hypothalamus and responsible for cyclic release of LH-releasing factor. These observations were in concert with the previous findings of Barraclough et al. that electrical stimulation or destruction of the preoptic anterior hypothalamus induces or abolishes ovulation, respectively, suggesting that the preoptic-suprachiasmatic region is intimately involved in the cyclic release of LH-RF necessary to induce ovulation.

LH-RELEASING ACTIVITY IN HYPOTHALAMIC EXTRACTS

S. M. McCann, S. Taleisnik and H. M. Friedman

Dept. of Physiology, School of Medicine, University of Pennsylvania, Philadelphia

Release of luteinizing hormone (LH) from the pituitary appears to be under hypothalamic neurohumoral control(1,2). Since convincing evidence is now available indicating that a corticotrophin-releasing factor and vasopressin can release adrenocorticotrophin from the pituitary(3-6), it seems of interest to examine hypothalamic and median eminence extracts to determine if a substance originating in these structures may regulate release of LH. Ovarian ascorbic acid depletion (OAAD) from heavily luteinized ovaries of suitably prepared immature rats has been shown by Parlow(7) to be an extremely sensitive and specific assay for LH, a finding that we have confirmed(2). In the present study this assay has been used to assess LH-releasing activity of hypothalamic extracts.

Methods. Assay animals were prepared by the following technic. Female rats, 26 days old, of the Wistar or Sherman strain were injected subcutaneously (sc.), first, with 75 International Units (IU) of pregnant mare's serum gonadotrophin (Equinex),§ and 58 to 67 hours later with 30 IU of human chorionic gonadotrophin. Five to 7 days later, under ether anesthesia the left ovary was removed for analysis of its ascorbic acid concentration, and the substance to be assayed was injected intravenously (IV) during one minute. One hour after removal of the first ovary, the right ovary was similarly removed and analyzed for its ascorbic acid concentration by the method of Mindlin and Butler(8). Results were expressed as percentage depletion (decrease) in ovarian ascorbic acid of the second ovary as compared to the first gland. Extracts of the stalk-median eminence

§ Kindly supplied by Dr. John B. Jewell, Ayerst Labs., N. Y.

(SME) region from adult male rats, normal or hypophysectomized (hypox.),∥ were made by grinding this tissue and adjacent ventral hypothalamus in 0.5 ml of 0.1 N HCl with sand and a stirring rod. Ten or more SME's were pooled, and the volume adjusted with 0.1 N HCl so that quantity to be injected into each assay rat was contained in 1 ml of the mixture. The diluted extract was then centrifuged at 3000 rpm for 15 minutes, and the supernatant assayed as described above. Extracts of rat cerebral cortex were prepared and assayed similarly. Hypox. assay rats were operated upon by the parapharyngeal approach and immediately used for assay as described above.

Results. The results (Table I) indicate that unilateral ovariectomy alone failed to elicit a significant OAAD. When an extract prepared from the SME region of 2 hypox. or normal (Table II) rats was injected into each assay rat, a highly significant OAAD resulted ($P<0.001$). On the contrary, an extract of rat cerebral cortex equivalent in wet weight to that from SME failed to elicit a significant OAAD.

A number of pharmacologically active agents known to exist in hypothalamic tissue was assayed to determine if the OAAD induced by the hypothalamic extract could be accounted for by any of these compounds. Epinephrine and Substance P were both inactive in these assay rats. Histamine and serotonin, on the other hand, in doses estimated to be about 1000 times greater than the amount expected to be present in the extracts of SME(9,10), evoked small but significant OAAD's which were much smaller ($P<0.001$) than that obtained with SME extract. Seventy mU of a commercial extract of vasopressin (Pitressin), corresponding to the quantity of vasopressin previously shown

∥ Obtained from Hormone Assay Labs., Chicago and used 24 hours post-hypox.

TABLE I. Ovarian Ascorbic Acid Depletion Induced by Hypothalamic Extracts and Various Pharmacological Agents.

Treatment	Ovarian ascorbic acid depletion (OAAD)	P vs control
Unilateral ovariectomy (control)	1 ± 1.8 (12)*	
Unilateral ovariectomy plus:		
A. Extract stalk-median eminence, hypox. rat, 2 SME's	22 ± 1 (6)	<.001
B. Extract rat cerebral cortex	1 ± 3 (5)	ns†
C. Serotonin creatinine SO₄, 25 µg	8 ± 1.9 (5)	=.05
D. Histamine, .3 mg	9 ± 0.9 (5)	<.05
E. Epinephrine, 2 µg	4 ± 3 (5)	ns
F. Substance P, 1 mg	2 ± 2 (5)	"
G. Pitressin, 70 mU	8 ± 1 (4)	>.05
H. Pitocin, 70 mU	7 ± 3 (6)	ns
I. Pitressin, 70 mU + Pitocin, 15 mU	6 ± 1 (5)	"

* Mean ± S.E. of mean (No. of rats/group).
† ns = no significant difference from control.

to be present in 2 hypox. rat SME's (6), induced an OAAD of borderline significance that was much less than that obtained with SME extract (P<0.001). Seventy mU of oxytocin (Pitocin) did not produce a significant OAAD and was not able to potentiate the activity of Pitressin when injected at a dose equivalent to that expected to be present in the injected extract (11).

Because the extract of SME might have contained LH, it was important to assay it in hypox. rats. These were used immediately after hypophysectomy because we found that if we used the rats 18-24 hours post-hypox., there was a very low ovarian ascorbic acid and decreased sensitivity to LH. Even during the one hour interval following removal of the first ovary a small decrease in ovarian ascorbic acid occurred (Table II).

The data in Table II show that the OAAD induced by LH or Pitressin was the same in both normal and hypox. rats. Two or 4 SME's from normal donor rats induced a small OAAD in the hypox. rats, significantly greater than the control value at the higher dose of 4 SME's; however, a significantly greater OAAD was obtained in normal rats at both the 2 and 4 SME dose than occurred in hypox. rats.

Discussion. The results indicate that rat SME or adjacent hypothalamic tissue contains substances which can deplete ovarian ascorbic acid. This is not a non-specific effect, nor can the activity of SME be explained by its content of certain known hypothalamic constituents.

The results with vasopressin and oxytocin are of particular interest since Martini et al. (12) have reported a gonadotrophin-releasing action of Pitocin and Pitressin in the rabbit. In contrast in the present experiments all activity of Pitressin was present in the absence of the hypophysis suggesting a direct action of this substance on the ovary.

Since SME extract evoked a greater OAAD in the normal than in the hypox. rat, a release of LH from the hypophysis of the normal assay animals appears to have occurred. The nature of the substance(s) responsible for this action remains to be determined. Further experiments are also required to ascertain if this substance, tentatively designated

TABLE II. Comparison of Effect of LH, Pitressin, and Hypothalamic Extract in Normal and "Acutely" Hypophysectomized Rats.

Treatment	Ovarian ascorbic acid depletion (OAAD) Normal	Hypophysectomized	P (hypox. vs normal)
Control (unilateral ovariectomy)	1.3 ± 1.8 (12)*	8.2 ± 2.9 (10)	=.05
Unilateral ovariectomy plus:			
A. LH, .2 µg	20 ± 2.3 (10)	17 ± 2.7 (8)	ns†
1.0 "	30 ± 2.5 (10)	29 ± 2.1 (8)	"
B. Pitressin, 0.5 U	21 ± 3.2 (9)	24 ± 2.4 (10)	"
C. Rat SME extract—2 SME's	18 ± 1.5 (14)	11 ± 1.4 (14)	<.005
4 "	22 ± 2.0 (9)	16 ± 1.9 (11)‡	<.05

* Mean ± S.E. of mean (No. of rats/group).
† ns = no significant difference from control.
‡ P <.05 when compared to response to uni-ovariectomy alone in the hypox. rat.

LH-releasing factor, acts directly on the adenohypophysis.

The residual OAAD produced by SME extract in the hypox. rat is presumably due to the presence of LH or vasopressin or a combination of the 2 in the extracts.

Since the difference between the OAAD in normal and hypophysectomized assay rats injected with SME extract was not large, it would appear that the extracts caused release of only a small amount of LH from the hypophysis. As we have shown that content of LH in the pituitary of these immature assay animals is very low, the amount of LH released by the extract is probably a very significant percentage of this total. Their low hypophysial LH content may constitute a major disadvantage to use of these immature rats for assay of LH-releasing activity. Nevertheless, the data show that a significant release of LH was produced by SME extracts in these assay animals.

Summary. Acid extracts of rat SME tissue evoked OAAD in immature rats pre-treated with gonadotrophins. Part of the activity in the extracts could be accounted for by their content of LH or vasopressin or both, whereas the remaining activity appeared to be due to release of LH from pituitary of assay rats. The substance(s) responsible for LH-releasing activity of extracts has been called LH-releasing factor. The nature of this material is unknown, but it appears to differ from histamine, serotonin, substance P, epinephrine, and vasopressin or oxytocin.

The technical assistance of Maria Smith is gratefully acknowledged.

1. Harris, G. W., *The Neural Control of the Pituitary Gland*, Arnold, London, 1955.
2. McCann, S. M., Taleisnik, S., Friedman, H. M., *Fed. Proc.*, 1960, v19, 292.
3. Saffran, M., Schally, A. V., Benfey, B. G., *Endocrinol.*, 1955, v57, 439.
4. Guillemin, R., Hearn, W. R., Cheek, W. R., Householder, D. E., *ibid.*, 1957, v60, 488.
5. Royce, P. C., Sayers, G., Proc. Soc. Exp. Biol. and Med., 1960, v103, 1.
6. McCann, S. M., Haberland, P., *ibid.*, 1959, v102, 319.
7. Parlow, A. F., *Fed. Proc.*, 1958, v17, 402.
8. Mindlin, R. L., Butler, A. W., *J. Biol. Chem.*, 1937, v122, 673.
9. Harris, G. W., Jacobsohn, D., Kahlson, G., *Ciba Foundation Colloquia (Endocrinology IV)*, 1952, 186.
10. Udenfriend, S., Shore, P. A., Bogdanski, D. F., Weissback, H., Brodie, B. B., *Recent Prog. Hormone Research*, 1957, v13, 1.
11. Van Dyke, H. B., Adamsons, K., Engel, S. L., in *The Neurohypophysis*, ed. Heller, H., 1957, 67.
12. Martini, L., Mira, L., Pecile, A., Saito, S., *J. Endocrin.*, 1959, v18, 245.

Received May 13, 1960.   P.S.E.B.M., 1960, v104.

26

Copyright © 1964 by the Physiological Society London

Reprinted from pages 474–475 and 484–485 of *J. Physiol.* **170**:474–486 (1964)

THE EFFECT OF INTRAPITUITARY INFUSION OF MEDIAN EMINENCE AND OTHER BRAIN EXTRACTS ON ANTERIOR PITUITARY GONADOTROPHIC SECRETION

By H. J. CAMPBELL, G. FEUER* AND G. W. HARRIS†

From the Department of Neuroendocrinology, Institute of Psychiatry, The Maudsley Hospital, London, S.E.5

(*Received* 7 *June* 1963)

It has been known since the time of Heape (1905) that the isolated female rabbit does not ovulate spontaneously but requires sensory stimuli, normally associated with coitus, to excite follicular rupture. The evidence indicates that the act of mating excites a nervous reflex pathway passing to the hypothalamus, which in turn stimulates the anterior pituitary gland to release increased amounts of luteinizing hormone (LH). Harris (1937, 1948), Haterius & Derbyshire (1937) and Markee, Sawyer & Hollinshead (1946) all found that electrical stimulation of the hypothalamus in the isolated female rabbit was followed by ovulation.

The mechanism by which the hypothalamus regulates gonadotrophin secretion by the anterior pituitary gland seems to involve the liberation of a humoral agent from the nervous tissue of the median eminence of the tuber cinereum into the hypophysial portal vessels, and thereby the transmission of this agent to the anterior pituitary gland. Evidence relating to this view is as follows (see Harris, 1955, for detailed discussion): (1) It is very doubtful whether nerve fibres, other than vasomotor, exist in the adenohypophysis. (2) All major vertebrate groups possess a vascular system carrying blood *from* the median eminence *to* the adenohypophysis (Green, 1951). (3) The evidence that electrical stimulation of the hypothalamus evokes ovulation in the rabbit, whereas similar stimulation applied directly to the anterior pituitary gland itself is ineffective (Markee *et al.* 1946; Harris, 1948), is compatible with the view of humoral stimulation of the gland cells. (4) Permanent interruption of the hypophysial portal vessels (by pituitary stalk section or pituitary transplantation) results in a permanent and severe loss of ovarian activity; temporary interruption followed by regeneration of the portal vessels is often associated with a post-operative return of normal ovarian function.

* Present address: BIBRA Laboratories, Carshalton, Surrey.
† Present address: Department of Human Anatomy, University of Oxford.

The present investigation was planned to see whether any material with excitatory actions on anterior pituitary cells could be extracted from the median eminence of the tuber cinereum. The median eminence is phylogenetically the most ancient part of the neurohypophysis. It is also the zone where hypothalamic nerve fibres enter into intimate association with the primary capillaries of the hypophysial portal vessels. Thus if the hypothalamic nerve tracts associated with ovulation in the rabbit contain some humoral agent concerned with gonadotrophic secretion, it would be reasonable to suppose that a more concentrated extract (per unit weight of tissue) could be obtained from the median eminence than from the hypothalamus. Extracts of median eminence have been tested for gonadotrophin-releasing properties by means of intrapituitary infusions, with a technique similar to that of von Euler & Holmgren (1956). Ovulation, as shown by the presence of ruptured follicles in histological sections of the ovaries removed 48 hr after infusion, was taken to indicate stimulation of secretion of gonadotrophic hormone.

[*Editor's Note:* Material has been omitted at this point.]

SUMMARY

1. Infusions of extracts of the median eminence of the tuber cinereum, obtained from the brains of rabbits, cattle and monkeys, into the anterior pituitary gland of isolated female rabbits was found to excite secretion of gonadotrophic hormone (presumably LH) as shown by consequent ovulation in 55 out of 90 cases.

2. Similar infusions into the pituitary gland of control brain extracts (cerebral cortex, corpus callosum, caudate nucleus), and other naturally occurring substances (synthetic vasopressin, synthetic oxytocin, synthetic vasotocin, adrenaline, histamine, serotonin, substance P), resulted in ovulation in only 6 out of 95 cases.

3. Intravenous infusions of median-eminence extracts (in a dose of 20 times that of the minimal effective dose given by intrapituitary infusion, or more) was found to evoke ovulation in 6 out of 23 rabbits.

4. After consideration of the possible role played by direct damage to the pituitary gland, or of hormonal contamination of the infused extracts, the conclusion is drawn that the median eminence contains some substance which excites the secretion of LH from the anterior pituitary gland of rabbits. It seems likely that the release of this substance into the hypophysial portal vessels forms part of the neurohumoral mechanism controlling LH secretion.

We wish to express our gratitude to Mr W. F. Piper for his skilled assistance in the construction of the cannulae, and to Messrs S. A. Williams and G. S. Garcha for their technical help. We wish also to thank Professor J. H. Gaddum, F.R.S., for the supply of substance P, Drs A. Cerletti and B. Berde of Sandoz Ltd, Basle, for the supply of synthetic vasopressin and synthetic vasotocin, and Drs A. J. Beale and A. C. Laurson of Glaxo Laboratories Ltd for making available the monkey material. Our gratitude is also due to the Ford Foundation for the support of one of us (G. F.), to the United States Air Force (contract No. AF 61(514)-953) and to the Maudsley Hospital Research Fund, for support of this work.

REFERENCES

Green, J. D. 1951. The Comparative Anatomy of the Hypophysis with Special Reference to Its Blood Supply and Innervation. *Am. J. Anat.* **88**:225–312.

Harris, G. W. 1937. The Induction of Ovulation in the Rabbit by Electrical Stimulation of the Hypothalamo-Hypophysial Mechanism. *R. Soc. London Proc.*, ser. B, **122**:374–394.

Harris, G. W. 1948. Electrical Stimulation of the Hypothalamus and the Mechanism of Neural Control of the Adenohypophyaia. *J. Physiol.* **107**:418–429.

Harris, G. W. 1955. *Neural Control of the Pituitary Gland.* London: Arnold.

Heape, W. 1905. Ovulation and Degeneration of Ova in the Rabbit. *R. Soc. London Proc.*, ser. B, **76**:260–268.

Markee, J. E., C. H. Sawyer, and W. H. Hollinshead. 1946. Activation of the Anterior Hypophysis by Electrical Stimulation in the Rabbit. *Endocrinology* **38**:345–357.

von Euler, C., and B. Holmgren. 1956. The Thyroxine "Receptor" of the Thyroid-Pituitary System. *J. Physiol.* **131**:125–136.

Copyright © 1965 by J. B. Lippincott Company

Reprinted from pages 282–283 and 286–289 of *Endocrinology*
76:282:289 (1965)

Fluctuations in Hypothalamic LH-RF (Luteinizing Hormone-Releasing Factor) During the Rat Estrous Cycle

V. DOMINGO RAMIREZ[1] AND CHARLES H. SAWYER

Department of Anatomy and Brain Research Institute, University of California, Los Angeles, California

ABSTRACT. A study has been made of changes in LH-RF content of the rat hypothalamus during the various phases of the estrous cycle. Normally cyclic female Sprague-Dawley rats under a regimen of 14 hr of light and 10 hr of darkness were killed at different times of day during each of the stages of the cycle. The stalk-median eminence region (SME) of the hypothalamus was quickly dissected out, extracted in 0.1N HCl and boiled for 10 min. The supernate was tested for LH-releasing activity in immature Holtzman rats by a variant of the Parlow LH method: the ovarian ascorbic acid depletion induced by the extract was considered the index of LH-RF. The amount of LH-RF present in the SME during late proestrus and early estrus was significantly lower than at other times during the cycle. The drop in SME LH-RF occurred later than the critical period of the day of proestrus, during which there is evidence for the release of pituitary LH. It is postulated that released pituitary LH in the plasma may exert a negative internal feedback action on the SME-secretion of LH-RF, inhibiting the synthesis of the neurohumor after it (LH) reaches a threshold level in the plasma. (*Endocrinology* 76: 282, 1965)

THE existence of a luteinizing hormone-releasing factor (LH-RF) in crude acidic extracts of stalk median eminence (SME) of the rat hypothalamus was reported by McCann *et al.* in 1960 (1). In an elegant study involving the direct infusion of rat SME extract into the pituitary, Nikitovitch-Winer was able to induce ovulation in the Nembutal-blocked proestrous rat (2). With a similar technique, Campbell *et al.* (3, 4) described the presence of an ovulation-inducing factor in the rabbit hypothalamus. Guillemin and his associates have described a partial purification of LH-RF (which he abbreviates "LRF"); the factor is distinct from vasopressin and other known hypothalamic neurohumors

Received July 30, 1964.
This study was supported by Grant NB 01162 from the National Institutes of Health and a Training Grant from the Ford Foundation.
[1] Ford Foundation Fellow on leave from the Department of Pathological Physiology, University of Chile, Santiago, Chile.

(5, 6). Recently, Ramirez *et al.* (7), using a G-25 Sephadex column, have also separated the LH-RF from vasopressin and CRF. Schally and his associates have quite recently confirmed the existence of this factor (8), and further purification was reported (9).

The demonstration of the so-called hypothalamic releasing factors that appear to control the output of pituitary hormones necessitates their chemical separation from other known hypothalamic agents (see Guillemin's paper for a precise definition of the criteria to be considered in establishing the existence of a specific neurohumor) (10). In addition to chemical purification the proof of the identity of such a factor requires the demonstration in the intact animal of physiological changes related to the function of this neurohumoral agent. The present paper deals with this approach. Fluctuations have been found in the LH-releasing capacity of crude acidic extract of rat SME tissue which may be correlated with release of LH during the rat estrous cycle.

Materials and Methods

Preparation of Crude SME Extract. As SME donor animals, female Sprague-Dawley (250-310 g body wt) rats were used. They were caged in groups of 8-10, fed Purina Lab Chow pellets and water *ad lib.*, and maintained under an artificial light regimen of 14 hr of light and 10 hr of darkness daily. Before the animals were sacrificed and used as SME donors, daily vaginal smears were taken for at least 2 weeks by vaginal lavage, except occasionally on Sunday. The estrous cycles were either 4 or 5 days in length. In general, 8-10 rats at the same stage in the estrous cycle were sacrificed with ether at the times indicated in the results. Before the skull was removed, each rat was exsanguinated by cutting the heart and great vessels with scissors, and the basal tuberal region of the hypothalamus including the SME was quickly dissected out.[2] The whole procedure did not take more than 1 min animal. The 8-10 SME's were placed immediately in 0.5 ml of 0.1N HCl in a plastic centrifuge tube at room temperature. They were then homogenized with a Teflon grinder and washed out with 2 ml of 0.1N HCl. The homogenate was centrifuged at 3500 rpm for 30 min; the precipitate was discarded, and the supernate (in general 2.2 ml) was kept frozen until the bio-assay date, from 1 to 5 days later. On the day of bio-assay the supernate was boiled for 10 min, and the very small precipitate which formed was taken out by centrifugation (3500 rpm for 30 min). This procedure destroys LH (11). In some cases the supernate was boiled on the day in which the sample was obtained and then kept frozen. There were no significant differences in the activities of samples treated in these 2 ways. On the day of the bio-assay the supernate was diluted with 0.1N HCl so that a final concentration of 1.6 SME ml was injected iv into each bio-assay animal.

Test for LH-RF Activity. The 1-hr, 2-ovary variant of the Parlow ovarian ascorbic acid depletion (OAAD) assay for LH (11) was used as an assay for LH-RF. The SME extracts were injected iv at a dose of 1 ml (1.6 SME) rat. Since the OAAD response is specific for LH (12-14), and since the extracts contained no active LH, OAAD was considered a response to LH-RF. Since no LH-RF Standard was available, LH-NIH-S1 was used as a standard. It was stored frozen, and tested at 2 dose levels in most of the experiments. The interval between successive dose levels was 5-fold. In each assay 4-5 rats were assigned to each dose of the standard and the SME extract. The results of replicate assays were combined according to the system of Sheps and Moore (15). In 2 cases in which the standards failed to meet biometric criteria of validity, the composite curve of the standard at doses 0.2 and 1 µg of LH was used (*cf* footnote† in Table 1); this procedure was legitimate, inasmuch as the mean responses and slopes of the different bio-assays did not differ significantly. The LH-releasing capacity of SME extract was calculated in terms of the LH Standard from this 3-point bio-assay design. Furthermore, late proestrous SME samples and early estrous ones were each tested simultaneously with diestrous SME samples obtained at the same time of day (*cf* colony time, Table 1).

As a test of the specificity and error of our assay and the possible contamination of the extract with blood LH, plasma from several sources (adult estrous and diestrous rats and immature 30-, 31- and 36-day-old female rats) was injected into bio-assay rats under the same experimental conditions as those used to test the extract. Plasma from 4-8 animals was pooled and used immediately or after being stored no more than 1 week in the frozen state. Two ml of plasma was injected iv into each immature Holtzman assay animal to test for LH or LH-RF activity.

[*Editor's Note:* Material has been omitted at this point, including figures 1, 2, and 3, and tables 1 and 2.]

---

[2] The mean wet wt of a proestrous SME in a group of 9 rats was 2.1 mg (range 1.5-2.4). In a diestrous group of 9 rats the SME wet wt was 1.9 (range 1.3-2.3).

Discussion

Cyclic variations in the LH-releasing capacity of the rat stalk-median eminence have now been added to the growing list of biochemical changes meshed with the estrous cycle and with mechanisms relating to ovulation. Rhythmic changes in LH-RF in the rat SME were reported independently at the 1964 Endocrine Meetings by our laboratory (16) and by Chowers and McCann (17).

Cyclic events related to ovulation in the rat generally show marked changes on the day of proestrus, and they can usually be fitted into a framework around the "critical period" during which the nervous system triggers the release of an ovulatory surge of gonadotropin from the hypophysis. Under con-

TABLE 3. Ovarian ascorbic acid depleting capacity (OAAD) of rat plasma

Plasma Source	Colony Time	Plasma Dose ml	OAAD % Mean ±SEM (No. assay rats)
Adult rats (D & E)*	—	2	1.9 (4)
Adult rats (D & E)*	—	2	0.7 (5)
Immature rats (30 days old)	—	2	4.4 (5)
Immature rats (36 days old)	—	2	3.1 (4)
Immature rats (31 days old)	—	2	0.9 (4)
Over-all Mean			2.2 ±0.9 (22)
Adult rats, proestrus	23:00	2	5.6 ±1.0 (5)
Adult rats, diestrus	23:00	2	4.0 ±0.5 (5)

* Mixed diestrous and estrous rats.

trolled lighting conditions with 14 hours of light daily, the time limits of the critical period have been defined with the use of blocking agents and anesthetics as lying between 2 and 4 PM (18, 19). With the use of hypophysectomy, Everett (20) subsequently demonstrated that not only is the hypophysis stimulated during the critical period but it also releases sufficient hormone prior to 4 PM to induce ovulation some ten hours later. With the ovarian ascorbic acid depletion method for LH, Schwartz and co-workers (21) found a reduced content of the tropin in the rat pituitary subsequent to the critical period. With the same technique, Ramirez and McCann (22) recently demonstrated an elevation in plasma LH on the day of proestrus. The rise appeared to start in the morning and to reach a peak in late afternoon, but it is not feasible to relate it to the critical period, since the latter has not been defined for the 12-hour lighting regimen employed. The same is true of the depression in hypothalamic LH-RF during proestrus reported by Chowers and McCann (17) on the same 12-hour lighting schedule. With careful attention to time relationships during proestrus in the 14-hour light regimen, we can report with confidence that hypothalamic LH-RF continues to rise for some time after the critical period and the release of an ovulating quantum of gonadotropin. It is some hours later that the SME LH-RF shows a depression, which is maintained into the morning of estrus. These relationships will be interpreted in terms of feedback mechanisms later.

Since vasopressin has a definite LH-releasing action, contamination of the SME extract with this neurohypophysial polypeptide might be a factor of importance in our results. However, recent studies have failed to reveal a cyclic variation in SME vasopressin content (Ramirez and Sawyer, unpublished results), so the fluctuations observed here must represent change in LH-RF. The amount of vasopressin extracted from one adult rat SME was found to be of the order of 10 mU.

The amount of LH-RF present in the SME and the amount of LH in the hypophysis at any one time must represent in each case a balance between synthesis and release. Even during diestrus there is adequate LH in the hypophysis to induce ovulation (23, 24), and sufficient LH-RF in the hypothalamus to trigger the process has been revealed in the present study and that of Chowers and McCann (17). Furthermore, Nedde and Nikitovitch-Winer reported (23) that the diestrous pituitary responded positively to infused LH-RF, though it may have required more than the minimal effective dose that ovulated the Nembutal-blocked proestrous rat. The latter had previously been estimated by Nikitovitch-Winer (2) to be 700 μg wet weight of rat SME or about 30% of the total weight of the SME. Another factor which must be taken into consideration is the sensitivity of the ovary during the various stages of the estrous cycle. Everett, following his demonstration that a greater preoptic stimulative lesion is required to induce ovulation during diestrus than during proestrus (24), has recently reported that more exogenous LH is needed to ovulate a diestrous ovary than a proestrous one (25). If accelerated secretion of LH prior to the critical period does in fact occur, as suggested by the results of Ramirez and McCann (22), its function might be to alter the sensitivity of the ovary and/or to stimulate preovulatory secretion of progestin, a process which may be a prerequisite to the neurogenous release of the ovulatory surge of gonadotropin. It should be remembered that, in five-day cyclic rats, treatment with exogenous progestin prior to 2 PM on the third day of diestrus will trigger ovulation that night, *i.e.*, 24 hours early (26).

From data in Fig. 2 and Table 1, it appears that on the day of proestrus synthesis of LH-RF becomes negligible after 17:30. Assuming this to be true, we can plot on semilog paper the level of LH-RF in the SME as a function of time. This yields a straight line, permitting us to estimate roughly the rate of release; it amounts to about 0.7%/min, or about 84% of the LH-RF present in the SME per 2 hours. If the same rate was in effect during the critical period, it would easily account for the ovulatory surge of LH release. Improved methodologies will be necessary to obtain a clear panorama of the dynamics involved in the nervous control of LH release during this period from onset of critical period to the time of ovulation.

It is of interest to speculate on the possible roles of LH itself as well as the ovarian hormones on the synthesis and release of LH-RF. It has been generally accepted that the synthesis and release of pituitary gonadotropins are controlled or influenced by the feedback actions of gonadal steroids exerted on the hypothalamus or the hypophysis directly (27). On the basis of electrophysiological evidence, Kawakami and Sawyer (28) proposed that pituitary ovulating hormone, discharged post coitum in estrogen-primed ovariectomized rabbits, might exert a feedback action on the nervous system to influence the further release of gonadotropin. It was not suggested that this internal feedback influence would replace the external feedback control exerted by the steroids, but might supplement it. Similarly, evidence for an internal feedback action of ACTH on the hypothalamus has been presented by Halász and Szentágothai (29). An internal negative feedback action of circulating LH on the synthesis of hypothalamic LH-RF is a concept consistent with our observations, and the postulation of such a scheme has recently been made by Chowers and McCann (17).

There is considerable evidence from the work of Everett (20), Schwartz and co-workers (21), and especially Ramirez and McCann (22), that LH has been released and has been circulating in the proestrous rat for some time before 17:30, the hour after which LH-RF synthesis appears to cease or to be sharply curtailed. It may be necessary for circulating LH to reach a certain threshold concentration to exert an internal negative feedback effect. Such a scheme would be consistent with the earlier electrophysiological observations of Kawakami and Sawyer in rabbits (30), in which exogenous gonadotropin actually lowered their "EEG after-reaction threshold" prior to elevating it. Biphasic effects on CNS thresholds are exerted by the ovarian steroids, especially the progestins (30), and it will be of interest to determine whether these changes are reflected in sequential LH-RF stimulation and inhibition in the rabbit. The possibilities exist that the ovarian hormones may exert direct influences on the LH-RF secretion mechanism or modify the sensitivity of pituitary gonadotropic cells to the LH-RF stimulus. Further studies will be needed to test these speculative hypotheses, and, regardless of the outcome, they should reveal additional valuable information on neuroendocrine interrelationships.

Acknowledgments

The Luteinizing Hormone Standard, Ovine (NIH-LH-S1), was generously supplied by the Endocrinology Study Section of the National Institutes of Health. The authors also wish to thank Miss Arlene Ross for technical assistance and Mrs. Christa Osterberg and Mr. Rudolph Sabbot for the preparation of illustrations.

References

1. McCann, S. M., S. Taleisnik, and H. H. Friedman, *Proc Soc Exp Biol Med* **104**: 432, 1960.
2. Nikitovitch-Winer, M. B., *Endocrinology* **70**: 350, 1962.
3. Campbell, H. J., C. Feuer, J. Garcia, and G. W. Harris, *J Physiol (London)* **157**: 30P, 1961.
4. Campbell, H. J., C. Feuer, and G. W. Harris, *J Physiol (London)* **170**: 474, 1964.
5. Courrier, R., R. Guillemin, M. Jutisz, E. Sakiz, and P. Ashheim, *C R Acad Sci (Paris)* **253**: 922, 1961.
6. Guillemin, R., M. Jutisz, and E. Sakiz, *C R Acad Sci (Paris)* **256**: 504, 1963.
7. Ramirez, V. D., R. Nallar, and S. M. McCann, *Proc Soc Exp Biol Med* **115**: 1072, 1964.
8. Schally, A. V., and C. Y. Bowers, *Endocrinology* **75**: 312, 1964.
9. Schally, A. V., C. Y. Bowers, W. Tommie, B. S. Redding, A. Kutoshima, and Y. Tshida, Program of the 46th Meeting of The Endocrine Society, 1964, p. 56.
10. Guillemin, R., *J Physiol (Paris)* **55**: 7, 1962.
11. McCann, S. M., *Amer J Med* **34**: 379, 1963.
12. Parlow, A. F., *In* Albert, A. (ed.), Human Pituitary Gonadotropins, Charles C Thomas, Springfield, Ill., 1961, p. 300.
13. Guiliani, G., L. Martini, A. Pecile, and M. Fochi, *Acta Endocr (Kobenhavn)* **38**: 1, 1961.
14. McCann, S. M., and S. Taleisnik, *Amer J Physiol* **199**: 847, 1960.
15. Sheps, M. C., and E. A. Moore, *J Pharmacol Exp Ther* **128**: 99, 1960.
16. Ramirez, V. D., and C. H. Sawyer, Program of the 46th Meeting of The Endocrine Society, 1964, p. 26.
17. Chowers, S., and S. M. McCann, Program of the 46th Meeting of The Endocrine Society, 1964, p. 27.
18. Everett, J. W., C. H. Sawyer, and J. E. Markee, *Endocrinology* **44**: 234, 1949.
19. Everett, J. W., and C. H. Sawyer, *Endocrinology* **47**: 198, 1950.
20. Everett, J. W., *Endocrinology* **59**: 580, 1956.
21. Schwartz, N. B., and D. Bartosik, *Endocrinology* **71**: 756, 1962.
22. Ramirez, V. D., and S. M. McCann, *Endocrinology* **74**: 814, 1964.
23. Nedde, N. R., and M. Nikitovitch-Winer, *Anat Rec* **148**: 317, 1964 (Abstract).
24. Everett, J. W., *In* Bajusz, E., and G. Jasmin (eds.), Major Problems in Neuroendocrinology, S. Karger, Basel/New York, 1964, p. 346.
25. ———, *Fed Proc* **23**: 151, 1964 (Abstract).
26. Everett, J. W., and C. H. Sawyer, *Endocrinology* **45**: 581, 1949.
27. Sawyer, C. H., *In* Cole, H. H. (ed.), Gonadotropins, W. H. Freeman and Co., San Francisco, 1964, p. 113.
28. Kawakami, M., and C. H. Sawyer, *Endocrinology* **65**: 631, 1959.
29. Halász, B., and J. Szentágothai, *Acta Morph Acad Sci Hung* **9**: 251, 1960.
30. Kawakami, M., and C. H. Sawyer, *Endocrinology* **65**: 652, 1959.

A Hypothalamic Follicle Stimulating Hormone-Releasing Factor

MASAO IGARASHI[1] AND S. M. McCANN

Department of Physiology, School of Medicine, University of Pennsylvania, Philadelphia, Pennsylvania

ABSTRACT. FSH activity in 1.5 ml of rat plasma was evaluated by a new sensitive mouse uterine weight method devised by the authors. No FSH activity was found in 1.5 ml of plasma from normal females, but it was readily determined in 1.5 ml plasma from chronically ovariectomized female rats. Treatment of ovariectomized females with single, subcutaneous doses of 50 µg estradiol benzoate and 25 mg progesterone significantly lowered plasma FSH activity on measurement 3 days later. Ten min after the intravenous injection of a crude acidic extract of 2 rat stalk-median eminences, a significant elevation in plasma FSH occurred in the ovariectomized, estrogen, progesterone-blocked rats, whereas cerebral cortical extract was without effect on plasma FSH in these animals. Furthermore, stalk-median eminence extract failed to alter plasma FSH in hypophysectomized rats. The extract was also ineffective when injected directly into the immature test mice for 3 days. These results indicate that contamination of the extracts with FSH cannot account for the FSH-releasing action observed. Stalk-median eminence extract also increased FSH activity in plasma of ovariectomized rats in which release of FSH had been blocked by electrolytic lesions in the median eminence, whereas cortical extract was ineffective under these conditions. It is concluded that an FSH-releasing factor resides in stalk-median eminence tissue. (*Endocrinology* 74: 446, 1964)

ACCUMULATED evidence indicates that the secretion of hypophysial gonadotrophins is under hypothalamic control, and there is strong support for the concept proposed by Harris and others (1–3) that the hypothalamus exerts its effect on the anterior pituitary not through purely nervous pathways, but through secretion of some neurohumoral substance(s) transmitted to hypophysial cells by means of the hypophysial portal circulation.

Until recently, there was little direct experimental evidence for the existence of hypothalamic substance(s) which might act to release gonadotrophins. Oxytocin was reported to have a possible effect on the release of luteotrophin (4), and Martini observed a rise in urinary gonadotrophin following intravenous injections of posterior pituitary preparations (5). Campbell and co-workers (6) demonstrated that direct infusion of median eminence extracts into the pituitary was effective in inducing ovulation in rabbits, and Nikitovitch-Winer (7) also succeeded in inducing ovulation in rats by direct intrapituitary infusion of median eminence extract. McCann and co-workers (8) were the first to demonstrate the presence of a hypothalamic luteinizing hormone-releasing factor (LH-RF) in stalk-median eminence extracts using the highly sensitive ovarian ascorbic acid depletion method of Parlow (9). Lastly, Kobayashi and co-workers (10) also have reported that crude median eminence extracts induce an increase in total

---

Received August 28, 1963.

Supported by Grant A-1236, C-6 from the National Institutes of Health.

[1] Postdoctoral Fellow of the Population Council.

gonadotrophin release from anterior pituitary cells cultured *in vitro*.

In the experiments presented here, direct evidence for the existence of a follicle stimulating hormone-releasing factor (FSH-RF) in hypothalamic extracts was sought with the use of a new sensitive method for assay of FSH (11).

[*Editor's Note:* Material has been omitted at this point.]

Discussion

It is well known that gonadectomy increases pituitary gonadotrophin content in animals and urinary gonadotrophin levels in man, but there are only a few reports of blood gonadotrophin levels in the castrate. Recently, plasma LH has been successfully assayed in ovariectomized rats by means of the ovarian ascorbic acid depletion test (13, 17). More recently, Parlow has found an elevated FSH titer in ovariectomized rat plasma with the Steelman-Pohley method (14). In the present work, the use of a more sensitive assay has made it possible to demonstrate elevated plasma FSH titers in a much smaller volume of plasma from ovariectomized rats than was previously required. Furthermore, a single injection of a large dose of both estrogen and progesterone was found capable of lowering plasma FSH activity in the ovariectomized rat. If it is assumed that the disappearance rate of FSH from plasma is unaltered by these procedures, the results can be interpreted to mean that removal of the ovaries results in increased rates of release of adenohypophysial FSH which can be inhibited by administration of ovarian steroids. The results therefore support the negative feedback hypothesis for the action of these steroids on FSH secretion.

The ovariectomized, estrogen, progesterone-blocked animal has previously

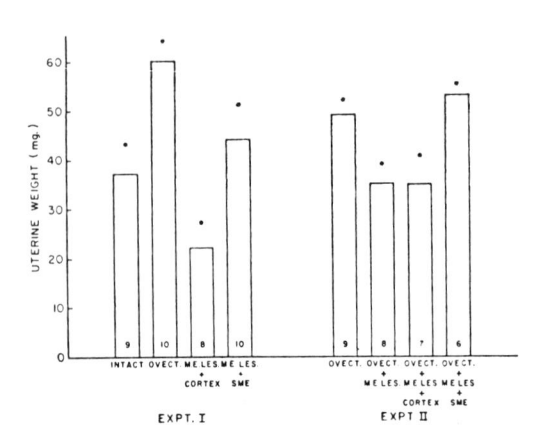

FIG. 6. Effect of stalk-median eminence and cortical extract on plasma FSH activity in ovariectomized rats with median eminence lesions. Treatment received by the mice is indicated by the legend at the base of each column.

been shown to respond to the iv injection of stalk-median eminence extract with an elevation of plasma LH levels (15). The present work demonstrates that injection of stalk-median eminence produces a similar increment in plasma FSH levels in these animals. Since comparable extract from the cerebral cortex was without effect on plasma FSH, the effect of stalk-median eminence cannot be explained as a nonspecific result of the injection of brain tissue. Since the effect of stalk-median eminence is absent in the hypophysectomized rat and cannot be demonstrated by direct injection into the test mice, it is clear that contamination of the extract with FSH cannot account for the results. It appears then that stalk-median eminence extract has evoked a release of adenohypophysial FSH which results in elevated plasma levels of the trophin.

The ability of median eminence lesions to lower plasma FSH dramatically in ovariectomized rats shows directly for the first time that such lesions can block hypophysial FSH secretion. The effectiveness of stalk-median eminence in elevating plasma FSH in ovariectomized rats with lesions tends to support our belief that the extract exerts a direct FSH-releasing action on adenohypophysial cells.

The chemical nature of this hypothalamic FSH-releasing factor is unknown, but it is intriguing to speculate on its similarity, or dissimilarity, to the LH-releasing and LtH-inhibiting factors (16) already found in stalk-median eminence extracts. Fractionation of hypothalamic extracts will be required to settle this point; however, since different conditions are thought to govern the secretion of FSH and LH, it would appear reasonable at the present stage to postulate discrete FSH- and LH-releasing factors to govern the release of these two trophins from the adenohypophysis.

Of course the results presented here are no better than the method upon which they rest. In tests with the ovine NIH-LH standard, no response was found with injection of LH to a dose of 200 μg; however, some inhibition of the response to FSH was found with doses of LH above 6 μg (11). Recently, tests with a purified rat LH preparation[5] have indicated that it may produce a small increment in uterine weight in doses equivalent to or greater than 2.5 μg of the NIH ovine LH standard. In this laboratory assays of plasma LH from ovariectomized rats of the present strain have yielded values as high as 10 μg LH/100 ml (17). Thus, there would be approximately 0.15 μg of LH in the dose of 1.5 ml of ovariectomized rat plasma used here, a value far below that which we have found to interfere with the assay of FSH by the present method.

Because of the ability of plasma from hypophysectomized rats to potentiate the response to FSH in the present test, we have been reluctant to express our results in terms of the NIH ovine FSH-S-1 standard. However, if such values are calculated, the mean of three determinations using 3- or 4-point assays in ovariectomized rats is 20.0 $\pm$ 2.5 μg of FSH/ml. In this laboratory the Steelman-Pohley assay has also been used for estimation of plasma FSH in ovariectomized rats, and the mean value obtained in four assays was 12.0 $\pm$ .8 μg of FSH/ml. If these values with the mouse assay are reduced by a factor to account for the potentiation of FSH by plasma of 1/3.7 (see Results), the mean value for plasma FSH obtained is 5.4 $\pm$ .7 μg/ml. The fact that this value is even lower than that

[5] Kindly supplied by Dr. A. F. Parlow, Department of Physiology, Emory University, Atlanta, Georgia.

obtained with the Steelman and Pohley method reinforces our conclusion that the present technique is specific for plasma FSH.

References

1. Harris, G. W., Handbook of Physiology, Washington, D. C., Amer. Physiol. Soc. Sect. I, vol. II, 1960, p. 1007.
2. Green, J. D., and G. W. Harris, *J Endocr* **5:** 136, 1947.
3. Hinsey, J. C., *Cold Spring Harbor Symposium on Quantitative Biology* **5:** 269, 1937.
4. Benson, G. K., and S. J. Folley, *J Endocr* **16:** 189, 1959.
5. Martini, L., L. Mira, A. Pecile, and S. Saito, *J Endocr* **18:** 245, 1959.
6. Campbell, H. J., G. Feuer, J. Garcia, and G. W. Harris, *J Physiol* **157:** 30, 1961.
7. Nikitovitch-Winer, M. B., *Endocrinology* **70:** 350, 1962.
8. (a) McCann, S. M., S. Taleisnik, and H. M. Friedman, *Proc Soc Exp Biol Med* **104:** 432, 1960.
   (b) McCann, S. M., *Amer J Physiol* **202:** 395, 1962.
9. Parlow, A. F., *Fed Proc* **17:** 402, 1958.
10. Kobayashi, T., T. Kobayashi, T. Kigawa, M. Mizuno, and Y. Amenomori, *Endocr Jap* **10:** 16, 1963.
11. Igarashi, M., and S. M. McCann, *Endocrinology* **74:** 440, 1964.
12. McCann, S. M., *Endocrinology* **60:** 664, 1957.
13. Parlow, A. F., Program of the 41st Meeting of The Endocrine Society, 1959, p. 46.
14. ——— (personal communication, 1963).
15. Ramirez, V. D., and S. M. McCann, *Endocrinology* **73:** 193, 1963.
16. Meites, J., P. K. Talwalker, and A. Ratner, Program of the 44th Meeting of The Endocrine Society, 1962, p. 19.
17. Ramirez, V. D., and S. M. McCann, *Endocrinology* **72:** 452, 1963.

Gonadotrophic Hormone Secretion in Female Rats After Partial or Total Interruption of Neural Afferents to the Medial Basal Hypothalamus

BÉLA HALÁSZ[1] AND ROGER A. GORSKI

Department of Anatomy and Brain Research Institute, UCLA School of Medicine, Los Angeles, California 90024

ABSTRACT. Neural connections to the medial basal hypothalamus (MBH) were partially or totally transected with a small knife. Ovulation, ovarian compensatory hypertrophy (OCH) and hypophysial response to castration were studied in the same animals. After complete deafferentation of the MBH, ovulation did not occur. Transection of the posterior and posterolateral connections to the MBH did not interfere with ovulation. If, in addition, lateral and superior afferents were also interrupted, 8 animals out of 12 still ovulated. Ovulation did not occur in 18 rats when only the anterior connections to the MBH were interrupted by an extended frontal cut just posterior to the optic chiasm, reaching 1.5 mm lateral from midline and extending from the base of the brain to the paraventricular nuclei above. A small frontal cut at the same level but extending only 0.6 mm lateral from midline was ineffective in blocking ovulation. When placed 1.5 mm behind the level of the optic chiasm this small frontal cut interfered with ovulation in 5 of 10 rats. OCH was blocked only in the animals with complete deafferentation of the MBH. In all rats with hypothalamic deafferentations, gonadectomy increased pituitary and serum LH content and castration cells developed in the pituitaries. The pituitary response to castration was diminished in the animals with complete deafferentation of the MBH. It is concluded that a) neural afferents which reach the MBH via the anterior hypothalamus are required for ovulation; b) above the optic chiasm these fibers are diffusely organized and converge toward the median eminence; c) at least 2 levels exist in the system for the negative feedback of gonadal steroids: one is represented by the MBH-pituitary complex, the other might be located in the anterior hypothalamus; d) the latter level can be independent of the neural afferents indispensable for ovulation; e) the MBH, which acts directly on the pituitary by its GTH releasing factors, is by itself capable of releasing these substances only in a tonic fashion; f) the nervous structures responsible for the cyclic release of the releasing factors (particularly LH-releasing factor) lie outside the MBH but influence the pituitary through it. (*Endocrinology* **80**: 608, 1967)

T HE MEDIAL basal hypothalamus (MBH), which includes the arcuate and periventricular nuclei and the medial part of the retrochiasmatic area, is capable of maintaining the structure and function of the transplanted anterior pituitary (1 3). This hypothalamic region was called the hypophysiotrophic area[2] (HTA) and has

Received August 30, 1966.
This work was supported by Grant HD-01182 from the USPHS.
[1] Ford Foundation Fellow on leave from the Department of Anatomy, University Medical School, Pécs, Dischka u 5, Hungary.
[2] Although the medial basal hypothalamus and hypophysiotrophic area both designate the same hypothalamic region, the more general form (MBH) will be used in the present report.

been assumed to produce the substances essential for normal pituitary structure and function. Further experiments (4), in which the MBH was completely cut around by means of a small knife, have suggested that this area is not merely the final common pathway which simply converts and conveys the influence of other hypothalamic structures to the pituitary but that it also exerts a regulatory influence on the anterior lobe. Target organ atrophy does not occur after complete neural deafferentation of the MBH. The pituitaries of such animals responded to methylthiouracil treatment or to surgical stress with an increased thyrotrophic or adrenocorticotrophic hormone secretion, respectively. At the same time, however, the data have clearly indicated that the MBH is not capable of maintaining completely normal pituitary function. In animals with complete deafferentation of the MBH fresh corpora lutea (CL) were not present in the ovaries and methylthiouracil-induced goiter did not reach the weight of that of intact treated controls.

Since this study of animals with hypothalamic deafferentation was preliminary (4), extensive studies were undertaken to obtain detailed information about the functional capacity of the deafferented MBH and to find out which neural afferents to the MBH are essential for normal pituitary function. Part of these studies is presented in this paper, which summarizes the data concerning pituitary GTH secretion as measured by ovulation, ovarian compensatory hypertrophy and pituitary response to castration. These results have been presented in preliminary form (5 7), and the observations regarding other pituitary hormones will be published elsewhere.

[*Editor's Note:* Material has been omitted at this point.]

Discussion

The proposal of Sawyer, Everett and Markee (11) that ovulation in the rat is brought about by a neural triggering mechanism is now well established. It is assumed that the neural trigger operates through the MBH by releasing neurohumors, particularly LH releasing factor (LH-RF), from this hypothalamic region. The LH-RF causes the release of the ovulating burst of LH from the pituitary (12).

The present findings clearly indicate that the MBH cannot, by itself, release LH-RF in amounts necessary for ovulation. Neural afferents from other parts of the CNS, but which reach the MBH from anterior, are indispensable for ovulation.[5] This observa-

---

[5] One of the authors has proposed that anterior

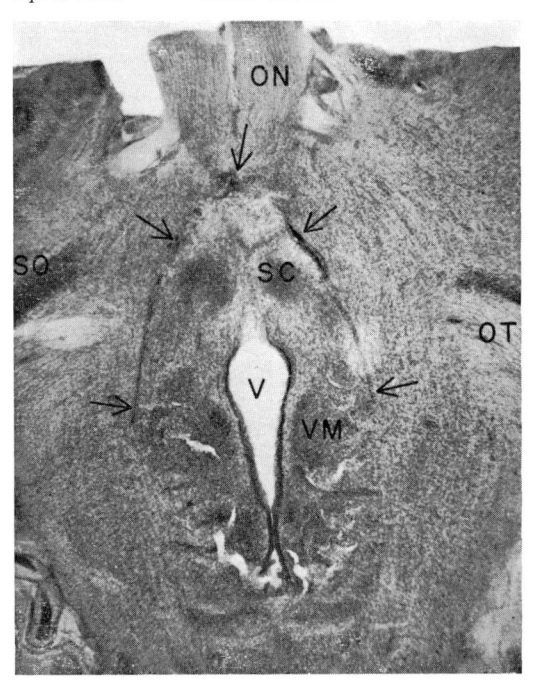

FIG. 6. Horizontal histological section which illustrates the position of the extended frontal cut which retained possible connections from the suprachiasmatic nuclei to the MBH.

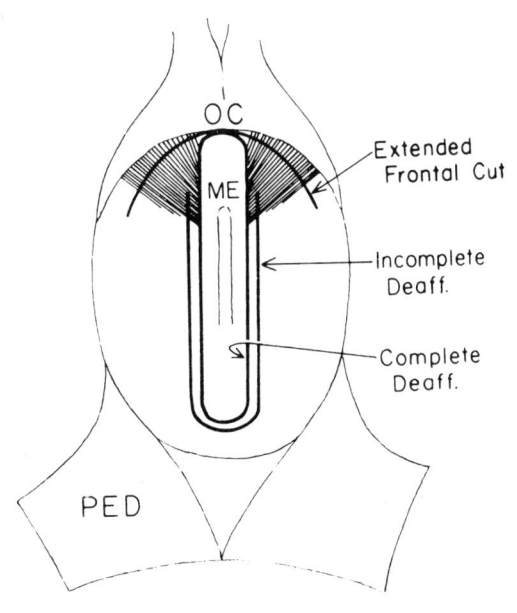

FIG. 7. Three basic types of deafferentations are superimposed on the ventral surface of the hypothalamus. Hatched region represents the area of the anterior hypothalamic nuclei which presumably plays an essential role in gonadal hormone feedback. The main part of this area was separated from the MBH by complete deafferentation, but not by incomplete deafferentation or the frontal cut.

tion is in good agreement with the findings that electrical stimulation (13, 15) or electrolytic destruction (16, and many others see 12) of the preoptic-anterior hypothalamic area induces or abolishes ovulation, respectively. Input from the mamillary peduncle, if critical for ovulation as has been proposed (17, but see 18), must reach the MBH indirectly.

The observations that (a) an extended frontal cut placed just behind the optic chiasm blocked ovulation, (b) a small frontal cut at the same rostral level inhibited "acute" but not "chronic" ovulation, (c) the same small frontal cut placed 1.5 mm behind the optic chiasm inhibited ovulation, and (d) long incomplete deafferenta-

input to the ventromedial-arcuate region of the tuberal hypothalamus is essential for ovulation (for discussion see 4). Presumably, the active components of this tuberal region are incorporated in the MBH.

tion which cut the anterolateral connections to the MBH blocked ovulation in 77% of the rats, suggest that the afferents essential for ovulation are spread over a large area superior to the optic chiasm, but converge toward the median eminence. This agrees with the observations of Hillarp (16) and the concept of Everett et al. (15) that the fibers concerned with ovulation are more widely dispersed in the septal region than near the median eminence.

With regard to the neural afferent system, two main questions arise: 1) Where are the neural afferents coming from, or where is the neural trigger for ovulation located? 2) Where do the afferent fibers end? The available data indicate that the fibers in question originate in a highly diffuse system throughout the septal complex (15). There is evidence that the preoptic-suprachiasmatic region is also profoundly involved in the timing of ovulation (see 12), but deafferentations as illustrated in Fig. 6, as well as the long incomplete deafferentation, suggest that the ScN themselves are dependent upon afferent input.

With regard to the second question, the following observations have to be considered: (a) The nerve endings around the capillary loops and in the surface zone of the median eminence belong to nerve cells of the MBH (19); (b) in rats the MBH is particularly rich in LH-RF (20); (c) only the MBH is capable of maintaining normal pituitary structure and function (including ovulation) if the pituitary is transplanted directly into the brain (1-3). Based on these findings, it can be assumed that the neural afferents in question do not terminate directly in the median eminence but end primarily on the neurons of the MBH. This assumption is in good agreement with the suggestion that at least two levels exist in the neural control of ovulation (5, 21-23). One level might be represented by the MBH, which produces the substances essential for pituitary activity. Since GTH secretion is fairly well maintained in male rats after complete deafferentation of the MBH (4), and, in contrast, the same intervention produces a blockade of ovulation without causing ovarian atrophy in the female, we can conclude that the MBH, by itself, can release the hypothalamic substances essential for pituitary GTH secretion in a tonic fashion. For a cyclic release of the hypothalamic factors (particularly LH-RF) nervous structures outside the MBH are required. These nervous elements which reach the MBH from anterior might represent the second level.

Although deafferentation of the MBH might disrupt many functions, the present interpretation that interruption of a relatively specific ovulation-regulating system has produced these results appears valid. No obvious behavioral defects were noted, and, although complete deafferentation did induce diabetes insipidus and occasionally obesity, the incomplete deafferentation, which denervated much of the MBH, was without effect. In addition, significant growth, and adrenal and thyroid function persist after deafferentation (unpublished observations).

The question whether gonadal steroids influence GTH secretion via the hypothalamus or act directly on the anterior pituitary is still unresolved, but data available at present strongly suggest that both sites are involved (for references see 12, 24). In our present studies we have found that complete deafferentation of the MBH has inhibited OCH. This finding supports the assumption that nervous elements are involved in gonadal feedback action. Since the medium incomplete deafferentation and the extended frontal cut placed just behind the optic chiasm did not interfere with OCH, we may conclude, as proposed initially by Flerkó and Szentágothai (25), that gonadal steroid sensitive nervous elements might be located in the area of the anterior hypothalamic nuclei. Apparently these structures were excluded from the deafferented region in the rats with complete deafferentation (hatched region in Fig. 7). This assumption is in good agreement with the findings that electrolytic lesions in the anterior hypothalamus interfere with OCH (10, 26-28), and estrogen inhibition of GTH secretion (29, 30).

Ovulation was blocked in the animals with the extended frontal cut, but at the same time OCH developed. A similar dissociation has been observed: OCH develops in the androgen sterilized rat (28) and anterior hypothalamic lesions which result in constant estrus do not alter OCH (31). The reports (10, 26-28) which demonstrate that anterior hypothalamic lesions prevent OCH seem to be in contradiction to the latter observation. In the light of present data we assume that the discrepancy probably is due to differences in the location of the lesions. It may be that those lesions which inhibited OCH were more posterior than those which did not. This assumption is supported by Gorski and Barraclough (28), who found that, while androgen sterilized constant estrous rats displayed marked ovarian hypertrophy following unilateral ovariectomy, there was little OCH when such rats also bore anterior hypothalamic lesions. The observations which indicate that ovulation can be blocked without inhibiting OCH suggest that there are nervous elements which are not involved in the estrogen feedback reaction following unilateral ovariectomy, but which play an essential role in the control of ovulation.

Complete deafferentation of the MBH which inhibited ovulation and OCH did not block the pituitary response to castration. Since castration changes in the pituitary are abolished when the anterior lobe is disconnected from the median eminence by heterotopic transplantation (32) or by stalk section (33), this observation suggests that the MBH is responsible for the pituitary response to castration. Although considerable evidence suggests that gonadal steroid sensitive nervous elements might be present in the MBH (34-43), perhaps the MBH simply maintained the normal structure and responsiveness of the pituitary and the castration changes occurred directly at the pituitary level. A third possibility is that the pituitary response was partly mediated by the hypothalamus and partly through the pituitary itself. This assumption is supported by the observation that implants of estradiol in either the median eminence or the anterior pituitary prevented the post-castration rise of plasma LH (41). However, implants in the median eminence also lowered hypophysial LH content. Palka et al. (43) reported that estradiol implanted into the median eminence or pituitary produced hypertrophy of the adenohypophysis. However, implants in the median eminence produced an elevation in plasma LH as well.

Although there was a pituitary response to castration in the animals with complete deafferentation, this response was below normal. The absence of a normal pituitary response in these rats is probably due to the fact that the gonadal steroid sensitive nervous structures postulated to exist in the anterior hypothalamus were excluded from the deafferented region.

Thus, two levels might exist in the system for gonadal feedback. One level might be represented by the MBH-pituitary complex and the other by the anterior hypothalamus. The assumption that the anterior hypothalamus may be more sensitive to gonadal steroids than the MBH-pituitary complex (22) is supported by our present observation that complete deafferentation of the MBH, which excluded the main part of the anterior hypothalamus from the deafferented region, blocked OCH, whereas castration changes did occur. Unilateral ovariectomy produces a less profound change in blood gonadal steroid titers than does castration.

Acknowledgments

Béla Halász would like to express his gratitude to Professor Charles H. Sawyer for the kind invitation to the Department of Anatomy and Brain Research Institute at the University of California, Los Angeles, where the present experiments were conducted, for the granting of a Ford Foundation Fellowship, and also for his interest in and discussion of this work.

The authors would like to thank B. Gibson and H. Abee for their expert technical assistance, and S. Sutherland, C. Rucker, A. Koithan, B. Bedard and S. Dorr for special services.

References

1. Halász, B., L. Pupp, and S. Uhlarik, *J Endocr* **25:** 147, 1962.
2. Halász, B., L. Pupp, S. Uhlarik, and L. Tima, *Endocrinology* **77:** 343, 1965.
3. Flament-Durand, J., *Endocrinology* **77:** 446, 1965.
4. Halász, B., and L. Pupp, *Endocrinology* **77:** 553, 1965.
5. Gorski, R. A., *J Reprod Fertil*, Suppl. **1:** 67, 1966.
6. Gorski, R. A., and B. Halász, *Fed Proc* **25:** 315, 1966 (Abstract).
7. Halász, B., and R. A. Gorski, *Excerpta Med, Inter. Cong. Series*, **111:** 194, 1966 (Abstract).
8. Gorski, R. A., and C. A. Barraclough, *Acta Endocr (Kobenhavn)* **39:** 13, 1962.
9. Parlow, A. F., *In* Albert, A. (ed.), Human Pituitary Gonadotropins, Thomas, Springfield, Ill., 1961, p. 300.
10. Critchlow, V., *In* Nalbandov, A. V. (ed.), Advances in Neuroendocrinology, University of Illinois Press, Urbana, 1963, p. 377.

11. Sawyer, C. H., J. W. Everett, and J. E. Markee, *Endocrinology* **44:** 218, 1949.
12. Everett, J. W., *Physiol Rev* **44:** 373, 1964.
13. ———, *In* Villee, C. A. (ed.), Control of Ovulation, Pergamon Press, New York, 1961, p. 101.
14. Gorski, R. A., and C. A. Barraclough, *Endocrinology* **73:** 210, 1963.
15. Everett, J. W., H. M. Radford, and J. Holsinger, *In* Martini, L., and A. Pecile (eds.), Hormonal Steroids, Academic Press, New York, 1964, vol. 1, p. 235.
16. Hillarp, N. Å., *Acta Endocr (Kobenhavn)* **2:** 11, 1949.
17. Critchlow, V., *Endocrinology* **63:** 596, 1958.
18. Pekary, A. E., and J M Davidson, *Anat Rec* **154:** 400, 1966 (Abstract).
19. Szentágothai, J., *J Progr Brain Res* **5:** 135, 1964.
20. McCann, S. M., *Amer J Physiol* **202:** 395, 1962.
21. Barraclough, C. A., and R. A. Gorski, *Endocrinology* **68:** 68, 1961.
22. Flerkó, B., *In* Szentágothai, J., B. Flerkó, B. Mess, and B. Halász (eds.), Hypothalamic Control of the Anterior Pituitary, Akadémiai Kiadó, Budapest, 1962, p. 192.
23. ———, *In* Nalbandov, A. V. (ed.), Advances in Neuroendocrinology, University of Illinois Press, Urbana, 1963, p. 211.
24. Bogdanove, E. M., *Vitamins Hormones (NY)* **22:** 205, 1964.
25. Flerkó, B., and J. Szentágothai, *Acta Endocr (Kobenhavn)* **26:** 121, 1957.
26. D'Angelo, S. A., and A. A. Kravatz, *Proc Soc Exp Biol Med* **104:** 130, 1960.
27. Flerkó, B., and V. Bárdos, *Acta Endocr (Kobenhavn)* **36:** 180, 1961.
28. Gorski, R. A., and C. A. Barraclough, *Proc Soc Exp Biol Med* **110:** 298, 1962.
29. Flerkó, B., *Endokrinologie* **34:** 210, 1957.
30. ———, *Arch Anat Micr Morph Exp* **46:** 159, 1957.
31. Desclin, L., J. Flament-Durand, and W. Gepts, *Arch Anat Micr Morph Exp* **50:** 329, 1961.
32. Hohlweg, W., and K. Junkmann, *Klin Wschr* **11:** 321, 1932.
33. Westman, A., and D. Jacobsohn, *Acta Obstet Gynec Scand* **18:** 99, 1938.
34. Lisk, R. D., *J Exp Zool* **145:** 197, 1960.
35. Davidson, J. M., and C. H. Sawyer, *Acta Endocr (Kobenhavn)* **37:** 385, 1961.
36. ———, *Proc Soc Exp Biol Med* **107:** 4, 1961.
37. Lisk, R. D., *Amer J Physiol* **203:** 493, 1962.
38. ———, *Acta Endocr (Kobenhavn)* **41:** 195, 1962.
39. Lisk, R. D., and M. Newlon, *Science* **139:** 223, 1963.
40. Kanematsu, S., and C. H. Sawyer, *Amer J Physiol* **205:** 1073, 1963.
41. Ramirez, V. D., R. M. Abrams, and S. M. McCann, *Endocrinology* **75:** 243, 1964.
42. Chowers, I., and S. M. McCann, *Endocrinology* **76:** 700, 1965.
43. Palka, Y. S., V. D. Ramirez, and C. H. Sawyer, *Endocrinology* **78:** 487, 1966.

Editor's Comments
on Papers 30 and 31

30A   MATSUO et al.
Structure of the Porcine LH- and FSH-Releasing Hormone. I. The Proposed Amino Acid Sequence

30B   BABA, MATSUO, and SCHALLY
Structure of the Porcine LH- and FSH-Releasing Hormone. II. Confirmation of the Proposed Structure by Conventional Sequential Analyses

31   BURGUS et al.
Primary Structure of the Ovine Hypothalamic Luteinizing Hormone-Releasing Factor (LRF)

The isolation and synthesis of luteinizing hormone–releasing hormone (LH-RH) was conducted independently in the laboratories of Schally and Guillemin. Matsuo et al. (Paper 30A) determined the correct amino acid sequence of porcine LH- and FSH-releasing hormone, using a combination of the Edman-dansyl procedure coupled with selective tritiation for C-terminal analysis. Additional evidence that LH-RH was a decapeptide with the structure (pyro) Glu-His-Trp-Ser-Tyr-Gly-Leu-Arg-Pro-Gly-NH$_2$ was obtained from the result of high and low resolution mass spectral fragmentation of natural porcine LH-RH.

Baba et al. (Paper 30B) confirmed the sequence of porcine LH- and FSH-releasing hormone, previously determined by Matsuo et al., using conventional degradation methods for sequential analysis involving the separation of chymotryptic and thermolytic digests after cleavage of the NH$_2$-terminal pyroglutamyl residue by pyrrolidonecarboxyl peptidase. Furthermore, they were able to synthesize the C-terminal pentapeptide amide of the proposed sequence using a solid phase synthetic procedure. The ability to synthesize LH-RH made it much easier to obtain adequate quantities for later physiological studies.

Burgus et al. (Paper 31) established the primary structure of ovine hypothalamic LH-RH to be p Glu-His-Trp-Ser-Tyr-Gly-Leu-Arg-Pro-Gly-NH$_2$ by hydrolyzing the decapeptide with chymotrypsin or pyrrolidone carboxylyl peptidase and by analysis of the products of an Edman-dansylation sequencing technique and by mass spectrophotometry. This study established that the structure of the ovine and porcine LH-RH is the same. Subsequently the structure has been found to be the same for all mammalian species.

30A

Copyright © 1971 by Academic Press, Inc.

Reprinted from *Biochem. Biophys. Res. Commun.* 43:1334-1339 (1971)

STRUCTURE OF THE PORCINE LH- AND FSH-RELEASING HORMONE. I. THE PROPOSED AMINO ACID SEQUENCE

H. Matsuo, Y. Baba, R.M.G. Nair, A. Arimura and A.V. Schally[1]

V.A. Hospital and Tulane University School of Medicine, New Orleans, La.

Summary. The complete amino acid sequence of porcine LH- and FSH- releasing hormone has been provisionally determined by the use on a micro-scale of the combined Edman-dansyl procedure coupled with the selective tritiation method for C-terminal analysis. These procedures were used directly on the digestion products of LH-RH with chymotrypsin and thermolysin, without separation of the fragments. Additional data were provided by high resolution mass spectral fragmentation of LH-RH. On the basis of these results, we propose the following decapeptide sequence for LH-RH: (pyro)Glu-His-Trp-Ser-Tyr-Gly-Leu-Arg-Pro-Gly-NH$_2$.

The hypothalamus regulates the release of luteinizing hormone (LH) and follicle-stimulating hormone (FSH) from the anterior pituitary gland by means of neurohumoral substance(s) designated LH-releasing hormone (LH-RH) and FSH-releasing hormone (FSH-RH) (1). Recently, we reported the isolation from porcine hypothalamic extracts of a polypeptide which has both LH-RH and FSH-RH activity (2, 3). FSH-RH activity could not be separated from LH-RH after 12 purification steps or by application of additional separation methods (2, 3). This paper describes the elucidation of the structure of porcine LH-RH/FSH-RH. Because of very limited amounts of material available for this structural work (less than 200 nmoles) and the blocked N-terminus as well as the C-terminus, many conventional methods for the sequential analyses of polypeptides were not applicable. After proteolytic digestion of LH-RH, the resulting reaction mixture, consisting of peptide-fragments along with the enzymes used, was submitted directly to terminal and sequential analyses. At each step, 1-5 μg amounts were analyzed by the selective tritiation method for the C-terminal analyses (4, 5) and Edman-dansyl degradation (6). Such a structural approach made it difficult to draw unambiguous conclusions about the structure. However, only one structure, (pyro)Glu-His-Trp-Ser-Tyr-Gly-Leu-Arg-Pro-Gly-NH$_2$ was consistent with the accumulated structural data.

MATERIALS AND METHODS

LH-RH/FSH-RH used in this work was isolated from pig hypothalami as described by Schally *et al.* (3). Analysis of Trp was performed after alkaline hydrolysis as well as after HCl hydrolysis in the presence of thioglycolic acid (7). Oxidation of LH-RH was carried out with performic acid (8).

---
[1] Supported by grants from V.A., USPHS AM-07467, and Population Council, New York, N.Y. to AVS.

Proteolytic digestion of LH-RH: LH-RH (5-20 nmole portions) was digested with chymotrypsin (Worthington, 2 x recryst. lot TRL 6259) or thermolysin (Calbiochem, 3 x recryst. lot 900382) in 10-50 μl of 0.1 M ammonium acetate buffer, pH 8.1 at 37° C for 16-19 hr. The S:E ratio was 20:1 in both cases. Thermolytic digestion was carried out in the presence of 0.001 M $MgCl_2$. After lyophilization, an aliquot representing one-fifth of the total was directly submitted to C-terminal analysis, while the remainder was analyzed by Edman-dansyl degradation. In both cases, control experiments were carried out under exactly the same conditions, except that LH-RH was omitted.

Sequence analyses: N-terminal residues of peptides were determined by the dansyl (DNS) method of Gray (6) with some modifications: generally 1 nmole of a peptide was treated with 2 μl of 0.25% DNS-chloride in acetone and 2 μl of 0.1 M $NaHCO_3$ in a small glass tube provided with a capillary (1-2 mm in diameter at the bottom). When arginine was expected as the N-terminal amino acids, 5-10 nmoles of peptide were dansylated to permit identification by TLC on silica gel. Dansylated peptides were hydrolyzed at 110° C in constant boiling HCl in sealed evacuated tubes. The time of hydrolysis was 16 hr. except that for the dansyl proline which was 3 hr. For DNS-Trp the conditions suggested by Matsubara and Sasaki (7) were utilized. DNS-amino acids were identified by TLC polyamide sheets (9) (Cheng Chin Trading Co.). DNS-Arg was further confirmed by TLC on silica gel (10). The Edman degradation was performed by scaling down a procedure proposed by Hartley (11). The N-terminal groups formed were identified by dansylation.

C-terminal analyses of thermolysin and chymotrypsin digests and their control samples were performed by a selective tritiation method recently improved by Matsuo and Narita (5), except that the specific activity of ^3H_2O used was 5 Ci/ml (Method A). The sample was dissolved in a mixture of pyridine (10 μl) and ^3H_2O (5 μl) and to this solution acetic anhydride (10 μl) was added. The mixture was kept at 0° C for 5 min and then at 20° C for 15 min. After another addition of pyridine (20 ul) and acetic anhydride (20 μl), the reaction mixture remained at 20° C for 1 hr, after which ^3H_2O (5 μl) was again added and it was left at 20° C for another hr. The resulting solution was then worked up in the same manner as previously described (4, 5). Acid hydrolyses of tritiated peptides were carried out in the presence of thioglycolic acid (7). After the addition of 0.1 umole of each constituent amino acid as a radioisotope-carrier to the hydrolysates, the separation of tritiated C-terminal amino acid was made on Whatman No. 1 filter paper by a combination of electrophoresis (2000 V for 1 hr), in 1 M formic acid (pH 1.8) and pyridine acetate buffer (pH 6.4), and paper chromatography (pyridine:acetone: NH_4OH: water = 50:20:5:50). The radioactivity was counted in a PPO-toluene mixture in a Tricarb liquid-scintillation counter.

Tritiation of LH-RH with $Ac_2O-^3H_2O$ (Method B) was carried out essentially as described for the tritiation of C-terminal proline (4, 12). LH-RH was heated at $60°$ C for 3 hrs. in a solution of acetic anhydride (40 μl) and ^3H_2O (5 ul). It was then worked up in the same way as in Method A.

High and low resolution mass spectra of natural LH-RH were obtained at $250-260°$ C in an AEI MS-9 mass spectrometer equipped with a PDP-8 computer and data reduction system MSDS-II.

RESULTS AND DISCUSSION

The amino acid composition of LH-RH was previously reported on the basis of a sample hydrolyzed with 6 N HCl (3). In addition, one Trp residue was detected by alkaline hydrolysis and by the method of Matsubara and Sasaki (7). The complete amino acid composition of LH-RH was then: Trp 1, His 1, Arg 1, Ser 1, Glu 1, Pro 1, Gly 2, Leu 1 and Tyr 1. When LH-RH was subjected to the Edman-dansyl procedure, the results showed that the amino-terminal group was blocked. High resolution mass spectral fragmentation pattern of LH-RH exhibited intense peaks at 83.0869 and 84.0936 mass units (pyrrolidone) , and 111.1181 and 112.1248 mass units [(pyro)Glu] , findings which supported the presence of pyro glutamyl residue at its N-terminus. C-Terminal tritiation of LH-RH by Method A gave no radioactive amino acid. Proline in LH-RH was not tritiated even by Method B, which would tritiate a C-terminal proline. Consequently, it was concluded that the C-terminal carboxyl group in LH-RH must be blocked. The lack of a free carboxyl terminus and the presence of pyroglutamyl residue at its N-terminus were also supported by the inactivation experiments of LH-RH previously reported (2, 3).

Sequence studies on LH-RH after digestion with chymotrypsin and thermolysin are summarized in Tables 1 and 2. Although in this case it was more difficult to draw unambiguous conclusions on the structure as compared with standard sequence analyses, only the structure proposed in Tables 1 and 2 was revealed to be consistent with the data obtained. LH-RH was cleaved at two sites by the chymotryptic digestion, as well as at three sites by the thermolytic digestion, as shown by the C-terminal analyses. The Edman degradation patterns were relatively simple, because the fragments with (pyro)Glu at their N-termini did not undergo degradation. The sequence Trp-Ser-Tyr-Gly-Leu was deduced from the data shown in Table 1. At the 3rd step of Edman degradation, Gly was detected, but Ser was not. Consequently, possibilities other than Trp-Ser-Tyr-Gly-Leu were excluded. For additional confirmation, N-terminal analyses was carried out on the chymotryptic digest of LH-RH, in which the Trp residue was oxidized by performic acid treatment. Only Gly was then detected as the main spot, while the Ser spot was minor. This confirmed the sequence mentioned above. As it can be seen in Table 2, the amounts of Tyr and

Table 1

SUMMARY OF THE SEQUENCE STUDIES AFTER DIGESTION OF LH-RH WITH CHYMOTRYPSIN

(pyro)Glu - His - Trp ↓ Ser - Tyr ↓ Gly - Leu - Arg - Pro - Gly - NH$_2$

Ch-1 ←→
Ch-2 ←→
Ch-3 ←→
Ch-4 ←→
Ch-5 ←→

Observed C-Terminal	Edman Degradation										
	Observed Results				Possible Pattern						
	1	2	3		1	2	3	4	5	6	7
				Ch-1	---	---	---				
Trp	Ser	Tyr	Gly	Ch-2	Ser	Tyr					
Tyr	Gly	Leu	Arg*	Ch-3	Gly	Leu	Arg	Pro	Gly		
				Ch-4	---	---	---	---	---		
				Ch-5	Ser	Tyr	Gly	Leu	Arg	Pro	Gly

*DNS-amino acid spot with weak fluorescence.

Leu which appeared at the 3rd step of degradation were minute as compared with that of Pro. This suggested that fragments Th-7, 8 and 9 must be minor and that Th-4 was the main component. Consequently, Gly detected at the 4th step, had to be derived from Th-4, which must be the C-terminal peptide. On the basis of these data, it was concluded that the structure of LH-RH is (pyro)Glu-His-Trp-Ser-Tyr-Gly-Leu-Arg-Pro-Gly-X. However, it must be admitted that the evidence for the linkage (pyro)Glu-His is not very strong. Similarly, the mode of blocking at C-terminal Gly still remains to be solved. The following information might be suggestive for the presence of glycine amide group at the C-terminus. When LH-RH was heated at 60° C for 3 hrs in the presence of acetic anhydride and ^{3}H$_2$O (Method B), glycine was tritiated, although the resulting radioactivity was low. This tritium incorporation into glycine suggests a new type of reaction not reported previously (4, 5, 12). Similar C-terminal tritiation was also observed in the case of both

Table 2

SUMMARY OF THE SEQUENCE STUDIES AFTER DIGESTION OF LH-RH WITH THERMOLYSIN

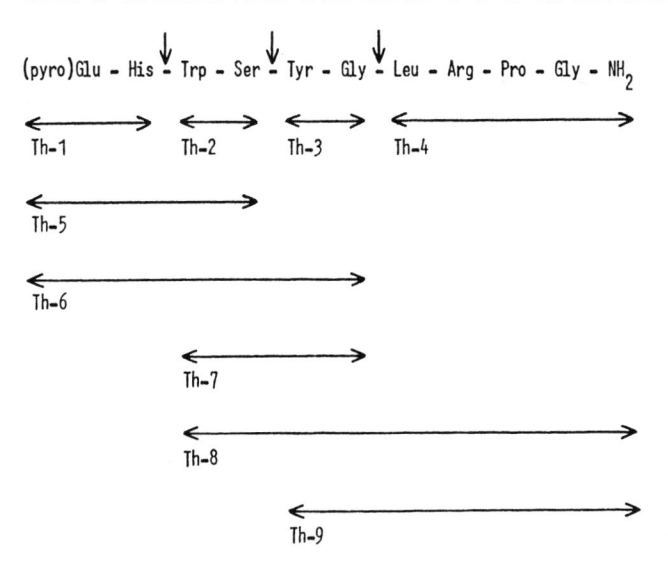

(pyro)Glu - His ↓ Trp - Ser ↓ Tyr - Gly ↓ Leu - Arg - Pro - Gly - NH$_2$

  ←——→ ←——→ ←——→ ←————————→
   Th-1   Th-2   Th-3   Th-4

  ←—————————→
    Th-5

  ←————————————————→
    Th-6

      ←——————————→
       Th-7

      ←——————————————————→
       Th-8

         ←——————————————→
          Th-9

Observed C-Terminal	Observed Results					Possible Pattern							
	1	2	3	4		1	2	3	4	5	6	7	8
					Th-1	---	---						
					Th-2	Trp	Ser						
His	Trp	Ser	Pro	Gly	Th-3	Tyr	Gly						
					Th-4	Leu	Arg	Pro	Gly				
Ser	Tyr	Gly	Tyr*		Th-5	---	---	---	---				
					Th-6	---	---	---	---	---	---		
Gly	Leu	Arg	Leu*		Th-7	Trp	Ser	Tyr	Gly				
					Th-8	Trp	Ser	Tyr	Gly	Leu	Arg	Pro	Gly
					Th-9	Tyr	Gly	Leu	Arg	Pro	Gly		

* DNS-amino acid spots with weak fluorescence.

Lysine-vasopressin and α-MSH, whose C-terminal groups are GlyNH$_2$ and ValNH$_2$, respectively. Thus, LH-RH probably has an amide group at the C-terminus. Although the strategy utilized in the present structural work on LH-RH led to only one possible amino acid sequence, this approach may not always be conclusive.

Synthesis of the proposed amino acid sequence of LH-RH which will be published separately, would verify the proposed structure. Preliminary results showed that the synthetic product has high degree of LH-RH activity.

ACKNOWLEDGMENTS

We are grateful to Dr. E. Daignaut, L.S.U. Medical School, New Orleans, La. for using his facilities for the tritiation experiments. We also wish to thank Professor Ralph C. Dougherty for permitting the use of the M.S. Center at Florida State University, Tallahasse, Fla.

REFERENCES

1. Schally, A.V., Arimura, A., Bowers, C.Y., Kastin, A.J., Sawano, S., and Redding, T.W.: Recent Progress in Hormone Research 24: 497, 1968.
2. Schally, A.V., Baba, Y., Arimura, A., Redding, T.W. and White, W.F.: Biochem. Biophys. Res. Commun. 42: 50, 1971.
3. Schally, A.V., Arimura, A., Baba, Y., Nair, R.M.G., Matsuo, H., Redding, T.W. and Debeljuk, L. Biochem. Biophys. Res. Commun. 43: 393, 1971.
4. Matsuo, H., Fujimoto, Y., and Tatsuno, T.: Biochem. Biophys. Res. Commun. 22: 69, 1966.
5. Matsuo, H. and Narita, K.: Abstr. of Symposium on Protein Structure (Japan) 1970, 45.
6. Gray, W.R.: "Method in Enzymology" vol. XI p. 139, Academic Press, 1967.
7. Matsubara, H. and Sasaki, R.: Biochem. Biophys. Res. Commun. 35: 175, 1969.
8. Hirs, C.H.W.: in "Method in Enzymology" vol. XI, p. 197, Academic Press, 1967.
9. Wood, K.R. and Wang, K.T.: Biochem. Biophys. Acta. 133: 369, 1969.
10. Gross, C. and Labouesse, B.: Europ. J. Biochem. 7: 463, 1969.
11. Hartley, B.S.: Biochem. J. 119: 805, 1970.
12. Matsuo, H., Fujimoto, Y., Kobayashi, H., Tatsuno, T. and Matsubara, H.: Chem. Pharm. Bull. (Japan) 18: 890, 1970.

30B

Copyright © 1971 by Academic Press, Inc.

Reprinted from *Biochem. Biophys. Res. Commun.* 44:459-463 (1971)

STRUCTURE OF THE PORCINE LH- AND FSH-RELEASING HORMONE. II. CONFIRMATION OF THE PROPOSED STRUCTURE BY CONVENTIONAL SEQUENTIAL ANALYSES.*

Yoshihiko Baba, Hisayuki Matsuo and Andrew V. Schally.

VA Hospital and Tulane University School of Medicine, New Orleans, La.

Summary. The proposed amino acid sequence of porcine LH- and FSH-releasing hormone (LH-RH/FSH-RH) was reinvestigated by Edman-dansyl degradation after the cleavage of N-terminal pyroglutamyl residue by pyrrolidonecarboxylyl (PCA) peptidase. A C-terminal fragment from chymotryptic digest of LH-RH/FSH-RH was found to be identical to synthetic Gly-Leu-Arg-Pro-Gly-NH$_2$. The results indicate that the structure initially proposed is correct. The amino acid sequence of porcine LH-RH/FSH-RH is thus (pyro)Glu-His-Trp-Ser-Tyr-Gly-Leu-Arg-Pro-Gly-NH$_2$.

In a previous communication (1) we proposed (pyro)Glu-His-Trp-Ser-Tyr-Gly-Leu-Arg-Pro-Gly-NH$_2$ as the amino acid sequence of LH and FSH releasing hormone (LH-RH/FSH-RH) isolated from porcine hypothalami. This structure was based mainly on the results of Edman-dansyl degradation and selective tritiation of the C-terminus which were applied directly to the chymotryptic and thermolytic digests of this hormonal polypeptide. A limited amount of the pure material (about 200 nmoles) and the blocked N-terminus as well as the C-terminus forced us to use this unconventional approach. After using less than half of the material, we were able nevertheless, to narrow down the possibilities to only one amino acid sequence. We tried to confirm this proposed amino acid sequence in two ways: (1) by conventional degradation methods for sequential analyses on the remainder of the pure natural material, (2) by the synthesis of the proposed structure. This report describes the results obtained following our first approach.

---

* Supported by grants from VA, USPHS grant AM-07467 and Population Council, New York, N.Y. to AVS.

MATERIALS AND METHODS

LH-RH/FSH-RH used in this study was isolated from pig hypothalami as described by Schally et al. (2).

Edman-Dansyl Degradation: Edman-dansyl degradation was performed as described in our previous communication (1). Polyamide sheets were used for the identification of DNS-amino acids. For DNS-histidine and DNS-arginine silica gel plates were also used and the developing solvent system consisted of benzene-2-chloroethanol-28% ammonia (8:10: 4). This modification of the solvent II described by Gross and Labouesse (3) was found to separate better these two basic amino acids.

PCA peptidase Digestion: Pyrrolidone carboxylyl (PCA) peptidase (4) (G-200 and A-25 preparations) was supplied by Dr. R.F. Doolittle. Generally, the enzyme preparations, precipitated by ammonium sulfate containing pyrrolidone as a stabilizer, were dialyzed twice against 0.05 M phosphate buffer pH 7.3, in presence of 0.01 M mercaptoethanol and 0.001 M EDTA just before use. The concentration of the enzyme was estimated by absorption at 280 mµ (4). Three digestions were made using this enzyme.

Digestion I. LH-RH/FSH-RH (3 nmoles) was digested by G-200 preparation of the enzyme at 30° C for 17 hours in 5 µl of the same buffer as used for the dialysis. The optical density (O.D.) of the enzyme in the reaction medium was 0.29 at 280 mµ. A control without LH-RH/FSH-RH was run simultaneously. After the digestion, the solution was evaporated and the residue was dansylated directly.

Digestion II. LH-RH/FSH-RH (6 nmoles) was digested in 10 µl buffer by A-25 preparation as in digestion I. The O.D. of the enzyme was 0.28 at 280 mµ.

Digestion III. LH-RH/FSH-RH (30 nmoles) was digested in 10 µl buffer by A-25 preparation (the same lot No. as used in Digestion II). The initial O.D. of the enzyme was 0.20 at 280 mµ. Further additions of 1 µl of the enzyme solution (OD_{280} = 1.00) were made after two and after four hours. The final volume of the reaction mixture was 12 µl, and the O.D. of the enzyme was found to be 0.33 at 280 mµ.

Synthesis of Gly-Leu-Arg-Pro-Gly-NH$_2$: Solid phase synthesis of the C-terminal pentapeptide amide of the proposed sequence was carried out by the procedure described by Stewart and Young (5). t-BOC-amino acids, and t-BOC- glycine resin ester were obtained from Mann Research Lab. For the removal of the solid support and the protecting groups, ammonolysis by methanol saturated with ammonia, followed by the catalytic reduction over palladium on charcoal and the treatment with trifluoroacetic acid in dichloromethane were employed. The resulting peptide was repurified by preparative TLC on cellulose. After hydrolysis, the amino acid ratios of this preparation were found to be: Pro 0.82, Gly 2.00, Leu 1.14, Arg 1.01.

Separation of Chymotryptic Fragments of LH-RH/FSH-RH: LH-RH/FSH-RH (80 nmoles) was digested by chymotrypsin (Worthington, 2 x recryst lot TRL 6259) in 200 µl of 0.1 M ammonium acetate buffer, pH 8.1 at 37° C for 16 hours. The E:S ratio was 1:20. After evaporation of the buffer, the resulting peptide fragments were separated by TLC on cellulose MN 300 HR, previously washed by the method of Haworth and Heathcote (6). The solvent system was 1-butanol-acetic acid-water (4:1:1). The sample was applied on half of the plate and the other half was used as a control, to subtract the amino acids contamination in cellulose. The guide regions were visualized by spraying with chlorine-tolidine reagent and the unsprayed bands were eluted by 0.2 N acetic acid. Amino acid analysis was performed as described previously (2).

RESULTS AND DISCUSSION

The N-terminal pyroglutamyl group of LH-RH/FSH-RH, proved by mass spectra (1, 2), was consistent with the failure to detect a free N-terminus by dansylation (2) as well as with the lack of inactivation by aminopeptidases (2). Except for the pyroglutamyl residue, no other glutamic acid or glutamine are present in this polypeptide. This indicated that LH-RH/FSH-RH was suitable for the application of Edman-dansyl degradation, if only the pyroglutamyl group could be removed, or if its pyrrolidone ring was opened. Attempts to use alkaline hydrolysis to open the pyrrolidone ring gave undesirable results. PCA peptidase was then tried for this purpose. The G-200 preparation of the enzyme was found unsatisfactory (Digestion I), because of the probable contamination with endopeptidases. Dansylation of the enzyme digest showed at least four new N-termini: Gly, Leu, Tyr, and His and/or Ser. However, only DNS-histidine was detected when a more purified A-25 preparation was used (Digestion II). This confirmed the (pyro)Glu-His linkage, previously unproven. This result suggested that the digestion of LH-RH/FSH-RH by A-25 enzyme followed by Edman-dansyl degradation would be successful. A larger amount of LH-RH/FSH-RH (30 nmoles) was then digested (Digestion III) under slightly different conditions from that of Digestion II. The volume of the reaction medium was reduced because the presence of large amounts of inorganic salts would disturb the identification of DNS-amino acids on polyamide layer, and particularly, of DNS-serine, DNS-arginine and DNS-histidine. On N-terminal analysis of the enzyme digest, DNS-histidine appeared as the major spot together with some DNS-serine. When Edman-dansyl degradation was continued up to ninth step, the amino acid sequence His-Trp-Ser-Tyr-Gly-Leu-Arg-Pro-Gly was confirmed clearly. At the attempted tenth step no DNS-amino acids were detected, other than a very faint spot of DNS-glycine. At the second, the third and the fourth steps, faint spots of DNS-tyrosine, DNS-glycine and DNS-leucine respectively were found in agreement with the unexpected cleavage of Trp-Ser linkage. Thus, the A-25 preparation of PCA peptidase proved to be useful for the sequential study on a micro scale of peptide whose N-terminus is pyroglutamic acid. However, more purified preparation of the enzyme to eliminate contaminating endopeptidase would have been preferable.

An attempt was also made to get further confirmation of the C-terminal amide group. After the digestion of LH-RH/FSH-RH by chymotrypsin, a fragment corresponding to synthetic Gly-Leu-Arg-Pro-Gly-NH$_2$ on TLC was found and eluted. The spot given by this fragment was strong and well separated and its mobility was exactly the same as that of the synthetic peptide. The amino acid ratios of this fragment were: Pro 1.21, Gly 2.20, Leu 1.00, Arg 0.94.

These results are in good agreement with the proposed amino acid sequence of porcine LH-RH/FSH-RH (1). The amino acid sequence of this decapeptide which stimulates the release of both LH and FSH from the pituitary is (pyro)Glu-His-Trp-Ser-Tyr-Gly-Leu-Arg-Pro-Gly (NH$_2$). The linkage Arg-Pro explains the lack of inactivation by trypsin (7). No acidic function was found in this polypeptide, nor in the other two hypothalamic hormones whose structures have been elucidated so far (thyrotropin-releasing hormone (8) and melanocyte-stimulating hormone-inhibiting hormone (9)). The synthesis of the amino acid sequence corresponding to LH-RH/FSH-RH will be reported shortly.

ACKNOWLEDGMENTS

We are grateful to Dr. R.F. Doolittle, University of California, San Diego, for generous gifts of PCA-peptidase and useful suggestions. We wish to thank Dr. C. Huggins, Tulane University School of Medicine, for the use of his synthetic facilities.

REFERENCES

1. Matsuo, H., Baba, Y., Nair, R.M.G., Arimura, A., and Schally, A.V.: Biochem. Biophys. Res. Commun. 43: #6, June 18, 1971.
2. Schally, A.V., Arimura, A., Baba, Y., Nair, R.M.G., Matsuo, H., Redding, T.W., and Debeljuk, L.: Biochem. Biophys. Res. Commun. 43: 393, 1971.
3. Gross, C., and Labouesse, B.: Europ. J. Biochem. 7: 463, 1969.
4. Doolittle, R.F. and Armentrout, R.W.: Biochemistry 7: 516, 1968.
5. Stewart, J.M. and Young, J.D., "Solid Phase Peptide Synthesis", W.H. Freeman, San Francisco, 1969.
6. Haworth, C. and Heathcote, J.G.: J. Chromatog. 41: 380, 1969.
7. Schally, A.V., Baba, Y., Arimura, A., Redding, T.W. and White, W.F.: Biochem. Biophys. Res. Commun. 42: 50, 1971.
8. Nair, R.M.G., Barrett, J.F., Bowers, C.Y. and Schally, A.V.: Biochemistry 9: 1103, 1970.
9. Nair, R.M.G., Kastin, A.J. and Schally, A.V.: Biochem. Biophys. Res. Commun. 43: June, 1971.

31

Reprinted from *Natl. Acad. Sci. Proc.* 69:278-282 (1972)

Primary Structure of the Ovine Hypothalamic Luteinizing Hormone-Releasing Factor (LRF)

(LH/hypothalamus/LRF/gas chromatography–mass spectrometry/decapeptide/Edman degradation)

ROGER BURGUS, MADALYN BUTCHER, MAX AMOSS, NICHOLAS LING, MICHAEL MONAHAN, JEAN RIVIER, ROBERT FELLOWS*, RICHARD BLACKWELL, WYLIE VALE, AND ROGER GUILLEMIN

The Salk Institute, La Jolla, California 92037; and *Department of Physiology, Duke University Medical Center, Durham, North Carolina 27706

Communicated by Robert W. Holley, November 5, 1971

ABSTRACT The primary structure of ovine hypothalamic hypophysiotropic luteinizing hormone-releasing factor, LRF, has been established as pGlu-His-Trp-Ser-Tyr-Gly-Leu-Arg-Pro-Gly-NH$_2$ by hydrolysis of the peptide with chymotrypsin or pyrrolidone-carboxylylpeptidase and by analysis of the products by an Edman-dansylation sequencing technique, as well as by mass spectrometry of the derived phenylthiohydantoins. A decapeptide with the proposed primary structure, prepared by total synthesis, gave the same result on sequencing. The synthetic decapeptide possesses the same biological activities as the native ovine LRF. The amino-acid sequence of ovine LRF is identical to that already published for porcine LRF.

Various areas of the central nervous system participate in the fine regulation of the secretion of all adenohypophysial hormones. The ultimate integrator of information originating in the central nervous system is the hypothalamus. The final information from the hypothalamus to the adenohypophysis is not transmitted in the form of nerve impulses, but is carried in the form of specific hypothalamic hypophysiotropic substances, the hypothalamic releasing factors, that are carried through the hypothalamo-hypophysial portal system of capillaries from the median eminence region of the ventral hypothalamus to the cells of the adenohypophysis. There is good physiological evidence that such a hypothalamic control is involved in the secretion of the gonadotropin, luteinizing hormone. In the early 1960s, several investigators reported experimental results that were best explained by proposing the existence of substances that specifically stimulated the secretion of luteinizing hormone, and that were probably polypeptides, in crude aqueous extracts of hypothalamic tissues of various mammalian species (1–3). Preparations of LRF, active at 1 μg per dose in animal bioassays, were obtained by gel filtration and ion-exchange chromatography on carboxymethylcellulose (4), an observation that was confirmed by similar methods by several investigators (5, 6). In spite of the vagaries of the various bioassay methods available, several laboratories reported preparations of LRF of increased potency (5, 6). Several of these early publications led to contradictory statements regarding purification and separation of LH-releasing factor (LRF), from a follicle-stimulating hormone releasing factor (5, 7). Two laboratories independently reported the isolation of porcine LRF (8) and ovine LRF (9), both groups concluding that LRF from either species was a nonapeptide containing, on the basis of acid hydrolysis, 1 His, 1 Arg, 1 Ser, 1 Glu, 1 Pro, 2 Gly, 1 Leu, 1 Tyr. Earlier results with the pyrrolidone-carboxylylpeptidase prepared by Fellows and Mudge (10) had led us to conclude (11) that the N-terminal residue of LRF was Glu in its cyclized pyroglutamic (pGlu) form, as in the case of hypothalamic TRF, (pGlu-His-Pro-NH$_2$).

While our own studies on the amino-acid sequence of ovine LRF were in progress, Matsuo *et al.* (12) reported that porcine LRF contained one residue of tryptophan (Trp), in addition to the other amino acids earlier observed by acid hydrolysis. On the basis of a series of elegant experiments, including enzymatic hydrolysis with chymotrypsin and thermolysin and analysis of the partial sequences of their decapeptide by Edman degradation-dansylation and selective tritiation of C-termini, Matsuo *et al.* proposed the sequence pGlu-His-Trp-Ser-Tyr-Gly-Leu-Arg-Pro-Gly-NH$_2$ for porcine LRF, a sequence that was confirmed by the same group using Edman degradation of a preparation of porcine LRF treated with a pyrrolidone-carboxylylpeptidase (13). Their studies were carried out with less than 200 nmol of peptide. They also stated that synthesis of that particular sequence gave a material with biological activity. We then reported synthesis by solid-phase methods of the decapeptide pGlu-His-Trp-Ser-Tyr-Gly-Leu-Arg-Pro-Gly-NH$_2$, which after isolation from the reaction mixture had the biological activity *in vivo* and *in vitro* of ovine LRF (14).

In this publication, we report the amino-acid sequence of ovine LRF obtained by analysis of hydrolysis products of LRF after digestion with chymotrypsin or pyrrolidone-carboxylylpeptidase, using Edman-degradation followed by determination of N- and C-termini by a quantitative dansylation technique. Confirmation of the positions of some of the amino-acid residues obtained by combined gas chromatographic–mass spectrometric analysis of phenylthiohydantoin (PTH) derivatives (15, 16) resulting from Edman degradations will also be described. We also report results obtained by degradation of synthetic LRF, since they confirm and clarify some peculiarities observed upon enzymatic cleavage of the native peptide.

A preliminary note describing these conclusions was published (17).

Abbreviations: LRF, luteinizing hormone releasing factor; Dns-, dimethylaminonaphthalene-5-sulfonyl-, (dansyl-); PTH, phenylthiohydantoin.

186

MATERIALS AND METHODS

The total amount of ovine LRF available for these studies was about 40 μg, or 30 nmol of peptide (measured by quantitative dansylation as described below); it was prepared as described by Amoss *et al.* (9) and represents about half of the total LRF yield from side fractions reserved from the early stages of the TRF isolation (18) from about 300,000 sheep hypothalamic fragments; the other half of the LRF fraction was used for the studies reported in ref 9.

Pure synthetic LRF decapeptide was prepared by solid-phase methods on a benzhydrylamine resin (14); the synthetic preparation had the biological activity *in vivo* and *in vitro* of ovine LRF.

Chymotrypsin A was 3× crystallized (Worthington, Lot CDI 8HD). Pyrrolidone-carboxylylpeptidase was obtained as described by Fellows and Mudge (10). Reagents used were reagent grade or analytical grade, some being further purified as described in the text.

Dansylation. Dansylation (19) of amino acids and peptides was conducted using [^{14}C]Dns-Cl (19–21). The sample, 50–100 pmol of hydrolyzate for direct amino-acid determination, 1–1.5 nmol for N-terminal analysis of peptides, was incubated at 37°C for 1 hr with 10 μl of 50 mM aqueous NaHCO$_3$ buffer (pH 9.3) and 10 μl of 7.7 nmol/μl of [^{14}C]Dns-Cl (45 Ci/mol Schwartz) in acetone.

Hydrolysis. Peptides were hydrolyzed in 6 × 50 mm Pyrex ignition tubes with 50 μl of triple-distilled 6 N HCl containing 0.5% thioglycolic acid (22). Tube contents were degassed by freezing and thawing at 50–100 μm (of Hg) pressure, and the sealed tubes were then incubated for 20–24 hr at 110°C. The same hydrolysis procedure was used for dansylated peptides, except that the hydrolysis time was reduced to 7.5 hr. When Dns-Pro was expected, hydrolysis was for 5 hr. Hydrolyzates were concentrated to dryness at 5–10 μm (of Hg) over NaOH.

Separation of Dns-Amino Acids. [^{14}C]Dns-amino acids were separated by two-dimensional thin-layer chromatography on 15 × 15 cm polyamide-coated sheets (Gallard Schlesinger) (23). The solvent for the first dimension was water–90% formic acid 200:3, and for the second dimension, benzene–glacial acetic acid 9:1. To further separate Dns-His, Dns-Arg, and Dns-Ser from each other and from other radioactive zones due to excess reagent, additional chromatography on the same sheet was conducted with chloroform–ethanol–glacial acetic acid 114:12:9 or *n*-heptane–*n*-butyl alcohol–glacial acetic acid 3:3:1.

Fluorescent zones were cut from the chromatogram and their radioactivity was determined in 10 ml of scintillation fluid (Beckman BBS3 scintillation-cocktail) with a Beckman LS 233 Liquid Scintillation Counter. In these experiments, only those zones corresponding to products of the amino acids present in significant quantities in hydrolyzates of LRF, i.e., Glu, His, Trp, Ser, Tyr (as *di*-Dns-Tyr), Gly Leu, Arg, Pro, and GlyNH$_2$, were counted. Dns-NH$_2$ and O-Dns-Tyr were not routinely counted. Determination of [^{14}C]Dns-Pro and [^{14}C]Dns-Leu obtained by dansylation of Leu and Pro in hydrolyzates or standard mixtures of free amino acids gave an average of 28 ± 5 cpm/pmol for five determinations each.

Hydrazinolysis. Determination of C-Termini. C-terminal determination of peptides was by hydrazinolysis without deamidation, by a modification of the method of Mesrob and Hollyeyšovský (24). Aliquots of 1–1.5 nmol of peptide were treated at 110°C for 6 hr with 50 μl of anhydrous hydrazine (Matheson, Coleman and Bell) in 10 × 75 mm heavy-walled Pyrex ignition tubes sealed at 50–100 μm (of Hg), while the tubes were immersed in liquid nitrogen. The hydrazine was removed under reduced pressure over sulfuric acid, and the residues were dissolved in 30 μl of deionized water and 30 μl of benzaldehyde [Matheson, Coleman and Bell, washed with aqueous NaOH, dried over CaCl$_2$, and redistilled at 35°C, 1 mm (of Hg)]. The tubes were covered with paraffin film and, after the mixtures were allowed to stand for 15 min with occasional agitation on a vortex mixer, the benzaldehyde phase was drawn off with a 100-μl microsyringe. The process was repeated three times. The benzaldehyde phase was discarded, and the remaining (C-terminal) amino acids in the aqueous phase were determined by dansylation. The benzaldehyde extraction step was omitted for the determination of Trp C-termini in separate aliquots of sample.

Edman Degradation. Sequential degradation of peptides was by the method of Edman (25), as modified by Gray (19), in which the peptide is converted to the *N*-phenylthiocarbamyl derivative by treatment with phenylisothiocyanate in aqueous pyridine, and the N-terminal amino acid is cleaved from the rest of the peptide as the 5-thiazolinone by treatment with anhydrous trifluoroacetic acid. The thiazolinone is extracted from the aqueous solution by butyl acetate. Reagents and procedures used in these experiments were exactly as described (19), except that 50 μl/liter of ethanedithiol was included in the butyl acetate to help preserve the Trp and Ser derivatives for subsequent mass spectrometric analysis of PTH derivatives. Test tubes with Teflon-lined screw caps were used to avoid interference by paraffin film with mass-spectrometric examinations. N-terminal determinations by dansylation were done on aliquots of the aqueous phase.

Mass Spectrometry. Combination gas chromatography–mass spectrometry was used to confirm the identity of some of the residues in the peptide sequences. The butyl acetate phase from each Edman cycle was concentrated to dryness under reduced pressure on a rotary evaporator, treated with 300 μl of 1 N HCl (1 μl/ml ethanedithiol) for 1 hr at 80°C to convert the thiazolinones to the PTH derivatives, concentrated to dryness, and treated for 1 min at 80°C with 50 μl of *N,O*-bis-trimethylsilylacetamide, (Pierce). The trimethylsilylated PTH derivatives were injected into the port of a gas chromatograph (Varian Aerograph model 1740-1) equipped with a 152 × 0.31 cm (diameter) stainless-steel column packed with 3% SE-30 on 100/120 mesh Varaport (Varian Aerograph). The oven temperature was initially set at 180°C. After injection, the oven temperature was programmed to increase at the rate of 2°C/min for the first 20 min, then at 10°C/min until it reached 275°C; the temperature was held at 275°C for the remainder of the run. The helium flow-rate was set at a back pressure of 1.2 atm at the start of the injection. A Biemann-Watson separator was used to remove the helium carrier gas in order to increase the sample concentration before it entered the ion source of the mass spectrometer (Varian Mat CH-5). As the sample was injected into the gas chromatograph, the mass spectrometer was set to sweep in a repetitive scan mode from mass 30 to mass 500 at a resolution of about 500, so that one spectrum was collected and stored

TABLE 1. *Analysis of trimethylsilylated PTH derivatives**

PTH derivatives	Retention time (min)	Major peaks in the mass spectrum†
Gly	11.3	264 (M+; 55), 249 (69), 86 (100)
Pro‡	13.6	232 (M+; 55), 203 (23), 135 (75), 119 (41), 69 (72)
Leu	16.6	320 (M+; 52), 305 (66), 277 (47), 264 (65), 249 (45), 142 (100)
Ser	18.5	366 (M+; 49), 351 (35), 336 (65), 321 (56), 276 (30), 261 (32), 188 (18), 103 (74)
Tyr	30.9	442 (M+; 5), 427 (16), 336 (55), 321 (9), 264 (16), 179 (100)
Trp	38.0	465 (M+; 2), 450 (4), 336 (49), 321 (6), 202 (94)

* 2-μl aliquots of standard solution containing 0.5 μg of each of the PTH derivatives (Mann) in 1 μl were injected for gas chromatography–mass spectrometry.

† Numbers in parentheses denote percent height of the peak relative to the base peak.

‡ PTH-Pro does not have any active proton for silylation.

automatically on the magnetic tape of the computer (Varian 620/i) every 11 sec. The PTH derivative emerged from the gas chromatograph at its specific retention time, which served as a qualitative identification of the amino acid; the identity of the derivative was then confirmed by its mass spectrum (Table 1). The method is not applicable to His or Arg, which do not extract as the thiazolinones into butyl acetate; also, the sensitivity of the method for Trp derivatives is low.

Digestion with Chymotrypsin. A 15 nmol (about 20 μg) aliquot of LRF (ovine or synthetic) was incubated 18 hr at 37°C in 50 μl of 0.1 M NH₄OAc buffer (pH 8.1) with 1 μg of chymotrypsin A. After incubation, aliquots of the digest were taken for C- and N-terminal analysis, the remainder was dried under reduced pressure and dissolved in 50% pyridine for sequencing by the Edman-dansylation procedure.

TABLE 2. *C-terminal determination by hydrazinolysis and dansylation of ovine LRF, with and without chymotrypsin treatment**

	Net cpm				
Dns-amino acid†	Synthetic LRF	Ovine LRF	Chymotrypsin-treated Ovine LRF	Control	n
Gly	23,939	12,164	11,434	3807 ± 1599	3
His	1,848	62	12,691	1809 ± 433	3
Leu	127	391	1,371	2004 ± 1828	3
Pro	2,850	0	1,929	773 ± 160	3
Ser	0	0	3,850	1150 ± 826	3
Tyr/2	1,089	582	7,592	1610 ± 790	3
Trp	2,993	1,528	—	2605 ± 503	3
Trp (no benzaldehyde)	—	—	4,599	2653	

* All values represent net cpm/nmol sample, corrected for mean control values. Controls are expressed as mean cpm ± standard error for n controls.

† Tyr is determined as O,N-di-Dns-Tyr; thus, the value observed is divided by two.

Digestion with Pyrrolidone-Carboxylylpeptidase. LRF (15 nmol, 20 μg) was incubated with 3 μg of pyrrolidone-carboxylylpeptidase for 22 hr at 37°C in 40 μl of buffer (0.05 M potassium phosphate (pH 6.5)–0.03 M 2-mercaptoethanol–1 mM EDTA). The digest was then dried and subjected to sequence analysis. Control samples of each enzyme were incubated and carried through the C- and N-terminal analyses and sequencing procedures.

RESULTS

Determination by [¹⁴C]dansylation of amino acids in ovine LRF after hydrolysis with 6 N HCl in the presence of thio-

TABLE 3. *Edman degradation plus dansylation of ovine LRF, with and without chymotrypsin treatment**

	Net cpm							
		Edman cycle after chymotrypsin						
Dns-amino acid	Untreated	0	1	2	3	4	Control	n
His	2995	—	—	—	—	—	—	—
Trp	0	8,177	0	66	911	2,828	1830 ± 418	6
Ser	240	26,249	1,692	—	400	3,684	1193 ± 538	3
Tyr/2	0	416	40,394	645	266	1,083	2332 ± 434	5
Gly	93	26,725	636	813	1,058	35,112	2266 ± 364	6
Leu	0	357	31,746	0	901	2,449	1580 ± 306	6
Arg	—	5,373	3,812	41,384	931	3,090	2033 ± 599	6
Pro	0	0	5,730	0	36,470	787	1540 ± 128	6
Gly-NH₂	—	—	—	—	—	34,339	3055	1
Total cpm	3328	67,297	84,010	42,908	40,937	49,033		
Total nmol amino acid†	0.1	2.4	3.0	1.5	1.5	1.8		

* Values of net cpm and controls were calculated as in Table 2.

† Calculated on the basis of 28 ± 5 cpm/pmol (see text).

188

TABLE 4. *Edman degradation plus dansylation of ovine LRF after treatment with PCA-peptidase**

Dns-amino acid	Net cpm Edman cycle									Control	n
	0	1	2	3	4	5	6	7	8†		
His	12,061	0	—	—	—	—	0	0	—	10,523 ± 6,394	6
Trp	0	4579	0	619	688	0	1141	2439	250	5,593 ± 1,262	8
Ser	0	713	10,483	0	0	191	0	0	—	2,954 ± 415	12
Tyr/2	619	233	2,682	3762	318	—	0	0	—	1,606 ± 213	12
Gly	4,604	0	0	209	8,430	0	0	2112	0	4,688 ± 699	12
Leu	0	3191	0	56	3,289	3710	454	0	0	713 ± 128	12
Arg	1,858	—	3,011	896	1,814	4591	4078	0	—	1,904 ± 615	7
Pro	0	0	0	2144	56	0	1517	2917	0	1,045 ± 264	12
Gly-NH$_2$	—	—	—	—	—	—	—	—	1625	1,191 ± 686	2
Total	19,142	8716	16,176	7686	14,595	8492	7190	7468	1922		
Total nmol amino acid	0.7	0.3	0.6	0.3	0.5	0.3	0.3	0.3	0.1		

* Legend as in Table 3, except that values for His and Arg were calculated by use of the appropriate control from each corresponding Edman cycle, because the cpm for these amino acids increased significantly with each cycle.
† Unhydrolyzed.

glycolic acid confirmed the presence of His, Arg, Ser, Glu, Pro, Gly, Leu, and Tyr, as reported earlier by Amoss *et al.* (9) and Schally *et al.* (8) for ovine and porcine LRF, respectively, plus the presence of Trp, as originally reported by Matsuo *et al.* (12) for porcine LRF.

Chymotryptic digestion of ovine LRF gave four major peptide fragments having as C-termini (Table 2): Gly, His, Trp, Tyr, and possibly a small amount of a peptide with C-terminal Ser. Hydrazinolysis–dansylation showed C-terminal Gly in untreated ovine and synthetic LRF. Since this Gly residue is amidated in the synthetic preparation, and was shown by sequencing to be amidated in ovine LRF (see below), there was probably some deamidation of the Gly-NH$_2$ residue during the hydrazinolysis procedure. Dansylation of the chymotryptic digest of ovine LRF revealed primarily N-terminal Ser and Gly, plus some Trp and Arg (Table 3). The major N-termini observed after the first Edman cycle were: Tyr and Leu, plus some Arg and Pro; after the second cycle: Arg; the third: Pro; and the fourth: Gly-NH$_2$; Gly-NH$_2$ was determined without hydrolysis by 6 N HCl as Dns-Gly-NH$_2$ (first dimension of polyamide thin-layer chromatography, R_f = 0.72; second dimension, R_f = 0.42); and, after hydrolysis, as Dns-Gly. Total recoveries of Dns-amino acids after each cycle were in good agreement with theoretical values. Mass spectral analysis of PTH derivatives showed Gly and Ser (trace of Leu) from the first Edman cycle and Pro from the fourth Edman cycle; the extract from the second Edman cycle was accidently destroyed; to be consistent with the dansylation results the third cycle should have given Arg, which is not detectable by this method. These results are consistent with the primary structure for LRF shown in Fig. 1, the major fragments from chymotryptic digestion being Ch I, Ch II, Ch III, and Ch IV, with smaller amounts of Ch V and Ch VI. Hydrolysis of peptides by chymotrypsin at His-, Ser-, and Leu-residues is not uncommon (26). The same principal cleavages occur upon digestion of synthetic LRF with chymotrypsin. The results of analysis of the chymotryptic digest do not rule out an alternative structure for ovine LRF, in which the Ser-4 and Gly-6 residues are interchanged; that is, pGlu-His-Trp-Gly-Tyr-Ser-Leu-Arg-Pro-Gly-NH$_2$. Moreover, the position of the His residue can only be obtained by inference, since it is not directly accounted for.

Digestion of ovine LRF with pyrrolidone-carboxylyl-peptidase, followed by the Edman–dansylation analysis (Table 4), however, confirms the sequence PCA I shown in Fig. 1. Again, synthetic LRF gave similar results. Consistent with the sequence shown in Fig. 1, mass-spectral analysis revealed trimethylsilylated PTH derivatives of Trp, Ser, Tyr, Gly, and Leu in the second to sixth Edman cycles, respectively, and Pro in the eighth cycle from pyrrolidone-carboxylylpeptidase-digested ovine LRF. Blanks occur in the first and seventh cycle, as would be expected, since the determination of His or Arg is not possible by the technique described above. All of the remaining degraded peptide after the eighth Edman cycle was dansylated because of the limited amount of material, so that the identity of the tenth residue could not be corroborated by our gas-chromatographic method. In contrast to the results with chymotrypsin, the total recoveries of Dns-amino acids were lower than expected after pyrrolidone-carboxylylpeptidase digestion of either ovine or synthetic LRF. Furthermore, there was some evidence for endopeptidase activity in the pyrrolidone-carboxylylpeptidase preparation used that gave

```
                        PCA I
                ←―――――――――――――――→
                               PCA II
                        ←―――――――――――――――→
    pGlu-His-Trp-Ser-Tyr-Gly-Leu-Arg-Pro-Gly-NH₂
      1    2   3   4   5   6   7   8   9   10
      Ch I        Ch II         Ch III
    ←――――――→ ←―――――X―――X―――――→
                                        Ch V
                                ←―――――――――――→
              Ch IV                    Ch VI
    ←―――――――――――→              ←―――――――――――→
```

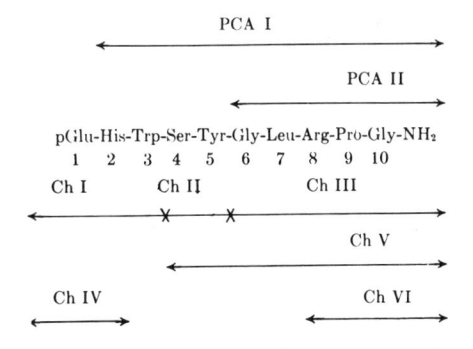

FIG. 1. Peptide fragments observed after treatment of ovine or synthetic LRF with chymotrypsin (Ch I–VI) or pyrrolidone-carboxylylpeptidase (PCA I-II).

rise to the fragment PCA-II, similar to Ch III (Fig. 1), since there is no evidence for this fragment in the undigested LRF preparations (Table 3). The batch of pyrrolidone-carboxylyl-peptidase used in these experiments does show more rapid loss of enzymatic activity upon storage than do batches of the enzyme used in our previous experiments (11) and, therefore, may contain some endopeptidase activity (R.F., unpublished data).

DISCUSSION

The amino-acid sequence of the hypothalamic releasing factor for luteinizing hormone is apparently the same in two different species (pig and sheep). A similar relationship has already been shown to exist in the case of the hypothalamic thyrotropin releasing factors of ovine and porcine origin, both of which have the amino-acid sequence pGlu-His-Pro-NH$_2$ (27–29). Of considerable physiological interest is the observation (12, 14, 30) that synthetic LRF stimulates the secretion of both luteinizing and follicle-stimulating hormones, thus reducing the probability that the follicle-stimulating hormone released by native LRF might have been due to a contaminant. These results do not settle the question of the possible existence of a follicle-stimulating hormone-releasing factor different from LRF (for a discussion of this point, see ref. 9).

LRF of ovine or porcine origin is biologically active in stimulating secretion of gonadotropins in several mammalian species (5, 6), including man (31). Knowledge of the structure of LRF from these species allows its synthesis in large quantities for possible use in testing pituitary capacity for gonadotropin secretion and as a means of inducing ovulation in farm animals, as well as in human beings. Synthetic analogues of LRF antagonistic to LRF would also be of interest as possible means of fertility control.

NOTE ADDED IN PROOF

After our initial communication describing chemical and biological properties of the purified LRF decapeptide synthesized on a benzhydrylamine solid support (See ref. 14, above), notes from other laboratories have appeared describing other routes of synthesis of the decapeptide: Sievertsson, H., Chang, J. K., Bogentoff, C., Currie, B. L., Folkers, K. & Bowers, C. Y., *Biochem. Biophys. Res. Commun.*, **44**, 1566–1571 (1971); Geiger, R., König, W., Wissman, H., Geisen, K. & Enzmann, F., *Biochem. Biophys. Res. Commun.*, **45**, 767–773 (1971); Matsuo, H., Arimura, A., Nair, R. M. G. & Schally, A. V., *Biochem. Biophys. Res. Commun.*, **45**, 822–827 (1971).

We thank H. Anderson, D. Erenea, T. Ewing, S. Garrison, R. Kaiser, E. Raines, R. Smith, and P. Wilson for excellent technical assistance. This research was supported by AID (csd-2785), the Ford Foundation, and the Rockefeller Foundation.

1. McCann, S. M. & Taleisnik, S. (1960) *Amer. J. Physiol.* **199**, 847–850.
2. Campbell, H. J., Feuer, G., Garcia, J. & Harris, G. W. (1961) *J. Physiol. (London)* **157**, 30–31.
3. Courrier, R., Guillemin, R., Jutisz, M., Sakiz, E. & Aschheim, P. (1961) *C. R. H. Acad. Sci.* **253**, 922–927.
4. Guillemin, R., Jutisz, M. & Sakiz, E. (1963) *C. R. H. Acad. Sci.* **256**, 504–507.
5. Schally, A. V., Arimura, A., Bowers, C. Y., Kastin, A. J., Sawano, S. & Redding, T. W. (1968) *Recent Progr. Horm. Res.* **24**, 497–581.
6. Burgus, R. & Guillemin, R. (1970) *Annu. Rev. Biochem.* **39**, 499–526.
7. Dhariwal, A. P. S., Watanabe, S., Antunes-Rodrigues, J. & McCann, S. M. (1967) *Neuroendocrinology* **2**, 294–303.
8. Schally, A. V., Arimura, A., Baba, Y., Nair, R. M. G., Matsuo, H., Redding, T. W., Debeljuk, L. & White, W. F. (1971) *Biochem. Biophys. Res. Commun.* **43**, 393–399.
9. Amoss, M., Burgus, R., Blackwell, R., Vale, W., Fellows, R. & Guillemin, R. (1971) *Biochem. Biophys. Res. Commun.* **44**, 205–210.
10. Fellows, R. E. & Mudge, A. (1970) *Fed. Proc.* **30**, 1078.
11. Amoss, M., Burgus, R., Ward, D. N., Fellows, R. E. & Guillemin, R. (June, 1970) *Progr. 52nd Meeting Endocrine Soc.* p. 61.
12. Matsuo, H., Baba, Y., Nair, R. M. G., Arimura, A. & Schally, A. V. (1971) *Biochem. Biophys. Res. Commun.* **43**, 1334–1339.
13. Baba, Y., Matsuo, H. & Schally, A. V. (1971) *Biochem. Biophys. Res. Commun.* **44**, 459–463.
14. Monahan, M., Rivier, J., Burgus, R., Amoss, M., Blackwell, R., Vale, W. & Guillemin, R. (1971) *C. R. H. Acad. Sci., Ser. D* **273**, 508–510.
15. Fales, H. M., Nagai, Y., Milne, G. W. A., Brewer, H. B., Bronzert, R. J. & Pisano, J. J. (1971) *Anal. Biochem.* **43**, 288–299.
16. Hagenmaier, H., Ebbighausen, W., Nicholson, G. & Vötsch, W. (1970) *Z. Naturforsch.* **25b**, 681–689.
17. Burgus, R., Butcher, M., Ling, N., Monahan, M., Rivier, J., Fellows, R., Amoss, M., Blackwell, R., Vale, W. & Guillemin, R., *C. R. H. Acad. Sci., Ser. D* **273**, 1611–1613.
18. Burgus, R. & Guillemin, R. (1970) in *Hypophysiotropic Hormones of the Hypothalamus*, ed. Meites, J. (Williams and Wilkins Co., Baltimore), pp. 227–241.
19. Gray, W. R. (1967) in *Methods in Enzymology*, ed. Hirs H. W. (Academic Press, New York), Vol. 11, pp. 469–475.
20. Chen, R. F. (1968) *Anal. Biochem.* **25**, 412–416.
21. Neuhoff, V., Haar, F. v. d., Schlimme, E. & Weise, M. (1969) *Hoppe-Seyler's Z. Physiol. Chem.* **350**, 121–128.
22. Matsubara, H. & Sasaki, R. M. (1969) *Biochem. Biophys. Res. Commun.* **35**, 175–181.
23. Woods, K. R. & Wang, K. T. (1967) *Biochim. Biophys. Acta* **133**, 369–370.
24. Mesrob, B. & Holleyšovský, V. (1967) *Collect. Czech. Chem. Commun.* **32**, 1976–1982.
25. Edman, P. (1956) *Acta Chem. Scand.* **10**, 761–768.
26. Hill, R. L. (1965) *Advan. Protein Chem.* **20**, 37–107.
27. Burgus, R., Dunn, T. F., Desiderio, D. & Guillemin, R. (1969) *C. R. H. Acad. Sci., Ser. D* **269**, 1870–1873.
28. Burgus, R., Dunn, T. F., Desiderio, D., Ward, D. N., Vale, W. & Guillemin, R. (1970) *Nature* **226**, 321–325.
29. Nair, R. M. G., Barrett, J. F., Bowers, C. Y. & Schally, A. V. (1970) *Biochemistry* **5**, 1103–1106.
30. Schally, A. V., Arimura, A., Kastin, A. J., Matsuo, H., Baba, Y., Redding, T. W., Nair, R. M. G., Debeljuk, L. & White, W. F. (1971) *Science* **173**, 1036–1038.
31. Fleischer, N. & Guillemin, R., in *Advances in Internal Medicine*, ed. Stollerman, G. H. (Year Book Medical Publishers, Chicago), in press.

Editor's Comments
on Papers 32 Through 35

32 SCHALLY et al.
    Gonadotropin-Releasing Hormone: One Polypeptide Regulates Secretion of Luteinizing and Follicle-Stimulating Hormones

33 ARIMURA et al.
    Immunoreactive LH-Releasing Hormone in Plasma: Midcycle Elevation in Women

34 PALKOVITS et al.
    Luteinizing Hormone-Releasing Hormone (LH-RH) Content of the Hypothalamic Nuclei in Rat

35 SOWERS et al.
    Pituitary Response to LHRH in Midtrimester Pregnancy

Schally et al. (Paper 32), on the basis of findings that natural preparations of LH-RH isolated from porcine hypothalami, as well as synthetic LH-RH, stimulated the release of FSH as well as LH, proposed that the decapeptide LH-RH controls secretion of both from the adenohypophysis. This proposal was strengthened by Schally's findings that FSH-releasing factor activity could not be separated from LH-RH activity after numerous purification steps. Schally concluded that natural LH-RH purified from porcine hypothalami and the synthetic preparation, having identical structures, represent a hypothalamic releasing hormone that exerts a specific and marked effect on the hypophysial secretion of gonadotropins. This proposal has gained wide acceptance by virtue of the fact that a separate FSH-releasing hormone has yet to be identified. The occurrence of discordant secretion of LH and FSH has been attributed to the modulating effect of gonadal steroids on the hypophysial gonadotropes. These results verified the conclusions of Igarashi and McCann (1964) that the hypothalamus controls the release of LH and FSH and that one hypothalamic substance from SME extracts was capable of stimulating release of both LH and FSH from the adenohypophysis.

Arimura et al. (Paper 33) raised antisera to LH-RH and developed a sensitive and specific radioimmunoassay for LHRH measurement in blood. They then demonstrated that LH-RH secretion is associated with the preovulatory surge in LH occurring in normally cycling women. They also postulated that endogenous LH-RH is secreted in a pulsatile manner similar to that previously described for LH secretion.

Palkovits et al. (Paper 34), utilizing a specific radioimmunoassay for LHRH and microdissection techniques developed in their laboratory, studied the precise location of LH-RH in small sections of the hypothalamus. The greatest concentration of LH-RH was found in the median eminence (ME), with lesser amounts in the arcuate nucleus and in the anterior (preoptic) area. These findings are in accord with the concept that the distribution of LH-RH corresponds to the tuberoinfundibular tract and that the releasing hormone is synthesized in the cell bodies of the arcuate nucleus and probably the preoptic nucleus and is subsequently transported to terminals in the ME by axonal flow from these nuclei. Thus, the LH-RH secretory neurons are scattered throughout the medial basal hypothalamus (MBH) as far anterior as the preoptic area, with one major area of concentration being the arcuate-ventromedial region (the axons of these cells contributing to the LH-RH tubero-infundibular tract) and another concentration existing in the preoptic-suprachiasmatic region. The arcuate nucleus is the primary locus of neuronal cells making up the LH-RH-tubero-infundibular system, which appears to be the site of negative gonadal hormone feedback. This is in concert with previous findings (Halász and Gorski, Paper 29) that complete differentiation of the MBH-median eminence region does not prevent postgonadectomy castration cell formation due to interception of direct negative feedback at the MBH exclusive of any other central nervous system circuit. It has been further demonstrated that neurons of the arcuate nucleus exhibit labeling following injection of tritiated estradiol or testosterone. Thus, it has been shown conclusively that LH-RH-tubero-infundibular neuronal cells within the arcuate nucleus are gonadal steroidal targets with the steroids inhibiting gonadotropin secretion.

The hypophysial stimulating effects of LH-RH in normal humans and animals have been found to be relatively specific for gonadotropin hormone release. Recently Sowers et al. (Paper 35) showed that there are marked prolactin (PRL) and lesser TSH and growth hormone (GH) responses to LH-RH administered during the second trimester of pregnancy. The markedly elevated basal PRL and nonspecific PRL responses to LH-RH during pregnancy are analogous to the elevated basal PRL and GH, and PRL and GH responses to LH-RH observed in the galactorrhea-amenorrhea syndrome associated with hypophysial microadenomas and in acromegaly, respectively. It was also noted in the study of Sowers et al. that there are absent LH and FSH responses to LH-RH in midtrimester pregnancy when a specific antibody raised against the beta subunits was employed to measure the gonadotropins. The inhibition of gonadotropin response and the high levels of basal PRL, as well as the nonspecific PRL response to LH-RH, were attributed by the authors to high levels of circulating estradiol exerting a marked negative feedback on gonadotropin secretion and stimulating lactotropic hyperplasia; the accompanying hypersecretion and nonspecific secretion of PRL is analogous to the situation that occurs with development of hyperplasia or an adenoma in the nonpregnant woman.

REFERENCE

Igarashi, M., and S. M. McCann. 1964. A Hypothalamic Follicle Stimulating Hormone Releasing Factor. *Endocrinology* 74:446.

GONADOTROPIN-RELEASING HORMONE: ONE POLYPEPTIDE REGULATES SECRETION OF LUTEINIZING AND FOLLICLE-STIMULATING HORMONES

A. V. Schally, A. Arimura, A. J. Kastin, H. Matsuo, Y. Baba, T. W. Redding, R. M. G. Nair, L. Debeljuk, and W. F. White

Abstract. *A polypeptide isolated from porcine hypothalami stimulates the release of both luteinizing hormone and follicle-stimulating hormone from the pituitaries of several species. This polypeptide has been structurally identified as (pyro)Glu-His-Trp-Ser-Tyr-Gly-Leu-Arg-Pro-Gly-NH$_2$ and synthesized. The natural and synthetic materials share biological properties. It appears that this peptide represents the hypothalamic hormone regulating the secretion of both luteinizing hormone and follicle-stimulating hormone.*

The hypothalamus controls the release of luteinizing hormone (LH) and follicle-stimulating hormone (FSH) [1]. The work of various investigators clearly demonstrated that there are, in hypothalamic extracts of animals, including man, substances, or one substance, capable of stimulating release of LH and FSH from the pituitary [1, 2]. Much evidence also exists that sex steroids are involved in this regulation. Initially, it was thought that two different substances designated luteinizing hormone-releasing hormone (LH-RH) and follicle-stimulating hormone-releasing hormone (FSH-RH) were responsible for stimulating release of LH and FSH, respectively [1]. However, it became necessary to question this belief when porcine LH-RH, obtained in a high state of purity, stimulated release of both LH and FSH in rats, chimpanzees, and human beings (*3–5*). Furthermore, after the addition of purified porcine LH-RH to an incubation system in vitro in which pituitaries of male rats were used, LH and FSH were released simultaneously with superimposable time courses (*3*). Stimulation of LH release by this material was also unequivocally established in sheep (*6*) and rabbits (*7*), but because of the unavailability of specific radioimmunoassays, it was difficult to test for the effect on FSH secretion in these two species.

It was not clear at first whether this FSH-releasing activity of porcine LH-RH was an intrinsic property of its molecule or whether it was due to a contamination with FSH-RH. Chemical or enzymatic inactivation of LH-RH was always accompanied by loss of FSH-releasing activity (*3, 4*). Moreover, during the fractionation of pig hypothalamic extracts, the location of FSH-RH activity always coincided with that of LH-RH (*8*). After porcine LH-RH was isolated in an essentially homogeneous state by a combination of 12 different purification steps or by countercurrent distribution, it was found that it too stimulated the release of FSH in vivo and in vitro in doses smaller than 1 ng (*8*). Further fractionation by partition chromatography in ten different solvent systems (*8*) did not result in separation of the LH-RH activity from the FSH-RH activity. In addition to stimulating the release of both LH and FSH, the pure natural LH-RH/FSH-RH significantly augmented the synthesis of these two pituitary hormones in tissue cultures (*9*), an effect that had been obtained with LH-RH of lesser purity (*10*).

As a result of the foregoing studies, we postulated that the isolated polypeptide represents the hypothalamic hormone that controls the secretion of both LH and FSH from the pituitary (*8*). However, we could not exclude the possibility, even by the use of most advanced fractionation methods, that two peptides with an identical amino acid composition and molecular weight but with a different amino acid sequence were present in this material, which we had assumed to be homogeneous. This final doubt was removed as a result of the recent determination of the structure of the hypothalamic polypeptide with both LH-RH and FSH-RH activities, but only one amino acid sequence: (pyro)Glu-His-Trp-Ser-Tyr-Gly-Leu-Arg-Pro-Gly-NH$_2$ (*11, 12*). This structure was confirmed by synthesis (*12*). When the synthetic LH-RH/FSH-RH was tested for its effect on the release of LH and FSH in vivo and in vitro, it showed the same spectrum of biological activities as the pure natural material. Thus, synthetic LH-RH/FSH-RH raised the concentration of LH in the plasma in ovariectomized rats that had received prior treatment with estrogen and progesterone (*8, 12*). Synthetic LH-RH/FSH-RH increased plasma FSH levels, as well as LH, in castrated male rats pretreated with testosterone propionate. A direct effect on the anterior pituitary gland was proven by stimulation of FSH and LH release in vitro from the pituitaries of male rats (*8, 12*). An example of these results is shown in Table 1. The FSH released was measured by the Steelman-Pohley assay (*13*). This system is considered at present the most specific for measuring stimulation of FSH release by hypothalamic materials (*14*). Furthermore, synthetic LH-RH/FSH-RH stimulated both the release and synthesis of FSH, as well as LH, in tissue cultures of rat pituitaries (*9, 10*). Preliminary results indicate that synthetic decapeptide also increased the plasma LH and FSH in humans (*15*). The response of one of these subjects can be seen in Fig. 1.

In summary then, it appears that the natural material purified from porcine hypothalami and the synthetic substance with the same structure represent a polypeptide that exerts a specific and profound effect on the pituitary secretion of hormones regulating the reproductive cycle. The overall control of FSH and LH secretion and the preferential release of one or the other of these gonadotropins may be mediated by the interplay of the hypothalamic polypeptide and sex steroids.

The availability of this hypothalamic hormone and its analogs should prove useful for studies on the enhancement or inhibition of fertility.

Table 1. The effect of natural and synthetic LH- and FSH-releasing hormones (LH-RH/FSH-RH) on the stimulation of release of FSH from rat pituitaries. Ten pituitary halves of male rats were incubated in 10 ml of Krebs-Ringer bicarbonate medium for 6 hours (*14*). The FSH released was measured by bioassay (*13*), and it is expressed in terms of NIH FSH-S-4 units.

Group	Addition	Dose (ng/ml)	Ovarian weight (mg ± S.E.)	P*	FSH (ng/ml)
1	Control		45.0 ± 2.6		19.7
2	Natural LH-RH/FSH-RH	2	77.9 ± 6.9	.005	29.7
3	Synthetic LH-RH/FSH-RH	2	71.4 ± 10.2	.05	27.2
4	Natural LH-RH/FSH-RH	8	93.6 ± 11.4	.005	35.9
5	Synthetic LH-RH/FSH-RH	8	86.8 ± 9.4	.005	33.4

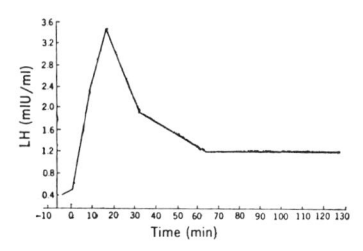

* Student *t*-test.

Fig. 1. Effect of an intravenous administration of an equivalent of 1.5 µg of synthetic LH-RH/FSH-RH in plasma LH concentrations in a woman who had been treated for 15 days with the oral contraceptive preparation Lyndiol. Plasma LH concentrations were measured by radioimmunoassay (*16*) and are plotted as milli-international units (*mIU*) of the 2nd IRP-HMP (second international research preparation of human menopausal gonadotropin) per milliliter of serum.

References and Notes

1. S. M. McCann and V. D. Ramirez, *Recent Progr. Hormone Res.* **20**, 131 (1964); A. V. Schally, A. Arimura, C. Y. Bowers, A. J. Kastin, S. Sawano, T. W. Redding, *ibid.* **24**, 497 (1968); G. W. Harris and F. Naftolin, *Br. Med. Bull.* **26**, 3 (1970).
2. A. V. Schally *et al.*, *J. Clin. Endocrinol. Metab.* **31**, 291 (1970).
3. W. F. White, in *Hypophysiotropic Hormones of the Hypothalamus*, J. Meites, Ed. (Williams & Wilkins, Baltimore, 1970), p. 249.
4. A. V. Schally, A. Arimura, A. J. Kastin, J. J. Reeves, C. Y. Bowers, Y. Baba, in *Mammalian Reproduction*, H. Gibian and E. J. Plotz, Eds. (Springer-Verlag, New York, 1970), p. 45; W. F. White, in *ibid.*, p. 84; A. V. Schally, Y. Baba, T. W. Redding, *Neuroendocrinology* **8**, 70 (1971); A. V. Schally, Y. Baba, A. Arimura, T. W. Redding, W. F. White, *Biochem. Biophys. Res. Commun.* **42**, 50 (1971).
5. A. J. Kastin, A. V. Schally, C. Gual, A. R. Midgley, Jr., C. Y. Bowers, A. Diaz-Infante, Jr., *J. Clin. Endocrinol. Metab.* **29**, 1046 (1969); ———, F. Gomez-Perez, *Amer. J. Obstet. Gynecol.* **108**, 177 (1970).
6. J. J. Reeves, A. Arimura, A. V. Schally, *J. Anim. Sci.* **31**, 933 (1970).

7. J. Hilliard, A. V. Schally, C. H. Sawyer, *Endocrinology* **88**, 730 (1971).
8. A. V. Schally, A. Arimura, Y. Baba, R. M. G. Nair, H. Matsuo, T. W. Redding, L. Debeljuk, W. F. White, *Biochem. Biophys. Res. Commun.* **43**, 393 (1971); *Endocrinology* **88**, A-70 (1971).
9. T. W. Redding, A. V. Schally, W. Locke, *Endocrinology* **88**, A-75 (1971).
10. J. C. Mittler, A. Arimura, A. V. Schally, *Proc. Soc. Exp. Biol. Med.* **133**, 1321 (1970).
11. Glu, glutamic acid; His, histidine; Trp, tryptophan; Ser, serine; Tyr, tyrosine; Gly, glycine; Leu, leucine; Arg, arginine; Pro, proline.
12. H. Matsuo, Y. Baba, R. M. G. Nair, A. Arimura, A. V. Schally, *Biochem. Biophys. Res. Commun.* **43**, 1334 (1971); Y. Baba, H. Matsuo, A. V. Schally, *ibid.* **44**, 459 (1971); R. M. G. Nair and A. V. Schally, in preparation; H. Matsuo, A. Arimura, A. V. Schally, in preparation.
13. S. L. Steelman and F. Pohley, *Endocrinology* **53**, 604 (1953).
14. J. C. Mittler and J. Meites, *ibid.* **78**, 500 (1966); A. V. Schally, J. C. Mittler, W. F. White, *ibid.* **86**, 903 (1970).
15. A. J. Kastin, C. Gual, A. Arimura, A. V. Schally, in preparation.
16. A. R. Midgley, Jr., *Endocrinology* **79**, 10 (1966).
17. Supported by grants from the Veterans Administration; by PHS grants AM-07467 and AM-09094; and by a grant from Population Council, New York. We thank Dr. W. Locke and Dr. E. Bresler for editorial suggestions.

24 June 1971

33

Copyright © 1974 by J. B. Lippincott Company

Reprinted from *J. Clin. Endocrinol. Metab.* 38:510-513 (1974)

IMMUNOREACTIVE LH-RELEASING HORMONE IN PLASMA: MIDCYCLE ELEVATION IN WOMEN*

A. Arimura, A.J. Kastin, and A.V. Schally
Department of Medicine, Tulane University School of Medicine, and Endocrine and Polypeptide Laboratories, VA Hospital, New Orleans, La. 70146

M. Saito, T. Kumasaka, Y. Yaoi, N. Nishi, and K. Ohkura
Department of Obstetrics and Gynecology, Tokyo Medical and Dental University, Tokyo

The influence of the brain upon ovulation and the menstrual cycle has been presumed to involve the release of luteinizing hormone-releasing hormone (LH-RH) from the hypothalamus at midcycle (1). Fink et al. reported that LH-RH activity in the portal blood of the pituitary measured by bioassay increased in the afternoon of proestrus in the rat (2). This has not been confirmed by other investigators, perhaps because of technical difficulties such as the influence of anesthesia. Measurement of LH-RH in peripheral blood has been desired by many investigators. Malacara et al. observed a rise of bioassayable LH-RH in the methanol extracts of plasma from some women at midcycle (3). Despite the use of 40 ml of plasma from each subject, the investigators were able only to perform semiquantitative determinations of LH-RH, so that such a method may not be practical for studying the secretory patterns of LH-RH in physiological and pathological conditions.

The availability of sufficient amounts of the synthetic LH-RH decapeptide (pyro) Glu-His-Trp-Ser-Tyr-Gly-Leu-Arg-Pro-Gly-NH$_2$ (4,5) made it possible to generate antiserum against LH-RH and establish radioimmunoassays for this hormone (6,7). Although several reports of immunoreactive LH-RH levels in the peripheral blood have appeared (7,8), no demonstration that the level rises prior or together with the midcycle elevation of plasma LH in women has yet been reported.

Since LH-RH released into the primary capillary plexus of the hypophysial portal vessels reaches the pituitary gland through these short channels without being diluted appreciably, a small increase in its release may lead to a sufficiently high concentration of LH-RH. The unused hormone which leaks into the general circulation may be immediately diluted and rapidly inactivated (9). In comparison with the elevation of serum LH levels at midcycle, the rise of LH-RH levels may be so meager that only an extremely sensitive assay method would detect it.

MATERIALS AND METHODS

"Paradoxical binding," such as has been used for determination of hormones like ACTH by radioimmunoassay (10), was utilized to establish a supersensitive radioimmunoassay for LH-RH in the serum (6).

---

*The results of this study were reported at the 55th Annual Meeting of the Endocrine Society, Chicago, in June, 1973. This study was supported in part by the Veterans Administration.
Submitted, November 16, 1973.

One of the antisera to unconjugated LH-RH which was generated in rabbits showed an increased binding with ^{125}I-labeled LH-RH in the presence of an unlabeled hormone in increasing doses, rather than ordinary inhibition of binding and thus could be used in this assay. At a 1:2100 dilution of the anti-LH-RH serum, this radioimmunoassay could detect 0.25 to 15 pg of LH-RH quantitatively (Fig. 1). The coefficient of within-assay variation was 6%. LH was determined by radioimmunoassay as described by Odell et al. using the NIH-human-LH Kit (11). LER 907 was used as the standard preparation.

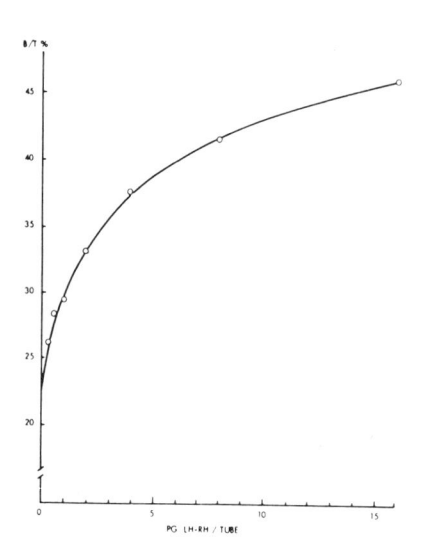

Fig. 1. Standard curve for LH-RH in the radioimmunoassay using paradoxical binding of labeled hormone to the rabbit anti-LH-RH serum. B/T increases as the dose of LH-RH increases up to 15 pg, where B and T represent bound and total radioactivities, respectively. The antiserum was diluted by 1:2100 and the reaction mixture was incubated for 48 hr at 4 C.

RESULTS AND DISCUSSION

Addition of human plasma or serum to the reaction mixture resulted in a dose-re-

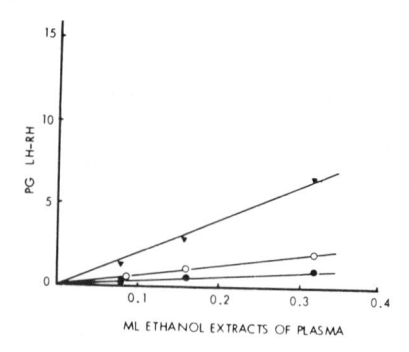

Fig. 2. Amounts of LH-RH determined as a function of the dilution of 3 human plasma extracts. The concentration of LH-RH in these plasma extracts falls linearly with dilution, indicating that the reactivities of LH-RH decapeptide and human plasma extracts are identical.

lated fall in bound hormone which may be due to some non-specific interaction of plasma proteins with this RIA (6). Deproteinization of acidified plasma with ethanol was found to eliminate this suppression. Our experience indicates that this step is essential for measuring LH-RH in serum. Thus, each plasma sample was acidified with 1N acetic acid and then deproteinized by adding dropwise 3 volumes of 100% cold ethanol. The deproteinized ethanol extract of plasma was concentrated in a flash evaporator and then lyophilyzed. The residue was dissolved in 1% egg white in phosphate buffered saline, pH 7.5, and assayed for LH-RH at 3 dose levels. All the samples were measured in the same assay. Mean recovery of known amounts of LH-RH added to human plasma was 81%. The amounts of immunoreactive LH-RH in all plasma extracts from various human subjects were in the range which showed paradoxical binding. The concentrations of LH-RH activity in the plasma extracts as determined by this RIA fell linearly with dilution (Fig. 2). This is equivalent to having superimposable curves for standard LH-RH and unknowns, and indicates that the immunoreactive substances in the human plasma extracts have similar immunological properties as the LH-RH decapeptide (12).

Fig. 3 illustrates the ranges of plasma LH and immunoreactive LH-RH levels during the early follicular stage, midcycle, or mid-luteal stage in 5 normal women with regular menstrual cycles. Day 0 indicates the day of LH surge. In the early follicular stage, from day -12 to day -7, LH-RH levels in the plasma were undetectable in 3 out of 5 women. The highest levels were 1.8 pg/ml. On day -3, LH-RH levels were detectable in 4 out of 5 women. On day -1 to day 0, LH-RH was detectable in all 5 samples, reaching as high as 17 pg/ml. At the mid-luteal stage, LH-RH returned to low levels in all but one woman. This woman also showed a concomitant but slight elevation of plasma LH and FSH levels. A similar phenomenon was found in other recent observations. In 2 out of 5 samples, LH-RH was detectable during the luteal stage.

The mean LH-RH level at midcycle was significantly higher than that in the follicular stage. In addition, in each individual, except for one subject, the LH-RH on day -3 was higher than the respective level in the early follicular stage. It is possible that endogenous LH-RH is secreted in a pulsatile manner similar to that described for LH secretion (13), so that any sample may reflect the level at only one moment in a fluctuating pattern. Nevertheless, our results suggest that LH-RH secretion reaches its peak level at approximately the same time as the LH peak. Thus, these findings may provide support for the concept that the preovulatory surge of LH is related to the increased secretion of endogenous LH-RH.

ACKNOWLEDGEMENTS

The authors wish to express their thanks to Miss Haruko Sato, Mrs. Joan Gauthier, and Mrs. Meredith Essinger for their technical help, to the National

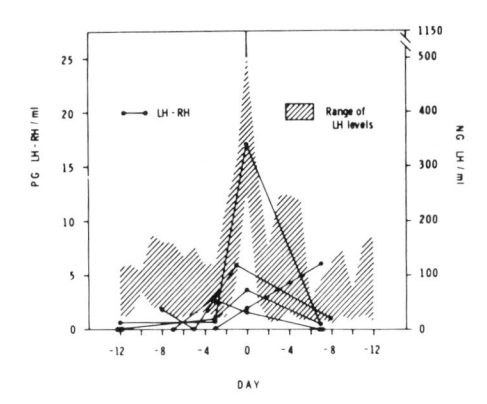

Fig. 3. Plasma LH and LH-RH levels measured by respective radioimmunoassays during the menstrual cycle in 5 women. Highest LH-RH levels were observed at the time of the LH surge at midcycle in 4 of the women. In all women except one, the level of LH-RH on day -3 was higher than that in the early follicular stage. LH and LH-RH levels were expressed in ng/ml in terms of LER 907 and pg/ml synthetic LH-RH (Sankyo Co., Tokyo), respectively.

Pituitary Agency for reagents of human LH radioimmunoassay, and to Dr. Y. Baba, Sankyo Co., for synthetic LH-RH.

REFERENCES

1. Evertt, J.W., Annu. Rev. Physiol. 31: 383, 1969.
2. Fink, G., R. Nallar, W.C. Worthington, Jr., J. Physiol. (London) 191: 407, 1967.
3. Malacara, J.M., L.E. Seyler, Jr., and S. Reichlin, J. Clin. Endocrinol. Metab. 34: 271, 1972.
4. Matsuo, H., A. Arimura, R.M.G. Nair, and A.V. Schally, Biochem. Biophys. Res. Commun. 45: 822, 1971.
5. Geiger, R., W. König, H. Wissman, K. Geisen, and F. Enzmann, Biochem. Biophys. Res. Commun. 45: 767, 1971.

6. Arimura, A., H. Sato, T. Kumasaka, R.B. Worobec, L. Debeljuk, J.D. Dunn, and A.V. Schally, Endocrinology 93: 1092, 1973.
7. Nett, T.M., A.M. Akbar, G.D. Niswender, M.T. Hedlum, and W.F. White, J. Clin. Endocrinol. Metab. 36: 880, 1973.
8. Keye, W.R. Jr., R.P. Kelch, G.D. Niswender, and T.B. Jaffe, J. Clin. Endocrinol. Metab. 36: 1263, 1973.
9. Redding, T.W., A.J. Kastin, D. Gonzalez-Barcena, D.H. Coy, E.J. Coy, D.S. Schalch, and A.V. Schally, J. Clin. Endocrinol. Metab. 37: 626, 1973.
10. Matsukura, S., C.D. West, Y. Ichikawa, W. Jubiz, G. Harada, and F.H. Tyler, J. Lab. Clin. Med. 77: 490, 1971.
11. Odell, W.D., G.T. Ross, and P.L. Rayford, J. Clin. Invest. 46: 248, 1967.
12. Yalow, R.S. and S.A. Berson, In "Principles of Competitive Protein-Binding Assays," W.D. Odell and W.H. Daughday (eds), J.B. Lippincott Co., Philadelphia, 1972, p. 374.
13. Yen, S.S.C., C.C. Tsai, F. Naftolin, G. Vanderberg, and L. Ajador, J. Clin. Endocrinol. Metab. 34: 671, 1972.

34

Copyright © 1974 by J. B. Lippincott Company

Reprinted from *Endocrinology* **96**:554–555, 557–558 (1974)

Luteinizing Hormone-Releasing Hormone (LH-RH) Content of the Hypothalamic Nuclei in Rat

M. PALKOVITS,[1] A. ARIMURA, M. BROWNSTEIN,
A. V. SCHALLY, AND J. M. SAAVEDRA

Laboratory of Clinical Science, National Institute of Mental Health, Bethesda, Maryland 20014, and Endocrine and Polypeptide Laboratories, Veterans Administration Hospital and Department of Medicine, Tulane University School of Medicine, New Orleans, Louisiana 70146

[*Editor's Note:* Table 1 has been omitted.]

ALMOST three decades ago, experiments were performed which suggested that cells present in the medial basal hypothalamus were responsible for release of luteinizing hormone (LH) from the pituitary (see ref. 1–5 for review). By 1960 extracts of hypothalamic tissue had been found to contain a substance which was capable of releasing LH (6). Subsequently investigators have sought the localization within the hypothalamus of cell bodies which produce that factor. Since the chemical nature of LH-RH was not known until recently, it was not possible to develop a sensitive and specific assay for it. Consequently, it was necessary to use bioassay methods in efforts to find the hypothalamic locus of LH-RH (7–11). Recently, the structure of LH-RH was reported to be (pyro) Glu-His-Tryp-Ser-Tyr-Gly-Leu-Arg-Pro-Gly-NH$_2$ (12,13). This decapeptide has been synthesized in many laboratories. The availability of synthetic LH-RH made it possible to generate an antiserum against LH-RH and to develop a radioimmunoassay (RIA) method for this compound (14). This RIA has allowed us to determine the amount of LH-RH present in small samples of tissue and to find the precise location of this molecule within the hypothalamus.

Materials and Methods

Female Osborne Mendel (NIH strain) rats weighing 150 g were used in these studies. The animals were killed by decapitation at 9:00 AM. The brains were removed and frozen on dry ice.

Microdissection. The size and shape of each nucleus must be known in order to remove individual nuclei from the hypothalamus of the rat. Studies of fixed and stained serial sections of the brain have been undertaken. These studies have provided information (Palkovits, in preparation) about the size and shape of the hypothalamic nuclei as well as information about the position of these nuclei in relation to landmarks which can be seen in frozen sections under the stereomicroscope.

The rostral border of the hypothalamus of the rat is at the level of the anterior commissure,

---

Received November 26, 1973.

[1] Present address: Department of Anatomy, Semmelweis Medical University, 1450 Budapest, Tuzoltou 58, Hungary.

Address correspondence to: Dr. M. Brownstein, Research Associate in the Pharmacology-Toxicology Program, National Institute of General Medical Sciences, National Institutes of Health, Bethesda, Maryland 20014.

the caudal border of this region is at the level of the mamillary peduncles. The rostral-to-caudal extent of the hypothalamus is 4.2 mm. Thus, fourteen 300 μ sections can be cut in the frontal plane through the hypothalamus (sections are cut perpendicular to the dorsal surface of the brain). The sections are cut in a cryostat at -10 C. Samples of the hypothalamic nuclei are removed from the frozen sections under stereomicroscopic control. The samples are obtained by use of small steel needles (15). The inner diameter of the needle which is used to remove any given hypothalamic nucleus never exceeds the cross-sectional diameter of the nucleus.

As an example of the use of the microdissection method, consider the removal of the supra-chiasmatic nucleus. This nucleus is present in the second and third sections (the most rostral section is numbered 1). It is found just dorsal to the chiasm and slightly lateral to the third ventricle. Its cross sectional diameter is 500 μ. It is removed from the point of intersection of the ventricle and the chiasm with a punch having an inner diameter of 300 μ. Care must be taken that the medial border of the sample not touch the wall of the ventricle in order to avoid contamination by tissue from the periventricular nucleus.

Table 1 contains a list of the nuclei which were removed for assay of LH-RH. The punch used, the sections from which each nucleus was removed, and the position of each nucleus relative to visible landmarks is presented. This method has been described in detail in a manuscript reporting the levels of norepinephrine and dopamine (16) in the hypothalamic nuclei of the rat. It is noteworthy that the distribution of catecholamines which was determined by combining microdissection and microassay techniques agrees well with that obtained by use of fluorescence histochemistry.

Assay. Two to 4 pellets of tissue 300–500 μ in diameter could be removed from each hypothalamic nucleus per animal. Similar nuclei from five animals were pooled. Tissue pellets were homogenized in 200 μl of 2N acetic acid and an aliquot of the homogenate was removed for protein determination according to the method of Lowry *et al*. (17) with bovine serum albumin as standard. The homogenates were then centrifuged and the supernatants were lyophylized.

The LH-RH content of the samples was determined by radioimmunoassay (14).

Results

The LH-RH contents of 16 hypothalamic nuclei and of the median eminence (Table 2) were determined in the first experiment. Each value in Table 2 is based on four separate determinations. In the second experiment the five subdivisions of the arcuate nucleus (Fig. 1) were taken out separately for LH-RH determination as described above. Since the volume of each subdivision of the arcuate nucleus has been determined (Palkovits, in preparation) the total amount of hormone in each subdivision could be estimated.

The concentration of LH-RH is highest in the median eminence (Table 2). The arcuate nucleus (NA) contains much more of the releasing factor than do the 15 other hypothalamic nuclei which were examined. Some LH-RH seemed to be present in the lateral part of the ventromedial nucleus (just lateral to the arcuate nucleus). The LH-RH content of the other hypothalamic nuclei was found to be less than 0.1 pg/μg protein (30 times less than that in the median eminence).

The concentration of LH-RH within the arcuate nucleus seemed not to be uniform. The highest level of the hormone was in the central part (NA III) of the nucleus (Fig. 1). The most rostral part of the arcuate nucleus (NA I) also contained a high concentration of the LH-RH. This subdivision is relatively small—it makes up only 9% of the total volume of the arcuate nucleus. When the sizes of the NA subdivisions are taken into account, 73% of the total LH-RH of the arcuate nucleus is found in the third subdivision of the NA. This is practically 73% of all the hypothalamic LH-RH other than that in the median eminence. The distribution of the remaining 27% is as follows: NA I = 7%; NA II = 7%; NA IV = 12%; NA V = 1%. (Palkovits *et al*. unpublished observations).

FIG. 1. Schematic drawing of a parasagittal section through the rat hypothalamus. The five subdivisions of the arcuate nucleus (I-V) are indicated. CO is optic chiasma; CM is mamillary body; NIST is nucleus interstitialis striae terminalis; Hy is pituitary gland; S is nucleus preopticus suprachiasmatis; V is nucleus premamillaris ventralis. The remainder of the abbreviations used appear in Table 2.

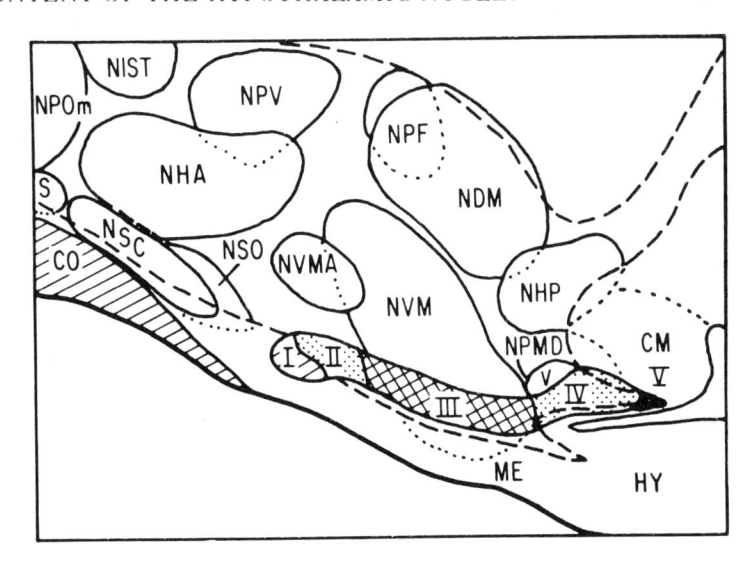

Discussion

Luteinizing hormone releasing hormone is unevenly distributed in the hypothalamus. It is present in a high concentration in the median eminence. Cell bodies producing LH-RH seem most likely to be in the arcuate nucleus, especially in its third subdivision which is directly above the median eminence. The concentration of LH-RH in the median eminence is 7.7 times higher than that in the arcuate nucleus. The volume of the arcuate nucleus, however, is 3.5 times larger than the volume of the median eminence (Palkovits, in preparation). Therefore, the amount of the LH-RH stored in the median eminence is only about twice that of the arcuate nucleus. It should be born in mind that the amount of LH-RH within hypothalamic regions might exhibit wide variation according to the age, sex, strain, phase of cycle, etc., of the rat.

Our data are in good agreement with various indirect observations which suggested that LH-RH containing cell bodies should be located in the medial basal hypothalamus, probably in the arcuate nucleus (1-5,18). Our data conflict with results of experiments using either the ovarian ascorbic acid depletion method (7) or the measurement *in vitro* of pituitary LH release (10,11). Although LH-RH was found in the median eminence by use of bioassay methods, such methods provided data which suggested that LH-RH activity of the hypothalamus extended from the area of the suprachiasmatic nuclei to the area of the median eminence and arcuate nuclei where the bulk of the activity was found. While immunohistochemical studies performed recently by Barry *et al.* (19) have also shown LH-RH to be present outside of the median eminence-arcuate region, those of Zimmerman *et al.* (20) are in agreement with our

TABLE 2. LH-RH content of the hypothalamic nuclei

		pg/µg protein
Nucleus preopticus medialis	(NPOm)	<0.05
Nucleus periventricularis	(NPe)	<0.05
Nucleus suprachiasmatis	(NSC)	trace (<0.1)
Nucleus supraopticus	(NSO)	trace (<0.1)
Nucleus hypothalamicus anterior	(NHA)	<0.05
Area hypothalamica lateralis anterior	(AHLa)	<0.05
Nucleus paraventricularis	(NPV)	<0.05
Median eminence	(ME)	22.4 ± 2.2
Nucleus arcuatus	(NA)	2.9 ± 0.8
Nucleus ventromedialis, pars medialis	(NVMm)	trace (<0.1)
Nucleus ventromedialis, pars lateralis	(NVMl)	0.6 ± 0.5
Nucleus dorsomedialis	(NDM)	<0.05
Nucleus perifornicalis	(NPF)	<0.05
Area hypothalamica lateralis posterior	(AHLp)	<0.05
Nucleus hypothalamicus posterior	(NHP)	trace (<0.1)
Nucleus premamillaris dorsalis	(NPMd)	<0.05
Nucleus premamillaris ventralis	(NPMv)	<0.05

findings. A very small amount of LH-RH seemed to be present in the suprachiasmatic and supraoptic nuclei (less than 0.1 pg/µg protein). (It should also be mentioned that the rostral tip of the first subdivision of the arcuate nucleus is about 500 µ caudal to the suprachiasmatic nuclei. This subdivision contains a high concentration of LH-RH). The anterior hypothalamic nucleus, the paraventricular nuclei (8), and the medial preoptic nuclei (10) contained little or no LH-RH. It might be supposed that the bioassay methods measured (7,9–11) a component present in hypothalamic extracts other than LH-RH which could mobilize LH from the pituitary.

It is well known that the medial preoptic nuclei play an important role in the regulation of LH release. Damaging these nuclei or severing their connection with the arcuate nucleus (8) might influence the synthesis or release of LH-RH in the arcuate nucleus.

The existence of cell bodies which bind estrogen in the medial preoptic, arcuate and lateral part of the ventromedial nuclei has been demonstrated autoradiographically (21–23). The fact that estrogen-addressed cells are present in the medial preoptic nucleus in large numbers suggests again that this region is important in the regulation of LH-secretion. Demonstration of ^{3}H-estradiol accumulation in the arcuate nucleus probably indicates an estrogen feedback effect directly on the LH-RH producing cell bodies.

References

1. Szentagothai, J., B. Flerko, B. Mess, and B. Halasz, Hypothalamic Control of the Anterior Pituitary, Akademiai Kiado, Budapest, 1968, p. 249.
2. McCann, S. M., A. P. S. Dhariwal, and J. C. Porter, Ann Rev Physiol 30: 589, 1968.
3. Sawyer, C. H., In Haymaker, W., E. Anderson, and W. J. H. Nauta (eds.), The Hypothalamus, Charles C Thomas, Springfield, Ill., 1969, p. 389.
4. Davidson, J. M., In Ganong, W. F., and L. Martini (eds.), Frontiers in Neuroendocrinology, Oxford University Press, New York, 1969, p. 343.
5. Flerko, B., In Martini, L., M. Motta, and F. Fraschini (eds.), The Hypothalamus, Academic Press, New York, 1971, p. 351.
6. McCann, S. M., S. Taleisnik, and H. M. Friedman, Proc Soc Exp Biol Med 104: 432, 1960.
7. ————, Am J Physiol 202: 395, 1962.
8. Mess, B., F. Fraschini, M. Motta, and L. Martini, Proc. 2nd Int. Congr. Horm. Steroids, Excerpta Medica Int. Congr. Ser. 132: 1004, 1967.
9. Schneider, H. P. G., D. B. Crighton, and S. M. McCann, Neuroendocrinology 5: 271, 1969.
10. Crighton, D. B., H. P. G. Schneider, and S. M. McCann, Endocrinology 87: 323, 1970.
11. Quijada, M., L. Krulich, C. P. Fawcett, D. K. Sandberg, S. M. McCann, Fed Proc 30: 197, 1971.
12. Matsuo, H., Y. Baba, R. M. G. Nair, A. Arimura, and A. V. Schally, Biochem Biophys Res Commun 43: 1334, 1971.
13. Baba, Y., H. Matsuo, and A. V. Schally, Biochem Biophys Res Commun 44: 459, 1971.
14. Arimura, A., H. Sato, T. Kumasaka, R. B. Worobec, L. Debeljuk, J. Dunn, and A. V. Schally, Endocrinology 93: 1092, 1973.
15. Palkovits, M., Brain Res 59: 449, 1973.
16. ————, M. Brownstein, J. M. Saavedra, and J. Axelrod, Brain Res. (In press).
17. Lowry, O. H., N. J. Rosebrough, A. L. Ferrel, and R. J. Randall, J Biol Chem 193: 265, 1951.
18. Flament-Durand, J., and L. Desclin, In Martini, L., M. Motta, and F. Fraschini (eds.), The Hypothalamus, Academic Press, New York, 1971, p. 245.
19. Barry, J., M. P. Dubois, P. Poulain, and J. Leonardelli, C R Acad Sci [D] (Paris) 276: 3191, 1973.
20. Zimmerman, E. A., K. C. Hsu, M. Ferin, and G. P. Kozlowski, Endocrinology (In press).
21. Stumpf, W. E., Science 162: 1001, 1968.
22. ————, Am J Anat 129: 207, 1970.
23. Attramadal, A., Z Zellforsch 104: 572, 1970.

Pituitary Response to LHRH in Midtrimester Pregnancy

JAMES R. SOWERS, MD, MARTA COLANTINO, BS, JAMIL FAYEZ, MD, FACOG, and HARRY JONAS, MD, FACOG

The effects of luteinizing hormone releasing hormone (LHRH) on serum luteinizing hormone (LH), follicle stimulating hormone (FSH), prolactin (PRL), thyroid stimulating hormone (TSH), and growth hormone (GH) were studied in 10 women in the second trimester of pregnancy. Serum LH was measured using the LHβ-RIA, with the anti-βLH serum being preabsorbed with purified hCG. This assay was unaffected by hCG levels up to 500 IU/ml. Basal serum levels of LH were undetectable and basal FSH levels were low in these 10 women. No release of LH or FSH was observed after administration of 100 μg of LHRH. However, there was a statistically significant rise in PRL from mean basal levels of 139.9 ng/ml to a mean peak level of 159.0 ng/ml at 30 minutes after LHRH administration. Both TSH and GH displayed small elevations at 15 minutes after LHRH administration; however, these elevations were not significant because of the wide range in responses. The results of this study indicate that gonadotropin release is inhibited during the second trimester of pregnancy. Finally, it appears that pregnancy is a condition in which LHRH administration results in a nonspecific release of several hormones.

DURING PREGNANCY the levels of serum follicle stimulating hormone (FSH) and luteinizing hormone (LH) are lower than in normally menstruating women.[1-8] Studies on the responses of FSH to luteinizing hormone releasing hormone (LHRH) in pregnant women are contradictory. Some investigators have reported an FSH response to LHRH,[2] while others have reported no such response.[3-7] Measurements of maternal serum LH levels and LH responses to LHRH have been hindered by cross-reactivity with human chorionic gonadotropin (hCG). Generation of antiserums to the β subunit of LH has made it possible to specifically measure LH in the presence of high levels of hCG present during pregnancy.[8] Studies performed using the βLH assay have reported small LH responses to LHRH.[7,5] However, in one of these studies it was found that the LH response to LHRH was progressively inhibited as pregnancy advanced, being abolished after 12 weeks of pregnancy.[9]

The pituitary stimulating effects of LHRH in normal subjects have been found to be relatively specific for gonadotropin hormone release. However, some patients with acromegaly display growth hormone (GH) release in response to LHRH.[10] In pregnancy the hypothalamic-pituitary axis is markedly altered with suppression of gonadotropin release and enhanced prolactin (PRL) synthesis and release.[11] The present study was conducted to determine if the pituitary stimulating effects of LHRH are specific for gonadotropin release in pregnancy. Second, we have further examined the FSH and LH responses to LHRH in the midtrimester of pregnancy.

MATERIALS AND METHODS

Subjects and LHRH Administration

Ten women, ages 20–31, undergoing second-trimester abortions volunteered for the study. The women ranged in gestational age from 17 through 22 weeks and were on no medication during gestation. The women fasted overnight and an IV bolus of 100 μg LHRH was given at 8:00 AM. Baseline samples of blood (−15 and 0 minutes) were drawn through an indwelling 19-gauge needle, and further blood samples were obtained at 15, 30, 45, 60, and 90 minutes after injection. Serum was stored at −20 C and all measurements of each hormone were performed in duplicate in one assay to avoid interassay variability.

Assay Methods

Luteinizing hormone was measured by means of a double antibody radioimmunoassay (RIA) using βLH[125]I, a rabbit anti-human βLH antiserum and human pituitary preparation LER-907 as the assay standard.[12] The anti-βLH serum was preabsorbed with purified hCG, 50 IU/ml, according to previously described methods.[12] The minimal detectable level of LH was 15

From the Departments of Medicine, Endocrine Section, and Obstetrics and Gynecology at the University of Missouri, Kansas City, Missouri.
Submitted for publication March 29, 1978.

TABLE 1. MEAN SERUM LH AND FSH RESPONSES IN 10 WOMEN RECEIVING 100 μg LHRH

| Hormone | Basal level | Levels after administration of LHRH (min) |||||
		15	30	45	60	90
LH (ng/ml)	< 15	< 15	< 15	< 15	< 15	< 15
FSH (ng/ml)*	36 ± 5	37.5 ± 5	36 ± 5	41.5 ± 5	35.5 ± 5	40.5 ± 5

* Mean ± SD.

ng/ml. No cross-reaction was observed with the addition of hCG, 500 IU/ml. Serum FSH was measured by a double antibody RIA procedure,[13] using LER-907 as the assay standard. The minimal detectable level was 15 ng/ml. Serum PRL was measured by a homologous RIA previously described.[14] The sensitivity of the assay was 3.12 ng/ml and the intraassay coefficient of variation (CV) was 6%. Serum TSH was measured by a sensitive double antibody RIA previously described;[15] the mean basal TSH in normal individuals was 2.5 ± 1.0 (SD) μU/ml. There is no appreciable effect of hCG in the TSH assay at hCG concentrations of less than 100 IU/ml. Serum GH was measured by a double antibody RIA using reagents prepared by S.A. Berson and R. Yalow and distributed by the NIAMDD; the lower limit of sensitivity for the GH assay was approximately 0.4 ng/ml and the mean interassay coefficient of variation was 8.5%.

Statistical comparisons of hormone responses were made using the Student t test for paired data.

RESULTS

The mean basal levels (average of −15 and 0) of LH and FSH and the mean levels after administration of LHRH in the 10 subjects are shown in Table 1. The basal and stimulated LH levels were below the limit of assay detectability, thus, no response to LHRH was observed. Mean basal FSH levels were low but measurable, 36 ± 5 ng/ml, in these 10 subjects. There was no observable FSH response to LHRH at any sampling time through 90 minutes.

The basal PRL levels ranged from 75.5 to 272.5 ng/ml. Even though mean post-LHRH levels through 60 minutes were higher than the mean basal level (139.9 ± 20.6 ng/ml) (Figure 1), only the 30-minute mean value (159 ± 21.3 ng/ml) was significantly elevated ($P < 0.05$) above basal. Seven of the 10 subjects demonstrated a ΔPRL of at least 20 ng/ml at either the 15- or 30-minute sampling times. The basal TSH levels ranged from 1.8 to 3.8 μU/ml. Although the mean post-LHRH levels at all sampling times through 90 minutes were elevated above the mean basal level (2.9 ± 0.4 μU/ml) (Figure 2), the elevations were not significant because of the relatively large variations in TSH responses in the 10 subjects.

The basal GH levels ranged from 0.4 to 6 ng/ml. The 15- through 45-minute mean GH levels were higher than the mean basal GH levels (2.2 ± 0.6 ng/ml) (Figure 3). However, because of the wide range of GH responses, the elevations were not significant. The peak GH responses were significantly ($\gamma = 0.62$, $P < 0.01$) correlated with the basal GH levels. The growth hormone response (ΔGH) to LHRH correlated ($\gamma = 0.50$, $P < 0.05$) with the ΔPRL.

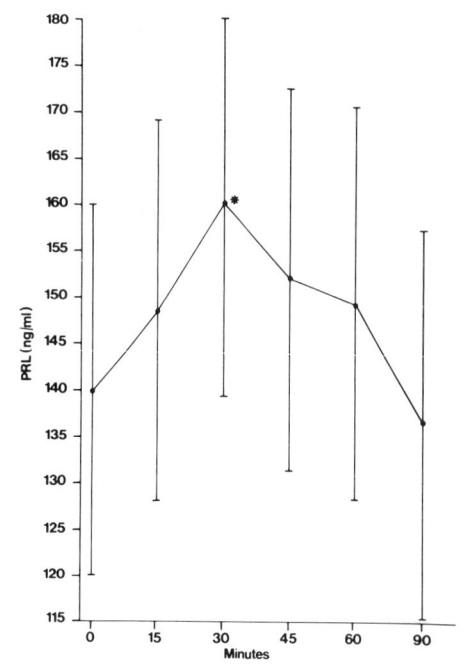

Fig 1. Mean (± SEM) serum PRL responses to LHRH (given at 0 time) in 10 women in midtrimester pregnancy; vertical bars show SEM. *A significant change from basal levels.

DISCUSSION

Results of the present study are in agreement with previous studies reporting low or undetectable basal levels of LH and FSH during the second trimester of pregnancy.[6,9] A higher level of immunoreactive serum FSH previously reported[2] is probably not of pituitary origin, since it does not behave like pituitary FSH on gel filtration or electrophoresis.[16] The absence of an FSH response to LHRH in the second trimester of pregnancy is in agreement with several previous studies.[4,6,7] Two previous studies have used a specific βLH assay to measure LH responses during pregnancy.[7,9] In both studies small, short-lived rises in LH levels were reported. However, when different stages of pregnancy were studied, it was found that LH responses to LHRH declined as pregnancy progressed, and were almost zero after 12 weeks of pregnancy.[17] The results of the present study also indicate an absence of LH response to LHRH after the first trimester of pregnancy. Thus, our findings, along with the observations of others, support the theory advanced over 40 years ago that increased circulating estrogen during pregnancy inhibits pituitary gonadotropin synthesis and secretion.[17] Similar diminutions in gonadotropin reserve have been observed in nonpregnant women and in men following estrogen administration.[18]

During pregnancy, the feedback mechanisms exerted by rising estradiol levels which result in diminished basal and LHRH stimulated gonadotropin levels also result in elevated basal PRL levels.[11] Women have higher basal levels of PRL and greater PRL responses to TRH[14] most likely related to a central estrogenic effect. Estrogen exerts both a direct PRL stimulatory effect on the pituitary and an indirect effect by depleting the hypothalamus of prolactin-inhibitory factor (PIF), thus removing hypothalamic inhibition of PRL release.[19] The nonspecific PRL response to LHRH observed in 7 of the 10 subjects in this study could possibly result from the abolition of the tonic inhibitory influence of PIF resulting from the high estradiol levels present during the midtrimester of pregnancy. The markedly elevated basal PRL and the nonspecific PRL response to LHRH during pregnancy is analogous to the elevated basal GH levels and the nonspecific GH response to TRH and LHRH observed in acromegalic subjects.[10,11] It is interesting that PRL responses to LHRH have also been observed in persons afflicted with acromegaly.[20]

Serum TSH responses to TRH are greater in women, probably because of the effects of estrogen.[21] Furthermore, the TSH response to TRH is highly correlated with basal TSH in euthyroid subjects.[21] In this study we observed a small elevation in TSH following LHRH in the midtrimester of pregnancy. This TSH response was not statistically significant because of the large range of responses in these 10 subjects. The small elevation of TSH cannot be accounted for on the basis of cross-reaction with hCG. There is essentially no cross-reaction

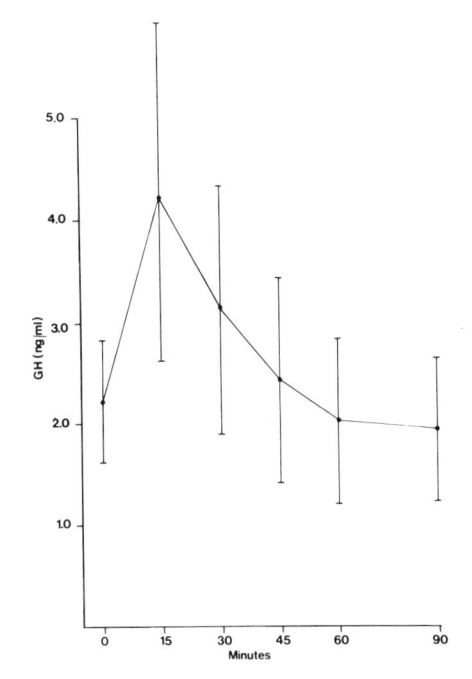

Fig 3. Mean ($\pm$ SEM) serum GH responses to LHRH (given at 0 time) in 10 women in midtrimester pregnancy; vertical bars show SEM.

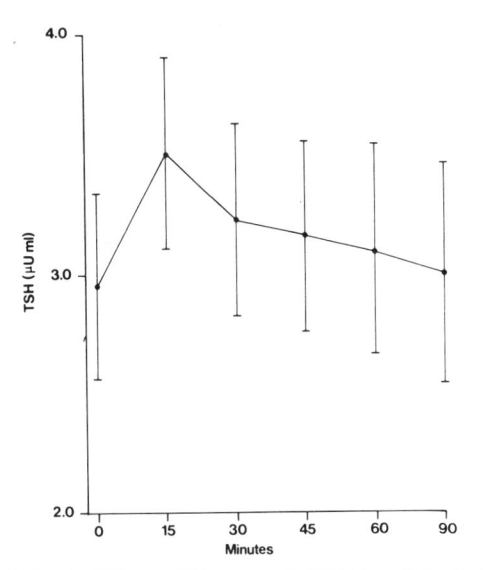

Fig 2. Mean ($\pm$ SEM) serum TSH responses to LHRH (given at 0 time) in 10 women in midtrimester pregnancy; vertical bars show SEM.

of hCG in our TSH assay at serum hCG concentrations of less than 100 U/ml. Furthermore, it has been previously shown that TRH does not cause release of hCG in pregnant women.[15] The small elevation in TSH following LHRH is more likely related to a nonspecific response of the pituitary thyrotropins due to an altered endocrine milieu during pregnancy.

Both basal and stimulated GH levels are reported to be lower in pregnancy than in nonpregnant women.[22,23] The mechanism of suppression of GH during pregnancy has been attributed to feedback inhibition by a structurally related substance, chorionic sommatomammotropin, produced by trophoblastic cells.[23] In view of the suppression of GH secretion that normally exists during pregnancy, it was interesting that there was a small elevation in serum GH during the first 45 minutes following administration of LHRH in 6 of our 10 subjects. The response of GH was significantly correlated with the PRL response to LHRH. In normal subjects estrogen pretreatment enhances both PRL and GH responses to a number of stimuli.[24] Thus, our finding of a small nonspecific GH response as well as a significant PRL response to LHRH during pregnancy might be explained by high levels of estrogen sensitizing pituitary cells to nonspecific releasing hormone stimuli.

REFERENCES

1. Mishell DR, Thorneycraft IH, Nagata Y, et al: Serum gonadotropin and steroid patterns in early human gestation. Am J Obstet Gynecol 117:631-639, 1973
2. Zarato A, Canales ES, Sorio J, et al: Pituitary responsiveness to synthetic luteinizing hormone-releasing hormone during pregnancy: Effect on follicle-stimulating hormone secretion. Am J Obstet Gynecol 116:1122-1123, 1973
3. Jeppson S, Rannevik G, Kullander S: Studies on the decreased gonadotropic response after administration of LH/FSH releasing hormone during pregnancy and the puerperium. Am J Obstet Gynecol 120:1029-1034, 1974
4. Nakano R, Kayashima F, Katayama K, et al: The radioimmunoassay of follicle-stimulating hormone (FSH) during human pregnancy; Serum concentration and response to luteinizing releasing factor (LRF). Acta Obstet Gynecol Scand 53:259-262, 1974
5. Soria J, Zarute A, Canales ES, et al: Serum FSH and synthetic LHRH response in pregnant women at term and in the newborn. Obstet Gynecol 47:80-82, 1976
6. Jeppson S, Rannevik G: Studies on the gonadotropin response after administration of LH/FSH-releasing hormone (LRH) during pregnancy and after therapeutic abortion in the second trimester. Am J Obstet Gynecol 125:484-490, 1976
7. Reyes FI, Winter JSD, Faiman C: Pituitary gonadotropin function during human pregnancy: Serum FSH and LH levels before and after LHRH administration. J Clin Endocrinol Metab 42:590-592, 1976
8. Varterkaitus JL, Ross GT, Reichert LE: Immunologic basic for within and between species cross-reactivity of luteinizing hormone. Endocrinology 91:1337-1342, 1972
9. Miyake A, Tanezawa O, Aono T, et al: Pituitary responses on LH secretion to LHRH during pregnancy. Obstet Gynecol 49:549-551, 1977
10. Faglia G, Beck-Peccoz P, Travaglini, et al: Elevations in plasma growth hormone concentration after luteinizing hormone-releasing hormone (LRH) in patients with active acromegaly. J Clin Endocrinol Metab 37:338-340, 1973
11. Martin JB, Reichlin S, Brown GM: Regulation of prolactin secretion and its disorders. Clinical Neuroendocrinology, FA Davis Company, 1977, pp 136-137
12. Dattatreyamurty B, Sheth AR, Purandare TV, et al: RIA of hLH in presence of hCG. Endocrinology 99:1554-1561, 1976
13. Midgley AR: Radioimmunoassay for follicle-stimulating hormone. J Clin Endocrinol Metab 27:295-299, 1967
14. Sowers JR, Hershman JM, Carlson HE, et al: Prolactin response to N^{3im}methyl-thyrotropin releasing hormone in euthyroid subjects. J Clin Endocrinol Metab 43:749-755, 1976
15. Hershman JM, Burrow GN: Lack of release of human chorionic gonadotropin by thyrotropin-releasing hormone. J Clin Endocrinol Metab 42:970-975, 1976
16. Talas M, Midgley AR, Jaffe RB: Regulation of human gonadotropins: XIV Gelfiltration and electrophorectic analysis of endogenous and extracted immuno-reactive human follicle-stimulating hormone of pituitary, serum and urinary origin. J Clin Endocrinol Metab 36:817-825, 1973
17. Van Dyke HB: The Physiology and Pharmacology of the Pituitary Body. Chicago, University of Chicago Press, 1936, pp 162
18. Thompson IE, Arfania J, Taymor ML: Effects of estrogen and progestrone on pituitary response to stimulation by luteinizing hormone releasing factor. J Clin Endocrinol Metab 37:152-155, 1973
19. Ratner A, Meites J: Depletion of prolactin inhibiting activity of rat hypothalamus by estradiol or suckling stimulus. Endocrinology 75:377-382, 1964
20. Catania A, Cantalamessa L, Reschini E: Plasma prolactin response to luteinizing hormone releasing hormone in acromegalic patients. J Clin Endocrinol Metab 43:689-691, 1976
21. Sowers JR, Hershman JM, Pekary AE: Effect of N^{3im} Methyl-thyrotropin releasing hormone on the human pituitary thyroid axis. J Clin Endocrinol Metab 43:741-748, 1976
22. Spellacy WN, Buhi WC, Birk SA: Human growth hormone and placental lactogen levels in midpregnancy and late postpartum. Obstet Gynecol 36:238-243, 1970
23. Mochizuki M, Morikawa H, Kawaguchi K, et al: Growth hormone, prolactin and chorionic somatomammotropin in normal and molar pregnancy. J Clin Endocrinol Metab 43:614-621, 1976
24. Merimee TJ, Rabinowitz D, Fineberg SE: Arginine-initiated release of human growth hormone. N Engl J Med 280:1434-1438, 1969

Part V
HYPOTHALAMIC-HYPOPHYSIAL CONTROL OF GROWTH HORMONE SECRETION

Editor's Comments
on Papers 36 Through 41

36   REICHLIN
Excerpts from *Growth and the Hypothalamus*

37   ROTH et al.
Secretion of Human Growth Hormone: Physiologic and Experimental Modification

38   BLACKARD and HEIDINGSFELTER
Excerpts from *Adrenergic Receptor Control Mechanism for Growth Hormone Secretion*

39   DEUBEN and MEITES
Excerpts from *Stimulation of Pituitary Growth Hormone Release by a Hypothalamic Extract* in Vitro

40   FROHMAN, BERNARDIS, and KANT
Hypothalamic Stimulation of Growth Hormone Secretion

41   WILBER and PORTER
Excerpts from *Thyrotropin and Growth Hormone Releasing Activity in Hypophysial Portal Blood*

    Reichlin (Paper 36) demonstrated that growth in rats in impaired following hypothalamic lesions. Lesions involving the median eminence, as well as ventral hypothalamic lesions, had the greatest effect on growth. This was the first significant direct evidence of hypothalamic regulation of growth hormone (GH) secretion. Although thyroidal and gonadal deficiencies were created by the lesions, these did not account for all growth retardation because physiological replacement with thyroxine and testosterone did not restore growth to normal.

    The concept of neural control of GH was further demonstrated by studies of stimulation and suppression of hypophyseal GH release. Roth et al. (Paper 37) established that GH secretion was stimulated by deprivation of intracellular glucose produced by absolute hypoglycemia or deoxyglucose administration, by exercise, as well as by falling blood glucose concentration. They also demonstrated that GH secretion is suppressed by glucose administration in normal subjects, but to a lesser extent in proven acromegalics. They suggested that the failure of GH to be lowered to normal levels after induction of hyperglycemia may be used as a specific test for acromegaly. They further demonstrated that, in a patient subjected to hypophyseal stalk section, induction of hyperglycemia failed to produce a normal reduction in plasma GH; marked hypoglycemia, induced by administration of insulin, failed to stimulate an increase in GH secretion. Thus, they showed that the integrity of neural or vascular connections between the hypothalamus and the hypophysis is necessary for responsiveness of GH secretion to changes in blood glucose concentration. These investigators developed and utilized a specific radioimmunoassay (RIA) of human GH for these studies. The development of the RIA for GH helped pave the way for development of the RIA technique for application in measurement of other hormones present in small quantities in the blood, with considerably greater sensitivity and specificity than could be achieved with other methods previously available.

Blackard and Heidingsfelter (Paper 38) demonstrated the existence of an adrenergic control mechanism for GH secretion, showing a stimulatory alpha- and inhibitory beta-adrenergic effect on GH secretion. Alpha-adrenergic blockade with phentolamine inhibited and beta-adrenergic blockade with propranolol enhanced GH response to insulin-induced hypoglycemia in normal subjects. They suggested that a number of GH-releasing stimuli, such as physical and mental stress, exercise, and hypoglycemia, may, at least in part, increase GH secretion through an alpha-adrenergic mediated mechanism.

Deuben and Meites (Paper 39) provided the first direct proof of the existence of an acid-extractable hypothalamic factor (GH-releasing factor) responsible for hypophyseal release of GH in vitro and in female rats. The crude acid extract of rat hypothalamus was found to stimulate release of four to six times as much GH from cultured rat hypophysis than the process of culturing the hypophyses without a hypothalamic extract or with a cerebral cortical extract. They found this acid extract of rat hypothalami to be relatively resistant to boiling and suggested that the GH-releasing factor was a small molecular weight polypeptide.

Frohman et al. (Paper 40) showed that electrical stimulation of the ventromedial nucleus, the arcuate nucleus, and the median eminence induced an increase in GH concentration in the plasma of rats. The same group of investigators had previously shown that destruction of the ventromedial hypothalamic nucleus (VMN) in weanling rats resulted in impaired growth associated with decreased GH levels in both the hypophysis and plasma. The results of these studies suggested that the

Editor's Comments on Papers 36 Through 41

hypothalamic locus involved in control of GH secretion is the ventromedial nucleus.

Wilber and Porter (Paper 41) used specific RIAs to measure GH and TSH released from adenohypophysial halves incubated with either portal or peripheral plasma. In comparison to peripheral plasma, the plasma from cut ends of hypophysial stalks caused a significantly greater release of GH and TSH, thus demonstrating the presence of GH- and TSH-releasing activities in portal plasma. In this study, unipolar electrode stimulation of the anterior hypothalamus did enhance TSH-, but not GH-, releasing activity in portal plasma.

36

Copyright © 1960 by J. B. Lippincott Company

Reprinted from pages 760, 769–773 of *Endocrinology*
67:760–773 (1960)

GROWTH AND THE HYPOTHALAMUS[1]

SEYMOUR REICHLIN

Departments of Medicine, Psychiatry and Preventive Medicine, Washington University School of Medicine, St. Louis, Missouri

ABSTRACT

Following certain hypothalamic lesions growth in rats is impaired. The localization of lesions responsible for this effect and the relation of growth impairment to well recognized lesion-induced endocrine deficiencies were studied in this experiment. Linear growth, tibial length and body weight change were measured in 71 male rats with hypothalamic lesions of various sizes and positions. Comparison was made with 71 paired control and 30 *ad libitum* fed animals. In certain subgroups "physiologic" replacement doses of L-thyroxine, corticosterone, DCA, testosterone propionate and Pitressin were administered. Relatively small lesions in any position were found to cause little growth disturbance, while large lesions reduced growth rate to levels significantly below that of paired controls. The most effective lesions were massive ones involving the anterior half of the median eminence. Although posterior lobe insufficiency and atrophy of the thyroid and the gonads were observed, lack of these hormones was not the cause of growth impairment since the defect persisted in spite of substitution treatment. Evidence was cited which suggests that adrenal dysfunction could also be excluded as a cause of poor growth. Based on this indirect evidence and on data in the literature the suggestion was advanced that growth hormone secretion is deficient in rats with hypothalamic lesions.

IN SEVERAL recent papers the suggestion has been made that the hypothalamus is involved in the regulation of growth hormone secretion in a manner analogous to the control it exerts over other anterior pituitary hormones. This view is based on a number of indirect lines of evidence from experiments in rats: growth impairment follows hypothalamic lesions (1–4), the insulin hypersensitivity caused by lesions is corrected by growth hormone administration (5) and the tibial epiphysial width is increased by treatment with Pitressin (6). Direct evidence of hypothalamic regulation of growth hormone secretion has not been adduced, however, nor has the anatomical region of the hypothalamus responsible for this effect been identified. This experiment, an extension of a previous study (4), was done in order to determine the localization of lesions responsible for growth impairment in rats, and the relation of growth impairment to the well established endocrine deficiencies that follow hypothalamic destruction.

[*Editor's Note:* Material has been omitted at this point, including tables 1 and 2 and figure 1.]

Received March 14, 1960.
[1] Supported by Grant B834, United States Public Health Service.

DISCUSSION

In these experiments it was found that certain hypothalamic lesions led to poor growth in rats. In some individuals poor growth was the result of reduced food intake, but reduced food intake could be only a contributory cause. In many animals the amount of food taken was enough to permit normal growth when given to unoperated animals, and in a number reduction in rate of body lengthening occurred in the face of increasing obesity. Furthermore, in lesion-bearing animals with slightly reduced food intake linear growth was less than that of normal animals whose diet had been similarly restricted. It must be concluded that rats with lesions have a distinct defect in growth independent of variations in diet. The defect is never as great as that found in hypophysectomized rats, for even with almost total hypothalamectomy, growth is seldom reduced by more than 50% of the normal rate. Thyroidal, gonadal and neurohypophysial deficiencies in rats with lesions may also contribute to poor growth. That they are not the sole cause of growth impairment is evident from the finding that physiological doses of thyroxine, testosterone and Pitressin did not restore growth to normal.

Lesion-induced adrenocortical deficiency as a cause of growth impairment, though not specifically studied in Experiments II and III, can probably be excluded for reasons summarized below. Evidence on this point must be cited in detail in view of the long recognized fact that adrenalectomized rats lose weight unless they are given sodium chloride or replacement steroid therapy (15). Close analysis of the growth failure of adrenalectomized rats indicates that the major handicap to growth in these animals is inadequate food intake. Adrenalectomized rats consume much less food than normal; when the intake of normal rats is restricted to the same degree by pair feeding, the normal rats lose even more weight than do the adrenalectomized animals (7). Saline replacement leads to an increase in the food intake of adrenalectomized rats though not to normal levels; the saline treated animals grow faster than do pair-fed normals (7), and have wider tibial epiphysial widths (16). When saline-treated adrenalectomized rats are force fed normal amounts of food they grow at a slightly greater than normal rate and have a normal body composition (17).

From the above data it may be concluded that if salt balance and food intake are maintained, rats with total adrenal deficiency grow at least as well if not better than do normal animals consuming equal amounts of food. This conclusion is pertinent to the present experiments because controls were offered the same amount of food as was consumed by the rats with lesions, and, in all pairs, the animals with brain damage ate as much as or more than the normal animals. Since food intake was controlled the other critical point is whether or not these animals were in salt balance. A number of studies of salt metabolism in animals with ventral hypothalamic lesions have been published (18, 19, 20) but the most specific answer to this question comes from experiments recently completed in this laboratory. In a group of 17 pairs of rats prepared and treated in a manner identical with Experiment III in the present study plasma sodium and potassium levels were determined at death; these values were found to be the same in the two groups. Although it would have been more elegant to conduct the experiments on all groups using adrenalectomized rats on replacement steroid treatment (as in Experiment I) the foregoing arguments make it highly unlikely that the poor growth observed in these animals could have been due to adrenocortical deficiency.

The anatomical location of lesions that affect growth was specifically sought in this experiment. The conclusion was drawn that the anterior half of the median eminence or the pituitary stalk must be destroyed or the infundibulum isolated from the hypothalamus in order to produce severe growth impairment (Fig. 1). Regions uniformly involved in rats with more severe degrees of growth reduction are the anterior half of the median eminence, the arcuate nuclei, and the supraoptic hypophysial tract as it courses through the median eminence. This region appears to be similar or identical with that controlling acute ACTH discharge following stress (21), and the great majority of animals with growth impairment have significant reduction in adrenal gland size also. Specific areas and structures can be excluded from consideration. These include: anterior commissure, fornix, preoptic area, mammillo-thalamic tract, and the following nuclei: supraoptic, paraventricular, suprachiasmatic, posterior, dorsal, anterior, ventromedial and mammillary. Destruction limited to the area between paraventricular nucleus and optic chiasm, the "thyrotrophic area" (4), does not necessarily prevent growth at a normal rate in rats given thyroxine.

Of the authors who have previously described growth impairment in rats with lesions, only Hinton and Stevenson (3) have noted a specific localization, and that to the anterior hypothalamus. Their studies differ further from the present experiment in that the onset of growth impairment was delayed for several weeks following operation. A different mechanism of growth reduction may be involved in the rats studied by these authors, one possibility being (in view of the position of the lesion and the delay in onset of the effect) that hypothyroidism was induced by the lesion. In Kennedy's experiments (2) no specific localization of lesions affecting growth was possible and localization was not mentioned by Bogdanove and Lipner (1). In a presumably related study by Spirtos and Halmi (5) in which insulin hypersensitivity in rats with lesions was observed, it is stated: "The most effective lesions were, in general, massive basal ones which extended rostro-caudally from the optic chiasm to the pre-mammillary region." These lesions are probably comparable to the ones found effective in reducing growth rate in this experiment. Spirtos and Halmi further note that ". . . smaller lesions, some of them even unilateral which damaged only the anterior or posterior hypothalamus also resulted in enhanced sensitivity to insulin." Growth impairment did not occur in this experiment with lesions of this distribution, but consideration must be given to the possibility that if growth impairment and insulin hypersensitivity are manifestations of a similar defect, the carbohydrate abnormality may be the more sensitive measure.

The most important problem raised by this localization of a growth-affecting hypothalamic lesion is that of distinguishing between a specific neural defect and non-specific damage to the major portion of the primary portal plexus through which in the rat passes most of the blood to the anterior pituitary (22). From India ink injections in this and a previous experiment (4), it is clear that the pituitary is well perfused even when lesions involve the median eminence, but there may be a physiologically important reduction in rate of hypophysial blood flow or disorganization of specific nerve terminals in this area. In one rat, the infundibulum had been isolated by the lesion, so that a flat vascular plate of median eminence tissue connected to the stalk was left. Growth in this animal was between 50 and 60% of the rate of its paired control despite a normal primary plexus. Reduced pituitary size as observed in this study cannot be taken as clear evidence of disturbed glandular blood flow since similar reduction followed lesions that did not affect any part of the pituitary vasculature in Experiment II (Table 1). If the impaired growth of rats with median eminence lesions is due simply to change in blood supply the animal preparation is then quite comparable to the rat with an extra-sellar pituitary transplant. Such animals may display a reasonable rate of growth as demonstrated by Hertz (23).

The relationship between disordered neurohypophysial function and growth impairment requires further comment. In rats whose lesions had caused growth impairment the supraoptic nuclei showed regressive changes and the supraopticohypophysial tract was invariably damaged. Vasopressin deficiency may be excluded as the cause of poor growth, nevertheless, by the failure of Pitressin in dosage controlling diabetes insipidus to influence rate of growth. Although a correlation exists between the degree of diabetes insipidus and the degree of growth impairment as was observed in this and a previous experiment (4), it is likely that the correlation arises because increasing damage to the median eminence also leads to increasingly severe damage to the neurohypophysial component of this area.

Neither this experiment nor others in the literature provide direct evidence for the suggestion that growth hormone secretion is influenced by the hypothalamus but the findings in this experiment are consonant with this hypothesis. Also in keeping with this hypothesis are the observations that regressive changes in the pituitary acidophils are observed in animals with lesions (5), and that the insulin sensitivity of these animals is corrected by STH more readily than by adrenocortical hormones (5). Of possible pertinence to the problem of hypothalamic regulation of STH secretion is the interesting observation by Del Vecchio *et al.* (6) that Pitressin injections induce an increase in tibial epiphysial width in the rat. Before one may conclude with certainty that hypothalamic lesions interfere with growth hormone secretion it would be essential to study production and release of the hormone directly and to demonstrate that the growth deficit is repaired by growth hormone treatment. Studies of this nature are underway at present in this laboratory.

Acknowledgment

The technical assistance of Joseph G. Brown and Mrs. Mary Ann Davies is gratefully acknowledged.

REFERENCES

1. Bogdanove, E. M., and H. L. Lipner: *Proc. Soc. Exper. Biol. & Med.* **81**: 410. 1952.
2. Kennedy, G. C.: *J. Endocrinol.* **16**: 9. 1957.
3. Hinton, G. G. and J. A. F. Stevenson: *Fed. Proc.* **18**: 69. 1959.
4. Reichlin, S.: *Endocrinology* **66**: 340. 1960.
5. Spirtos, B. N. and N. S. Halmi: *Endocrinology* **65**: 669. 1959.
6. Del Vecchio, A., E. Genovese and L. Martini: *Proc. Soc. Exper. Biol. & Med.* **98**: 641. 1958.
7. Reichlin, S. and J. G. Brown: *Am. J. Physiol.* 199: 217. 1960.
15. Hartman, F. A. and G. W. Thorn: *Proc. Soc. Exper. Biol. & Med.* **28**: 94. 1930.
16. Buffett, R. F. and L. C. Wyman: *Am. J. Physiol.* **180**: 16. 1955.
17. Cohn, C., E. Shrago and D. Joseph: *Am. J. Physiol.* **180**: 503. 1955.
18. Daily, W. J. R. and W. F. Ganong: *Endocrinology* **62**: 442. 1958.
19. Davis, J. O., R. C. Bahn, N. A. Yankopoulos, B. Kliman and R. E. Peterson: *Am. J. Physiol.* **197**: 380. 1959.
20. Keeler, R.: *Am. J. Physiol.* **197**: 847. 1959.
21. McCann, S. M.: *Am. J. Physiol.* **175**: 13. 1953.
22. Worthington, W. C., Jr.: *Endocrinology* **66**: 19. 1960.
23. Hertz, R.: *Endocrinology* **65**: 926. 1959.

Secretion of Human Growth Hormone: Physiologic and Experimental Modification

By Jesse Roth, Seymour M. Glick, Rosalyn S. Yalow
and Solomon A. Berson

Human growth hormone (HGH) in plasma was measured by radioimmunoassay. In normal subjects, the rate of secretion of HGH was markedly stimulated by (a) hypoglycemia; (b) intracellular deprivation of glucose produced by administration of deoxyglucose; (c) (occasionally) during a rapid fall in blood sugar concentration even in the absence of hypoglycemia; (d) after prolonged fasting; (e) after muscular exercise. In markedly obese subjects, (c), (d) and (e) were without notable effect but insulin-induced hypoglycemia was associated with a striking increase in plasma HGH. Administration of glucose to normal subjects suppresses HGH secretion.

EMPLOYING a sensitive and specific immunoassay for human growth hormone (HGH) in plasma, we have shown[1] that insulin-induced hypoglycemia in normal adults is followed shortly by a marked increase in plasma HGH concentration and that plasma HGH rises significantly on prolonged fasting and falls after feeding.

Further studies have revealed (table 1):

(1) Hypoglycemia induced by fructose in a sensitive subject was accompanied by high plasma HGH concentrations, although plasma insulin was low or undetectable. Similar findings in patients with hypoglycemia associated with nonpancreatic mesenchymal tumors were reported previously.[1]

(2) Administration of glucose to normal subjects produced an abrupt fall in plasma HGH from levels observed after an overnight fast. The subsequent decline of blood sugar concentration was followed by a striking increase in plasma HGH; in some cases the secondary rise in plasma HGH occurred while the blood sugar was falling rapidly but had not yet fallen to or below fasting levels.

(3) Inhibition of cellular utilization of glucose in a normal subject by means of 2-deoxy-D-glucose was followed by hyperglycemia and a marked increase in plasma HGH.

From the Radioisotope Service, Veterans Administration Hospital, Bronx, New York. Received for publication May 14, 1963.

PLASMA HGH (mμg/ml.) IN LARGE BOLD FIGURES
BLOOD GLUCOSE (mg / 100ml.) IN SMALL LIGHT FIGURES

EXPERIMENTAL CONDITION	SUBJECT	0	30	60	90	120	180	240	300	360
GLUCOSE 100 gm P.O. AT 0 MINUTES	NORMAL (4)	3 88 1 88 50 82 1.5 80	1 128 <1 122 6 102 1 115	<1 138 <1 121 3 90 <1 65	<1 97 3 97 2 78 91	<1 100 3 120 1 87 <1 91	<1 90 2 72 2 76 <1 71	2 79 14 83 15 84 1 71	4 82 40 76 12 80 45 76	2 70 3 85 2 87 25 92
	MILD DIABETES (1)	3 94	2 118	<1 174	1 131	2 128	2 134	1 110	14 60	>50 79
	MARKED OBESITY (2)	<1 80 <1 90	<1 111 <1 117	<1 130 <1 129	<1 132 <1 126	<1 107 <1 125	1 101 <1 117	<1 102 <1 64	1 68 <1 74	<1 64 <1 76
	ACRO-MEGALY (1)	195 96	240 161	200 208	120 170	250 115	180 64			
GLUCOSE I.V. 1gm/min. FOR 90 MINUTES & GLUCAGON 1mg I.V. AT 30 MIN. & AT 60 MIN.	NORMAL (4)	<1 71 4 78 5 78 <1 84	1 167	1 194 2 364 2 312 <1 200	294 <1 406 330 <1 239	3 169 3 300 3 124 <1 101	>50 42 >50 98 >50 54 >50 42	>50 61 >50 43 50 61 >50 48		
GLUCOSE & GLUCAGON IV (as above) INSULIN 0.1 U/kg at 120 min.	STALK SECTION (1)	3 80	2 336	3		1 592	1 336	<1 66	1 42	
GLUCOSE 100 gm P.O. at 0 min. - GLUCOSE & GLUCAGON I.V. (as above) from 180-270 min.	ACRO-MEGALY (1)	170 82	120 176	85 112		110 120	80 108	140 218	150 53	50
2 DEOXY-D-GLUCOSE 60 mg/kg. I.V. 0-30 min.	NORMAL (1)	4 78	14 78	>40 105	>40 105	>40 200				
FRUCTOSE 60 gm. P.O.	FRUCTOSE INDUCED HYPO-GLYCEMIA (1)	8 86	7 63	25 56	13 47		• (140 min. = >50 82) ▲ (150 min. = >50 167)			

Table 1.

(4) In normal subjects, moderate exercise, unaccompanied by detectable changes in blood sugar concentration, was followed by a significant increase in plasma HGH concentration and by the subsequent appearance of acetonuria.

(5) In 2 markedly obese subjects, neither prolonged fasting nor exercise was followed by significant changes in plasma HGH. The appearance of acetonuria was delayed during prolonged fasting; acetonuria was not detected after exercise. In contrast to normal subjects there was no late rise in plasma HGH following ingestion of glucose. Insulin-induced hypoglycemia did, however, produce an increase in plasma HGH comparable to that observed in normal subjects.

(6) Unlike 22 patients subjected to total hypophysectomy for nonpituitary disorders, none of whom had measurable plasma HGH, a woman subjected to pituitary stalk section showed HGH concentrations in the range 2 to 5 mμg./ml. on repeated analyses of several plasma samples. Sustained hyperglycemia produced only a sluggish reduction in plasma HGH; marked hypoglycemia, induced by insulin, failed to stimulate an increase in plasma HGH concentration.

(7) Insulin-induced hypoglycemia in acromegalic subjects produced a rise in HGH levels beyond the high basal levels.

(8) Hyperglycemia following the administration of glucose to acromegalic subjects was followed by a fall in plasma HGH, which, however, failed to reach normal levels. Failure

of plasma HGH to reach normal levels after prolonged hyperglycemia may be a specific test for acromegaly.

In summary, the mechanism responsible for stimulating secretion of growth hormone is sensitive not only to a) obvious deprivation of intracellular glucose produced by absolute hypoglycemia or deoxyglucose administration but also to b) a rapidly falling blood glucose concentration, c) fasting and d) muscular exercise. Conversely, GH secretion is abruptly suppressed by glucose administration.

The integrity of neural or vascular connections between the hypothalamus and the pituitary appears to be necessary for responsiveness of growth hormone secretion to changes in blood glucose.

Taking cognizance of Raben's demonstration that administration of growth hormone results in rapid release of fatty acids from adipose tissue,[2] we interpret the results presented here as follows: endogenous plasma growth hormone concentrations are strikingly increased in a variety of physiologic and experimental conditions known to be associated with high concentrations of unesterified fatty acids in plasma. Thus, hypoglycemia, exercise, fasting and interference with glucose utilization by means of deoxyglucose are all followed by secretion of growth hormone, a response that provides for increased availability of a noncarbohydrate source of oxidizable substrates, namely, fatty acids. The observations presented here also suggest that consideration be given to the possibility that the diabetogenic and protein-anabolic effects of growth hormone are likewise concerned with the day to day and even hour to hour regulation of metabolic activities.

Marked obesity is associated with, and possibly conditioned by, a deficient secretory response of pituitary growth hormone to certain physiologic stimuli, a defect that is expressed in the failure to metabolize fat normally.

REFERENCES

1. Roth, J., Glick, S., Yalow, R. S., and Berson, S. A.: Hypoglycemia: A potent stimulus to secretion of growth hormone. Science In press.
2. Raben, M. S., and Hollenberg, C. H.: Effect of growth hormone on fatty acids. J. Clin. Invest. 38:484, 1959.

Adrenergic Receptor Control Mechanism for Growth Hormone Secretion

WILLIAM G. BLACKARD and SYLVIA A. HEIDINGSFELDER

From the Department of Medicine, Louisiana State University School of Medicine, New Orleans, Louisiana 70112

ABSTRACT The influence of catecholamines on growth hormone secretion has been difficult to establish previously, possibly because of the suppressive effect of the induced hyperglycemia on growth hormone concentrations. In this study, an adrenergic receptor control mechanism for human growth hormone (HGH) secretion was uncovered by studying the effects of alpha and beta receptor blockade on insulin-induced growth hormone elevations in volunteer subjects.

Alpha adrenergic blockade with phentolamine during insulin hypoglycemia, 0.1 U/kg, inhibited growth hormon elevations to 30–50% of values in the same subjects during insulin hypoglycemia without adrenergic blockade. More complete inhibition by phentolamine could not be demonstrated at a lower dose of insulin (0.05 U/kg). Beta adrenergic blockade with propranolol during insulin hypoglycemia significantly enhanced HGH concentrations in paired experiments. The inhibiting effect of alpha adrenergic receptor blockade on HGH concentrations could not be attributed to differences in blood glucose or free fatty acid values; however, more prolonged hypoglycemia and lower plasma free fatty acid values may have been a factor in the greater HGH concentrations observed during beta blockade. In the absence of insulin induced hypoglycemia, neither alpha nor beta adrenergic receptor blockade had a detectable effect on HGH concentrations. Theophylline, an inhibitor of cyclic 3'5'-AMP phosphodiesterase activity, also failed to alter plasma HGH concentrations.

These studies demonstrate a stimulatory effect of alpha receptors and a possible inhibitory effect of beta receptors on growth hormone secretion.

INTRODUCTION

Many of the stimuli for growth hormone secretion such as physical and surgical stress (1, 2), psychic stress (2), exercise (2), 2-deoxyglucose (1), hypoglycemia (1), histamine (3), vasopressin (4), and pyrogen (5) result in increased catecholamine concentrations in blood and tissues (2, 6–10). The control of pituitary growth hormone secretion by the hypothalamus is now widely accepted and recent evidence has shown that at least one of the above mentioned stimuli caused a discharge of growth hormone–releasing factor from the hypothalamus (11). As the catecholamine content of the hypothalamus is higher than that of any other central nervous system structure (12), the possibility that the effect of these stimuli on growth hormone secretion may be mediated by catecholamines must be considered.

The role of epinephrine in the control of growth hormone secretion has been controversial. Two groups of investigators (13, 14) have detected a stimulatory effect of epinephrine on growth hormone secretion while other investigators have been unable to demonstrate elevated growth hormone concentrations after epinephrine administration (2, 6, 15, 16). Perhaps epinephrine-induced hyperglycemia masked a stimulatory effect of the hormone on growth hormone secretion in the negative studies since hyperglycemia suppresses plasma growth hormone concentrations (1).

The present investigation was performed (a) to determine the effect of catecholamines on growth hormone secretion under conditions in which hyperglycemia could not mask a stimulatory effect, (b) to characterize any observed effect in terms of alpha and beta adrenergic receptors, and (c) to assess the role of endogenous catecholamines on the plasma growth hormone response to insulin hypoglycemia. Administration of alpha and beta adrenergic blocking agents during insulin hypoglycemia to determine their effect on plasma human growth hormone (HGH) elevations proved a suitable experimental design for these purposes.

[Editor's Note: Material has been omitted at this point.]

DISCUSSION

The effect of catecholamines on growth hormone secretion has been controversial (2, 6, 13–16). In the present study, partial inhibition of the growth hormone response to hypoglycemia by alpha adrenergic blockade with phentolamine would tend to indicate a stimulatory effect of catecholamines on growth hormone secretion. In previous investigations showing no effect (6, 15) or even some inhibition (2, 16) of growth hormone concentrations in response to epinephrine, catecholamine-induced hyperglycemia may have suppressed growth hormone secretion. By utilizing endogenous catecholamines released as a result of hypoglycemia for the blocking experiments in this investigation, we avoided the possible masking effect of hyperglycemia on plasma HGH concentrations.

The influence of catecholamines on growth hormone secretion might be exerted anywhere along the hypothalamic-hypophyseal axis and even perhaps at higher centers, but the hypothalamus seems the most likely site. Although the effect of hypoglycemia on growth hormone secretion may be only partially mediated by catecholamines, present evidence suggests that hypoglycemia initiates a growth hormone response by stimulating a discharge of growth hormone–releasing factor (GHRF) from the hypothalamus. Hypoglycemia depresses GHRF content in the rat hypothalamus (11) and increases plasma GHRF in hypophysectomized rats (21). The hypothalamus is rich in adrenergic neurons (22) for which catecholamines are the neurohumoral transmitters and it is tempting to postulate that the neurons which detect depression of blood glucose and stimulate release of GHRF are adrenergic. Although there is no complete agreement as to the site of GHRF production, recent data suggest that the ventromedial nucleus of the hypothalamus is essential for growth hormone secretion (23). The fact that the ventromedial nucleus is one of the few catecholamine-poor areas of the hypothalamus (22) makes it unlikely that this nucleus is stimulated directly by adrenergic neurons. However, the adrenergic tone of other areas of the hypothalamus may influence the ventromedial nucleus if indeed this is the source of GHRF. As the blood brain barrier for catecholamines present in most areas of the brain does not exist in the hypothalamus (24), circulating catecholamines from the adrenal medulla and other peripheral sources may be at least partly responsible for the growth hormone response during hypoglycemia.

It can not be concluded from the present experiments that the effect of hypoglycemia on growth hormone secretion is entirely mediated by catecholamines since complete inhibition of HGH response could not be achieved with phentolamine. The growth hormone secretory mechanism is apparently sensitive to changes in blood glucose and not just to catecholamines released by hypoglycemia since elevations of blood glucose suppress HGH secretion (1). Catecholamines may merely modify the stimulatory effect of hypoglycemia on HGH release. Investigations by Sutin have shown an effect of insulin hypoglycemia on the evoked electrical potential recorded from a probe in the ventromedial nucleus of the hypothalamus after stimulation of the amygdala and septal nuclei (25). These changes in electrical potential from the ventromedial nucleus could be reproduced by injection of norepinephrine into the nucleus (26). Norepinephrine modified the amplitude of electrical response in the ventromedial nucleus to stimuli from other nuclei but did not initiate a response.

The stimulatory effect of catecholamines on growth hormone secretion has important implications as practically all of the recognized stimuli for growth hormone secretion, with the exception of amino acid infusion and estrogens, invoke a catecholamine response. Even small decreases in blood glucose (less than 10 mg/100 ml) which have been reported to elevate plasma HGH are accompanied by increased urinary catecholamines (6). In addition, the sympathetic tone in the hypothalamus may be important in the secretory regulation of other pituitary hormones. Hypothalamic catecholamine-depleting agents such as reserpine have been shown to influence gonadotropin secretion (27) as well as to inhibit the growth hormone response to hypoglycemia (28). Vasopressin secretion also is probably modified by adrenergic tone in the hypothalamus (29).

The present study characterized the growth hormone response to catecholamines in terms of alpha and beta adrenergic receptors. During insulin hypoglycemia the inhibitory effect of alpha blockade on growth hormone secretion was pronounced while the stimulatory effect of beta blockade was less impressive and was associated with more prolonged hypoglycemia and lower plasma FFA concentrations. More prolonged hypoglycemia probably was not responsible for the enhanced HGH response during beta blockade as studies in monkeys during insulin hypoglycemia have shown that growth hormone hypersecretion occurs while blood glucose concentrations are falling but return to normal even though plasma glucose concentrations remain depressed (30). Limited data on the effect of plasma FFA on growth hormone levels are available. Schalch and Kipnis were unable to demonstrate an effect of plasma FFA elevations on plasma HGH concentrations in three subjects given a fat meal followed by heparin (31). However, preliminary data from Dr. K. Shizume in Tokyo (personal communication) have suggested that elevations of plasma growth hormone concentrations by nicotinic acid may be related to the fall in plasma FFA. Data by Abramson, Arky, and Woeber, which showed a modest increase in hypoglycemia-induced plasma HGH elevations during beta adrenergic blockade, support our findings (32).

The present studies demonstrate a definite stimulatory effect of alpha adrenergic receptors and a possible inhibitory effect of beta adrenergic receptors on growth hormone secretion. This pattern is the opposite of the adrenergic control mechanism for insulin secretion where it has been shown that alpha receptors inhibit (33) and beta receptors stimulate (34) insulin release. Since the predominant effect of catecholamines on hormonal regulation appear to be through alpha receptors, another remarkable homeostatic mechanism to maintain the constancy of the internal milieu is observed. During hypoglycemia, catecholamines inhibit insulin secretion and assist in promoting a rise in plasma HGH which antagonizes the action of insulin and also increases plasma FFA which may be used for energy requirements.

The lack of effect of adrenergic blockade or theophylline, an inhibitor of cyclic 3'5'-AMP phosphodiesterase activity, on plasma HGH concentrations in the absence of hypoglycemia probably negates a significant role of the adrenergic nervous system in control of resting plasma HGH levels.

ACKNOWLEDGMENTS

We would like to acknowledge the capable technical assistance of Miss Thelma Cameron.

This paper was supported by grant AM-10151-01 from the National Institutes of Health.

REFERENCES

1. Roth, J., S. M. Glick, P. Cuatrecasas, and C. S. Hollander. 1967. Acromegaly and other disorders of growth hormone secretion. *Ann. Internal Med.* 66: 760.

2. Schalch, D. S. 1967. The influence of physical stress and exercise on growth hormone and insulin secretion in man. *J. Lab. Clin. Med.* 69: 256.
3. Meyer, V., and E. Knobil. 1966. Stimulation of growth hormone secretion by vasopressin in the Rhesus monkey. *Endocrinology*. 79: 1016.
4. Gagliardino, J. J., J. D. Bailey, and J. M. Martin. 1967. Effect of vasopressin on serum-levels of human growth hormone. *Lancet*. 1: 1357.
5. Kohler, P. O., B. W. O'Malley, P. L. Rayford, M. B. Lipsett, and W. D. Odell. 1967. Effect of pyrogen on blood levels of pituitary trophic hormones. Observations on the usefulness of the growth hormone response in the detection of pituitary disease. *J. Clin. Endocrinol. Metab.* 27: 219.
6. Luft, R., E. Cerasi, L. L. Madison, U. S. von Euler, L. D. Casa, and A. Roovete. 1966. Effect of a small decrease in blood-glucose on plasma-growth-hormone and urinary excretion of catecholamines in man. *Lancet*. 2: 254.
7. Statt, W. H., and M. B. Chenoweth. 1966. Release of catecholamines by vasopressin into the cavernous sinus blood of the dog. *Proc. Soc. Exptl. Biol. Med.* 123: 785.
8. Sanford, J. P., J. A. Barnett, and C. Gott. 1960. A mechanism of the glycogenolytic action of bacterial endotoxin. *J. Exptl. Med.* 112: 97.
9. Laszlo, J., W. R. Harlan, R. F. Klein, N. Kirshner, E. H. Estes, Jr., and M. D. Bogdonoff. 1961. The effect of 2-deoxy-D-glucose infusions on lipid and carbohydrate metabolism in man. *J. Clin. Invest.* 40: 171.
10. Kellaway, C. H., and S. J. Cowell. 1922. On the concentration of the blood and the effects of histamine in adrenal insufficiency. *J. Physiol.* 57: 82.
11. Katz, S. H., A. P. S. Dhariwal, and S. M. McCann. 1967. Effect of hypoglycemia on the content of pituitary growth hormone (GH) and hypothalamic growth hormone-releasing factor (GHRF) in the rat. *Endocrinology*. 81: 333.
12. Carlsson, A. 1959. The occurrence, distribution, and physiological role of catecholamines in the nervous system. *Pharmacol. Rev.* 11: 490.
13. Gagliardino, J. J., and J. M. Martin. 1967. Mechanism of growth hormone secretion. *In* Program of the 49th Meeting. The Endocrine Society. 74. (Abstr.)
14. Meyer, V., and E. Knobil. 1966. The acute elevation of plasma growth hormone concentration in response to various stimuli. *Federation Proc.* 25: 379. (Abstr.)
15. Roth, J., S. M. Glick, R. S. Yalow, and S. A. Berson. 1963. Hypoglycemia: a potent stimulus to secretion of growth hormone. *Science*. 140: 987.
16. Rabinowitz, D., T. J. Merimee, J. A. Burgess, and L. Riggs. 1966. Growth hormone and insulin release after arginine: indifference to hyperglycemia and epinephrine. *J. Clin. Endocrinol. Metab.* 26: 1170.
17. Saifer, A., and S. Gerstenfeld. 1958. The photometric microdetermination of blood glucose with glucose oxidase. *J. Lab. Clin. Med.* 51: 448.
18. Trout, D. L., E. H. Estes, Jr., and S. J. Friedberg. 1960. Titration of free fatty acids of plasma: a study of current methods and a new modification. *J. Lipid Res.* 1: 199.
19. Schalch, D. S., and M. L. Parker. 1964. A sensitive double antibody immunoassay for human growth hormone in plasma. *Nature*. 203: 1141.
20. Frohman, L. A., E. Z. Ezdinli, and R. Javid. 1967. Effect of vagotomy and vagal stimulation on insulin secretion. *Diabetes*. 16: 443.
21. Krulich, L., and S. M. McCann. 1966. Evidence for the presence of growth hormone-releasing factor in blood of hypoglycemic hypophysectomized rats. *Proc. Soc. Exptl. Biol. Med.* 122: 668.
22. Shute, C. C. D., and P. R. Lewis. 1966. Cholinergic and monoaminergic pathways in the hypothalamus. *Brit. Med. Bull.* 22: 221.
23. Bernardis, L. L., and L. A. Frohman. 1967. Plasma and pituitary growth hormone levels in rats with hypothalamic lesions. Program of the 49th Meeting. The Endocrine Society. 86. (Abstr.)
24. Weil-Malherbe, H. 1960. The passage of catechol amines through the blood-brain barrier. Adrenergic mechanisms. CIBA Foundation Symposium. J. R. Vane, G. E. W. Wolstenholme, and M. O'Connor, editors. Little, Brown and Co., Boston. 421.
25. Sutin, J. 1963. An electrophysiological study of the hypothalamic ventromedial nucleus in the cat. *Electroencephalog. Clin. Neurophysiol.* 15: 786.
26. van Orden, L. S., and J. Sutin. 1963. Differential effects of norepinephrine on responses evoked in the hypothalamic ventromedial nucleus. *Electroencephalog. Clin. Neurophysiol.* 15: 796.
27. Lippmann, W., R. Leonardi, J. Ball, and J. A. Coppola. 1967. Relationship between hypothalamic catecholamines and gonadotrophin secretion in rats. *J. Pharmacol. Exptl. Therap.* 156: 258.
28. Müller, E. E., S. Sawano, A. Arimura, and A. V. Schally. 1967. Blockade of release of growth hormone by brain norepinephrine depletors. *Endocrinology*. 80: 471.
29. Rothballer, A. B. 1959. The effects of catecholamines on the central nervous system. *Pharmacol. Rev.* 11: 494.
30. Abrams, R. L., M. L. Parker, S. Blanco, S. Reichlin, and W. H. Daughaday. 1966. Hypothalamic regulation of growth hormone secretion. *Endocrinology*. 78: 605.
31. Schalch, D. S., and D. M. Kipnis. 1965. Abnormalities in carbohydrate tolerance associated with elevated plasma nonesterified fatty acids. *J. Clin. Invest.* 44: 2010.
32. Abramson, E. A., R. A. Arky, and K. A. Woeber. 1966. Effects of propranolol on the hormonal and metabolic responses to insulin-induced hypoglycaemia. *Lancet*. 2: 1386.
33. Porte, D., Jr. 1967. A receptor mechanism for the inhibition of insulin release by epinephrine in man. *J. Clin. Invest.* 46: 86.
34. Porte, D., Jr. 1967. Beta adrenergic stimulation of insulin release in man. *Diabetes*. 16: 150.

39

Copyright © 1964 by J. B. Lippincott Company

Reprinted from pages 408–409 and 412–414 of *Endocrinology*
74:408–414 (1964)

Stimulation of Pituitary Growth Hormone Release by a Hypothalamic Extract *in Vitro*[1]

ROGER R. DEUBEN AND JOSEPH MEITES

Michigan State University, Department of Physiology and Pharmacology, East Lansing, Michigan

ABSTRACT. Anterior pituitaries from mature female virgin rats were cultured in synthetic medium 199 at 35 C in an atmosphere of 95% O_2–5% CO_2. At the end of 18 days of culture, 167% more growth hormone (STH) activity was recovered from the medium than was originally present in fresh anterior pituitary, as determined by the standard tibia assay in young hypophysectomized rats.

In 2 separate trials, addition of an acid extract of rat hypothalamus to the medium during a 6-day culture period increased pituitary STH release 4- to 6-fold. These differences were highly significant statistically. An equivalent amount of extract of rat cerebral cortex had no effect on pituitary STH release. When an extract of rat hypothalamus was boiled for 15 min, $\frac{2}{3}$ of the STH-releasing activity still remained in the extract, whereas boiling has been reported to destroy pituitary STH activity. Injections of hypothalamic extract directly into assay rats had no significant effect on cartilage width, also indicating that the extract *per se* was free of STH activity.

Since acid extracts of rat hypothalamus inhibit pituitary prolactin release *in vitro*, and prolactin injections into assay rats produced only a slight increase in cartilage width, prolactin is not believed to have contributed significantly to the STH activity recovered from the culture medium. These results are believed to demonstrate the existence of an STH-releasing factor in rat hypothalamus. (*Endocrinology* 74: 408, 1964)

THE RELATION of the hypothalamus to growth hormone release has received little attention thus far. Reichlin (1) reported that placement of massive ventral lesions in the hypothalamus reduced body weight gains of intact rats and lowered the pituitary content of growth hormone (STH) to approximately 15% of that found in sham-operated controls. Spirtos *et al.* (2) noted that rats with hypothalamic lesions showed an increased sensitivity to insulin identical with that seen in hypophysectomized rats, suggesting that the hypothalamic lesions resulted in reduced STH release. When exogenous STH was administered, the increased sensitivity to insulin was lost.

We previously reported that the rat pituitary can release growth hormone *in vitro* (3). Pituitaries cultured for six days apparently released as much STH into the medium as was present in fresh rat pituitary, and differences were observed in the capacity of pituitaries from rats of various age groups to release STH. Franz *et al.* (4) recently reported the presence of a growth hormone-releasing factor in a crude extract of hog hypothalamus. However, their results cannot be considered convincing since standard assay procedures were not followed and increases in cartilage width of less than 40 μ were reported to be significant.

Hypothalamic extracts have been reported to stimulate the release of ACTH (5), TSH (6) and LH (7) and to inhibit the release of prolactin (8). It was of interest to determine whether extracts of rat hypothalamus could increase re-

---

Received August 8, 1963.

[1] This work was supported in part by NIH Grant AM-04784-03. Published with the approval of the Michigan Agricultural Experiment Station as Journal Article No. 3215.

225

lease of STH by rat anterior pituitary when cultured *in vitro*. A preliminary report of these results has been published elsewhere (9).

[*Editor's Note:* Material has been omitted at this point.]

Discussion

These *in vitro* results demonstrate that acid extracts of rat hypothalamus can produce a 4- to 6-fold increase in STH release by cultured rat anterior pituitary. This activity could not be demonstrated in an acid extract of rat cerebral cortex, indicating that this area of the rat brain does not contain STH-releasing activity. When rat hypothalamic extract was boiled, STH-releasing activity was reduced by about one third. Further work is necessary to determine whether boiling can alter STH-releasing activity in the hypothalamus. These results indicate that STH *per se* was not present in the hypothalamic extract, since STH is destroyed by boiling (13). A further indication that rat hypotha-

TABLE 5. Effects of acid extract of hypothalamus on epiphysial cartilage width in hypophysectomized assay rats

Group	No. of Assay Animals	Dose Total Hypothalamus /Assay Animal /4 day	Response $\mu \pm \text{SE}$
(1) Acid extract of hypothalamus	5 5 5	0.4 1.2 2.4	145 ±5 137 ±1 156 ±4
(2) Controls	5	None	124 ±2

lamic tissue does not contain STH is our observation that injections of acid extract of hypothalamus into young hypophysectomized rats did not significantly increase epiphysial cartilage width.

Consideration must be given to the other anterior pituitary hormones which may influence the tibia test. Both ACTH and the gonadotropins have been reported to reduce epiphysial cartilage width in young hypophysectomized rats (13). Since hypothalamic extracts can stimulate the release of these hormones (5, 7, 15, 16) their presence may have partially counteracted the full activity of STH released into the medium, and more STH may actually have been present than is reported here. TSH and prolactin enhance the epiphysial cartilage response in young hypophysectomized rats (13). Although TSH release into the medium was not measured, Geschwind and Li (13) expressed the view that relatively large amounts of TSH are required to influence epiphysial cartilage width in hypophysectomized rats. Prolactin is not believed to have influenced our results for the reasons previously discussed (Experiment 4).

More STH activity was recovered from the pituitary culture system *in vitro* than was originally placed into it. The increase of 167% in STH activity during an 18-day culture period is much less than for prolactin, since 1000% more prolactin was recovered daily from the medium than was originally placed into the culture system (17). However, the hypothalamus chronically depresses prolactin release under most conditions (18), whereas hypothalamic stimulation is required for normal growth hormone release (1, 19, 20).

The nature of the STH-releasing factor(s) in the rat hypothalamus remains to be established. Its relative resistance to boiling suggests that it is a small molecule, perhaps a polypeptide like the other hypothalamic factors extracted thus far (5, 7, 21, 22). Preliminary experiments in our laboratory with hypothalamic extracts from cattle, sheep and swine indicate that these can also induce STH release *in vitro* by the cultured rat pituitary.

Addendum

Recently, Martini, Mueller and Pecile (private communication) demonstrated *in vivo* release of pituitary STH in the rat by a rat hypothalamic extract. A single intracarotid injection of extract, followed by sacrifice of the animal 15 min later and removal of the pituitary for assay by the standard tibia test, caused a marked depletion of pituitary STH content. A cerebral cortical extract was inactive. We have confirmed this observation, finding approximately a 50% decrease in rat pituitary STH content after a single intracarotid injection of an extract equivalent to 2 rat hypothalami.

References

1. Reichlin, S., *Endocrinology* 69: 225, 1961.
2. Spirtos, B. N., W. R. Ingram, E. M. Bogdanove, and N. S. Halmi, *J Clin Endocr* 14: 790, 1954 (Abstract).

3. Meites, J., T. F. Hopkins, and R. Deuben, *Fed Proc* **21** (2): 196, 1962 (Abstract).
4. Franz, J., C. H. Haselbach, and O. Libert, *Acta Endocr (Kbh)* **41**: 336, 1962.
5. Guillemin, R., *In* Fields, W. S., R. Guillemin, and C. A. Carton (eds.), Hypothalamic-Hypophysial Interrelationships, Charles C Thomas, Springfield, Illinois, 1956.
6. Schreiber, V., M. Rybak, and V. Kmentova, *Experientia* **18**: 338, 1962.
7. McCann, S. M., *Amer J Physiol* **202**: 395, 1962.
8. Talwalker, P. K., A. Ratner, and J. Meites, *Amer J Physiol* **205**: 213, 1963.
9. Deuben, R., and J. Meites, *Fed Proc* **22**(2): 571, 1963 (Abstract).
10. Nicoll, C. S., and J. Meites, *Endocrinology* **72**: 544, 1963.
11. Greenspan, F. S., C. H. Li, M. E. Simpson, and H. M. Evans, *In* Emmens, C. W. (ed.), Hormone Assay, Academic Press, New York, 1950.
12. Pugsley, L. I., *Endocrinology* **39**: 161, 1946.
13. Geschwind, I. I., and C. H. Li, *In* Smith, R. W., Jr., O. H. Gaebler, and C. M. H. Long (eds.), The Hypophyseal Growth Hormone, Nature and Actions, McGraw-Hill, New York, 1955.
14. Srebnik, H. H., M. M. Nelson, and M. E. Simpson, *Proc Soc Exp Biol Med* **101**: 97, 1959.
15. Igarashi, M., and S. M. McCann, *In* Program, 45th Ann. Meeting, Endocrine Soc., Atlantic City, N. J., 1963, p 29 (Abstract).
16. Kobayashi, T., T. Kobayashi, T. Kegawa, M. Mizuno, and Y. Amenomori, *Endocr Jap* **8**: 223, 1961.
17. Nicoll, C. S., and J. Meites, *Endocrinology* **70**: 272, 1962.
18. Meites, J., C. S. Nicoll, and P. K. Talwalker, *In* Nalbandov, A. V. (ed.), Advances in Neuroendocrinology, chapter 8, University of Illinois Press, Urbana, Ill., 1963.
19. Bernardis, L. L., B. M. Box, and J. A. F. Stevenson, *Endocrinology* **72**: 684, 1963.
20. Harris, G. W., Neural Control of the Pituitary Gland, Edward Arnold Ltd., London, 1955.
21. Schreiber, V., A. Eckertova, Z. Franc, M. Rybak, I. Gregorova, V. Kmentova, and V. Jirgl, *Physiologia Bohemoslovenica* **12**: 1, 1963.
22. Schally, A. V., H. S. Lipscomb, and R. Guillemin, *Endocrinology* **71**: 164, 1962.

HYPOTHALAMIC STIMULATION OF GROWTH HORMONE SECRETION

Lawrence A. Frohman, Lee L. Bernardis, and Kenneth J. Kant

Abstract. *Stimulation of the ventromedial hypothalamic nucleus in rats resulted in increased plasma growth hormone levels within 5 minutes, as measured by radioimmunoassay. Stimulation of the cerebral cortex was without effect. These observations confirm previous results involving destructive lesions and establish the ventromedial nucleus as a hypothalamic locus involved in the control of growth hormone secretion.*

Evidence for the hypothalamic control of growth hormone secretion has been based primarily on experiments involving destructive hypothalamic lesions. In most studies, however, large areas of the ventral hypothalamus, including the median eminence, have been destroyed (1), thus precluding the specific localization of the site of control of growth hormone secretion. Recent studies from our laboratory (2) have demonstrated that destruction of the ventromedial hypothalamic nucleus (VMN) in weanling rats results in impaired growth associated with decreased growth hormone levels in both the pituitary and plasma. Since the median eminence was undamaged in these animals, we suggested that the hypothalamic control of growth hormone secretion resides in the VMN. The present report offers evidence of a different nature to support this hypothesis.

Female Holtzman rats weighing 180 to 220 g were anesthetized with pentobarbital, tracheotomized, and a catheter was inserted in the carotid artery. The animals were then positioned in a Horsley-Clarke stereotactic instrument. Burr holes were made, and a 0.25-mm unipolar stainless steel electrode, insulated with spar varnish except at the tip, was inserted in the VMN. The coordinates have been previously described (3). Stimulation was in the form of biphasic square wave pulses of 1 ma intensity, 5 msec duration, and 50 cycle/sec. The stimulation was applied for 3 minutes, and the current intensity was monitored with an oscilloscope. The stereotactic instrument served as the indifferent electrode. Control animals were stimulated in a similar manner except that the tip of the electrode was positioned in the cerebral cortex.

Heparinized blood samples (0.2 ml) were removed through the catheter immediately prior to stimulation and at several intervals after stimulation was begun (3, 5, 10, and 15 minutes). Plasma was separated at 4°C and stored at −20°C for the subsequent assay of growth hormone.

After the last blood sample was obtained, an anodal direct current of 1.0 ma intensity and of 5 seconds duration was used to produce a lesion, thereby identifying the site of the electrode tip. The rats were then killed. The brains were fixed in formalin, serially sectioned, and stained with cresyl violet, and the location of the lesions (stimulation sites) was identified.

Plasma growth hormone was measured by a double antibody radioimmunoassay method previously described (2); rat growth hormone-I^{131} and guinea pig anti-porcine growth hormone serum were used. No immunologic cross-reaction has been observed with rodent thyroid-stimulating hormone or prolactin, porcine adrenocorticotropin, or bovine follicle-stimulating hormone or luteinizing hormone. Plasma levels in hypophysectomized rats range from under 2 to 9 mμg/ml. In rats with transplantable pituitary tumors producing growth hormone, plasma levels as high as 40 μg/ml have been observed and correlate well with bioassay results (4).

Thirteen of 14 rats in which stimulation of the VMN was performed had elevated plasma growth hormone levels within 15 minutes of the start of stimulation, as shown in Fig. 1. No elevation of plasma growth hormone occurred by the end of the 3-minute stimulation period, but a rise occurred in over half of the group of rats 2 minutes later. With the exception of the one animal which did not respond, all plasma samples measured at 10 and 15 minutes contained growth hormone levels greater than in the prestimulation samples.

There was a tendency for the prestimulation growth hormone level to influence the response to stimulation. The animals with initial levels of less than 50 mμg/ml (seven rats) had a twofold (absolute) and a 4½-fold (percentage) greater rise following stimulation than those (seven rats) with initial values of greater than 50 mμg/ml. The one nonresponder had the highest prestimulatory growth hormone value (143 mμg/ml). The difference in the initial growth hormone levels of the VMN-stimulated (65 ± 9) and cortex-stimulated (38 ± 7) rats was not significant. A similar phenomenon has been reported in human subjects where the growth hormone response to several stimuli (insulin, arginine, endotoxin) was impaired by elevated prestimulatory values (5). This appears to be a manifestation of a general biological phenomenon, Wilder's Law of the Initial Value (6). Control rats which were stimulated in the cerebral cortex showed a gradual decline in plasma growth hormone levels.

Figure 2 illustrates the electrolytic lesion in a rat in which the tip of the electrode was in the VMN. Elevations of plasma growth hormone were observed only in those rats in which the electrode tip was within the VMN. Rats which received stimulation in the lateral hypothalamus or the fornix failed to show any rise in plasma growth hormone levels after stimulation. In preliminary studies four rats were stimulated in the VMN for 1 minute. Only one showed a rise in growth hormone levels.

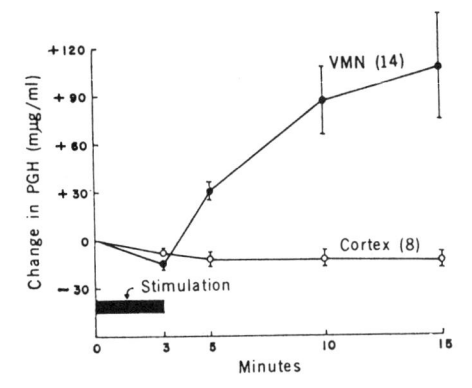

Fig. 1. Changes in plasma growth hormone (PGH) levels after stimulation of either ventromedial nucleus (VMN) or cerebral cortex in rats. Shown are the mean ± standard error. The number of animals in each group is shown in parentheses.

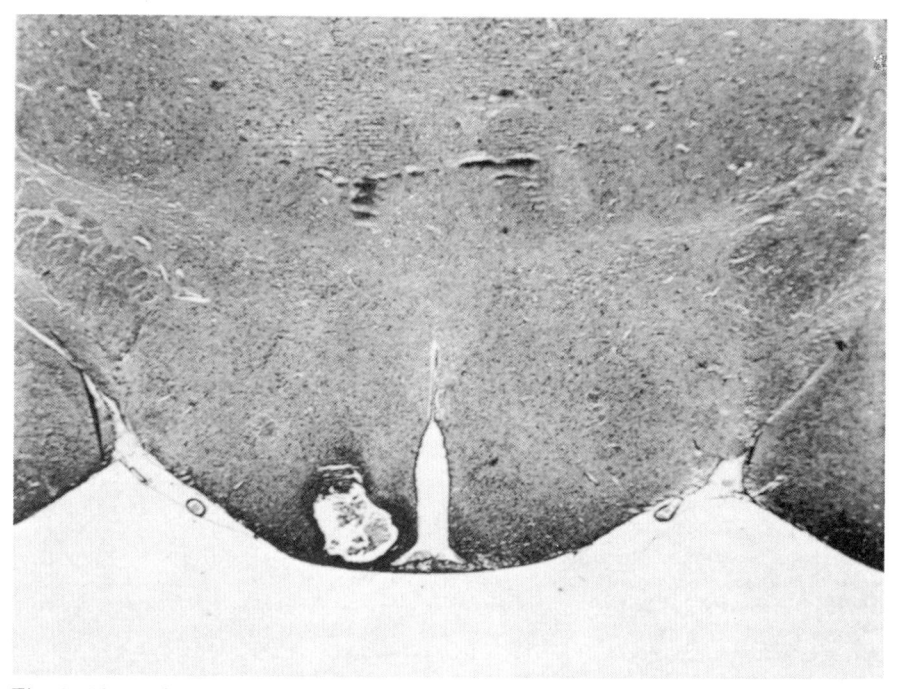

Fig. 2. Photomicrograph showing a coronal section of the hypothalamus of a rat which was stimulated in the ventromedial nucleus. The electrolytic lesion identifies the site of stimulation.

These observations give support to the previous study (2) which identified the VMN as the hypothalamic locus responsible for the control of growth hormone secretion. Whether growth hormone releasing factor is formed in the VMN and transported into the portal hypophyseal capillary plexus which originates in the median eminence or whether neural connections from the VMN stimulate formation of growth hormone releasing factor in the median eminence is not yet known.

References and Notes

1. S. Reichlin, *Endocrinology* **69**, 225 (1961).
2. L. A. Frohman and L. L. Bernardis, *ibid.* **82**, 1125 (1968).
3. L. L. Bernardis and F. R. Skelton, *Am. J. Anat.* **116**, 69 (1965).
4. L. A. Frohman and R. W. Bates, in preparation.
5. L. A. Frohman, T. Aceto, Jr., M. H. MacGillivray, *J. Clin. Endocrinol. Metab.* **27**, 1409 (1967).
6. J. Wilder, *Z. Ges. Neurol. Psychiat.* **137**, 317 (1931).
7. Supported by PHS grant HD-03331 and United Health Foundation of Western New York grant GG67UB6, We thank Maureen Mills, Jane Asmus, and Michael Bahorsky for their technical assistance.

41

Copyright © 1970 by J. B. Lippincott Company

Reprinted from pages 807 to 810-811 of *Endocrinology* 87:807-811 (1970)

Thyrotropin and Growth Hormone Releasing Activity in Hypophysial Portal Blood

JOHN F. WILBER,

Department of Medicine, Northwestern University School of Medicine, Chicago, Illinois,

AND JOHN C. PORTER,

Department of Physiology, University of Texas, Southwestern Medical School, Dallas, Texas

ABSTRACT. Studies of TSH and GH releasing activities in plasma from pituitary stalk blood have been conducted. TSH and GH released from anterior pituitary halves incubated *in vitro* with either portal or peripheral plasma were measured by means of specific radioimmunoassays. Relative to peripheral plasma, portal plasma resulted in 161% increase in TSH secretion and 149% increment in GH secretion. Electrical stimulation of the anterior hypothalamus further augmented TSH release to 201%, but no further GH release was observed after electrode stimulation. Prior treatment with triiodothyronine did not abolish the influence of electrical stimulation upon TSH releasing activity. Both TSH and GH were also identified in portal plasma. It was estimated that these tropic hormones, presumed to originate from pars tuberalis, could contribute as much as 5% of circulating TSH and GH in the periphery of intact rats. (*Endocrinology* **87**: 807, 1970)

OVERWHELMING evidence supports the importance of hypothalamic neurohumors in the regulation of pituitary function (1). Documentation that these substances are present in the hypophysial portal circulation, however, has been meager. Thyrotropin releasing activity has been described in one report under conditions of hypothalamic electrical stimulation only (2). Growth hormone releasing activity was not found in the studies of Worthington and his associates (3). The recent development of new methodology has provided a tool for the selective collection of portal blood, free of contamination from other blood sources (4). This method has now been applied to initial studies of thyrotropin and growth hormone stimulators in this circulation. The demonstration of thyrotropin and growth hormone releasing activities in portal plasma, and their differential enhancement by electrical stimulation, forms the substance of this report.

Received March 17, 1970.

Supported in part by NIH Research Grants AM-01237, AM-10699, and Training Grant AM-05071 from the National Institute of Arthritis and Metabolic Diseases, USPHS, Bethesda, Md.

[*Editor's Note:* Material has been omitted at this point.]

Discussion

Our studies provide documentation that TSH and GH releasing activities are present in portal plasma. Previously, thyrotropin release was reported to be augmented in five out of nine rabbits following the intrapituitary administration of portal plasma obtained from electrically stimulated rats (2). However, statistical analyses performed by several techniques have failed to confirm this demonstration of portal TRF activity (10). One possible explanation for this result is that test samples were injected directly into the anterior pituitary, a technique which has not proved to be satisfactory in our hands (10). In this study, in addition, portal plasma from unstimulated rats inhibited TSH release in rabbits, and the possibility of hypothalamic "thyrotropin inhibiting factor" was raised. No support for this concept is provided by the present investigation.

The magnitude of thyrotropin releasing activity in portal plasma appears to be small relative to *in vivo* requirements. Base line TSH secretion observed *in vitro*, for example, approximated 10% of the estimated *in vivo* TSH production rate.[2] Yet portal plasma increased medium TSH only 61%, whereas medium TSH would have to have been raised 1000% to equal the performance of the intact pituitary. Several considerations may be relevant to this discrepancy.

First, the pituitary may not possess full *in vivo* secretory potential under *in vitro* conditions. Secondly, anesthesia is capable of lowering plasma TSH in the intact rat (7). In our preparation, animals used for portal plasma collection are subjected not only to barbiturate anesthesia, but also to the stress of surgery, which may exert additional inhibitory influence upon TSH release (12). Thirdly, TRF can be inactivated by plasma at 37 C (5), and a latent interval of three to four minutes occurs between entry of portal plasma into the distal

---

[2] This estimate is calculated from our observed plasma concentration of TSH by immunoassay in the euthyroid rat (mean 41 μU/ml) (7), the TSH $t_{1/2}$ disappearance in the euthyroid rat (mean 12 min), and the extrapituitary distribution space for TSH (mean 4.8% body weight). The latter 2 data were obtained from Bakke and Lawrence (11).

end of the collection tubing and its passage into the refrigerated chamber (2 C). Some destruction of TRF undoubtedly takes place during this interval and possibly also during the thawing process, prior to incubation with pituitary tissue.

Previous studies by Worthington and associates have not demonstrated growth hormone releasing activity in portal plasma (3). However, in these experiments GH *depletion* from the intrapituitary compartment was the parameter measured, rather than GH *released* from the pituitary. Since the amount of growth hormone released by portal plasma in the present investigation never exceeded 2% of one hemipituitary GH content, no depletion could have been measurable by present assay methods.

Unipolar electrode stimulation of the anterior hypothalamus resulted in enhancement of TSH but not GH releasing activity in portal plasma. This result confirms the previous work of Averill and associates (2) and provides a mechanism for the activation of TSH release *in vivo* when the anterior hypothalamus has been subjected to electrical stimulation (13). That GH release, in contrast, was not increased is compatible with the observation of Frohman that a region of the hypothalamus posterior to our electrode placement is involved in the control of rat GH secretion (14). Moreover, the selective enhancement of TSH releasing activity demonstrates that TSH and GH secretion are controlled by separate neurohumoral substances. Studies with electrodes placed more posteriorly in the ventromedial hypothalamus are in progress.

The failure of triiodothyronine to suppress electrode activation of TSH releasing activity in portal plasma provides added support to the concept that thyroid hormones do not alter the hypothalamic secretion of TRF (15). Further studies are required, however, to determine whether thyroid hormones also inhibit the TSH releasing activity in unstimulated portal plasma.

Both TSH and GH were identified in the portal circulation, and the concentrations in portal plasma were comparable to what has been found in the peripheral plasma of intact animals (7, 8). If one assumes that the very low concentrations of TSH and GH observed in the peripheral plasma from hypophysectomized animals originated exclusively from this suprahypophysial source, as much as 5% of circulating GH and TSH could originate from the pars tuberalis, and the presence of TSH in the stalk-median eminence region has been reported by Bakke (16).

Acknowledgment

The authors are grateful to Miss Jayne Martin for technical assistance.

References

1. McCann, S. M., and J. C. Porter, *Physiol Rev* **48**: 240, 1969.
2. Averill, R. L. W., P. F. Salaman, and W. C. Worthington, Jr., *Nature (London)* **211**: 144, 1966.
3. Worthington, W. C., J. D. Fulmer, P. C. Kansal, and M. G. Buse, Abstracts to the Third International Congress of Endocrinology, p. 93.
4. Porter, J. C., and K. R. Smith, *Endocrinology* **81**: 1182, 1967.
5. Redding, T. W., and A. V. Schally, *Proc Soc Exp Biol Med* **131**: 415, 1969.
6. Porter, J. C., M. F. M. Hines, K. R. Smith, R. L. Repass, and A. J. K. Smith, *Endocrinology* **80**: 583, 1967.
7. Wilber, J. F., and R. D. Utiger, *Endocrinology* **81**: 145, 1967.
8. Schalch, D., and S. Reichlin, *Endocrinology* **79**: 275, 1966.
9. Worcester, J., *New Eng J Med* **274**: 27, 1966.
10. Porter, J. C., B. D. Goldman, and J. F. Wilber, In Meites, J. (ed.), Hypophysiotropic Hormones of the Hypothalamus, Williams and Wilkins Co., Baltimore, Md., 1969.
11. Bakke, J. L., and N. L. Lawrence, *Endocrinology* **71**: 43, 1962.
12. Ducommun, P., E. Sakiz, and R. Guillemin, *Proc Soc Exp Biol Med* **121**: 921, 1966.
13. D'Angelo, S. A., J. Snyder, and J. M. Grodin, *Endocrinology* **75**: 417, 1964.
14. Frohman, L. A., L. L. Bernardis, and K. J. Grant, *Science* **162**: 580, 1968.
15. Reichlin, S., *New Eng J Med* **269**: 1182, 1963.
16. Bakke, J. L., and N. L. Lawrence, *Neuroendocrinology* **2**: 315, 1967.

Editor's Comments
on Papers 42 Through 45

42 KRULICH, DHARIWAL, and McCANN
    Excerpts from *Stimulatory and Inhibitory Effects of Purified Hypothalamic Extracts on Growth Hormone Release from Rat Pituitary* in Vitro

43 BRAZEAU et al.
    Hypothalamic Polypeptide That Inhibits the Secretion of Immunoreactive Pituitary Growth Hormone

44 VALE et al.
    Excerpts from *Effects of Somatostatin on the Secretion of Thyrotropin and Prolactin*

45 BROWNSTEIN et al.
    The Regional Distribution of Somatostatin in the Rat Brain

The existence of a hypothalamic GH-release-inhibiting hormone (GHRIH) was first suggested by Krulich et al. (Paper 42) on the basis of the results of studies on the effects of hypothalamic extracts on GH release by rat hypophysial incubates. They noted that gel filtration of sheep and rat hypothalamic extracts on sephadex G-25 yielded two distinct zones. The first zone increased GH release sevenfold and the second zone decreased GH release to approximately 50 percent of that in control hypophysis incubated in the presence of elution buffer. They suggested that GHRIH may have physiological significance and that its secretion may be regulated in a reverse manner to that of GH-releasing factor, thus suggesting a dual control mechanism for hypothalamic control of GH secretion.

Brazeau et al. (Paper 43) elucidated the structure of GHRIH as being a cyclic tetradecapeptide, upon isolation from half a million ovine hypothalami, and found it to inhibit the release of GH from rat and human hypophysial cells in vitro and rats in vivo. They were able to synthesize a linear form of the tetradecapeptide by solid-phase methodology with purification by gel filtration, which was found to have biological activity similar to that of the natural compound in vitro and in vivo. They proposed the name *somatostatin* for this GHRIH and suggested that it might have a potential clinical significance, particularly in the treatment of acromegaly and the management of insulinopenic diabetes mellitus.

Vale et al. (Paper 44) reported that somatostatin inhibits the TRH-mediated release of TSH in a dose-response-dependent manner. Somatostatin did not inhibit the TRH-mediated release of PRL in rats. However, in vitro somatostatin inhibited the spontaneous release of TSH and, to a lesser extent, PRL in adenohypophyseal cultures. A degree of specificity was shown by its inability to inhibit the LH-RH-induced secretion of LH. Additionally, they showed that somatostatin and thyroid hormone exhibited summation in their inhibition of TSH in vivo and in vitro studies. They suggested that their data indicate that somatostatin acts in conjunction with thyroid hormones and TRH to modulate TSH secretion physiologically.

Brownstein et al. (Paper 45) used a specific radioimmunoassay developed in their laboratory to study the distribution of somatostatin in rat brain. Highest concentrations were found in the hypothalamus, especially in the median eminence and arcuate nucleus. However, since somatostatin was found in all hypothalamic nuclei, the authors postulated that it may be synthesized in cell bodies in several hypothalamic nuclei, reaching neuronal terminals in the median eminence by axonal flow. They also suggested that, in view of its widespread distribution throughout the brain, somatostatin may function as a neurotransmitter in areas of the brain remote from the median eminence, where it acts as a release inhibitory hormone when secreted into the portal circulation. They were able to detect immunological, but not biological, somatostatin activity in the ventromedial nucleus (VMN). They interpreted this finding to suggest that there is as much or more GH-releasing activity in the VMN as there is somatostatin activity. This corroborates the findings of Frohman et al. (Paper 40) that lesions of the VMN cause a decrease in plasma GH levels and that electrical stimulation of the VMN causes a prompt increase in plasma GH levels.

42

Copyright © 1968 by J. B. Lippincott Company

Reprinted from pages 783 and 789-790 of Endocrinology 83:783-790 (1968)

Stimulatory and Inhibitory Effects of Purified Hypothalamic Extracts on Growth Hormone Release from Rat Pituitary in Vitro[1]

L. KRULICH,[2] A. P. S. DHARIWAL, AND S. M. McCANN[3]

Department of Physiology, University of Texas Southern Medical School, Dallas, Texas 75235

ABSTRACT. Male rat anterior pituitaries were incubated in vitro for 5 hr in Krebs-Ringer bicarbonate medium and the growth hormone (GH) released from the glands was estimated by the tibial epiphyseal cartilage assay. Addition of crude sheep or rat hypothalamic extract to the pituitaries increased the GH concentration in the medium on comparison to either diluent or cortical extract-treated controls. The ovine extracts also depleted pituitary GH concentration when injected into male rats in vivo. Gel filtration of either sheep or rat hypothalamic extract on a column of Sephadex G-25 resulted in the elution from the column of 2 zones which influenced the release of GH in vitro on addition to the incubated pituitaries. The first zone of activity to be eluted increased the release of GH from the glands severalfold, whereas the second zone inhibited the release of GH to levels about one half of that released by control glands incubated in the presence of the eluting buffer. Increasing the dose in the inhibitory zone resulted in a further decrease in GH release. The addition of either the stimulatory or inhibitory fractions to the incubation medium at the termination of the incubation failed to affect the value for GH obtained on assay. This result indicates that neither fraction altered the assay of GH. Consequently, the results obtained are attributable to altered rates of release of GH from the incubated glands. The findings are consistent with the hypothesis that hypothalamic extracts of rat and sheep origin contain a GH-inhibiting factor (GIF) in addition to the GH-releasing factor (GRF). The GH-releasing activity of crude extracts is explained by assuming that the relative concentration of GRF exceeds that of GIF. (Endocrinology 83: 783, 1968)

SEVERAL publications have appeared recently which have demonstrated the presence of a growth hormone-releasing factor (GRF) in crude or purified hypothalamic extracts from several animal species. These extracts were active both in vivo, where they caused depletion of GH from the pituitary of the rat (1, 2) or increased plasma levels of GH as detected by radioimmunoassay in the sheep (3) or monkey (4-6), and in vitro, where they increased output of GH from incubated rat pituitaries (7, 8) or the GH content in pituitary tissue cultures (9). This GRF has been purified and separated from other hypothalamic releasing factors (10-12).

In the present communication, data are presented which indicate that an inhibitor of GH release is also present in hypothalamic fractions obtained by gel filtration on Sephadex of crude extracts from sheep or rat hypothalami. Preliminary communications of a part of these results have already been published (13-15).

Received April, 1, 1968.

[1] Please address reprint requests to Dr. S. M. McCann, Dept. of Physiology, Southwestern Medical School, Dallas, Texas 75235.

[2] Present address: Praha II, Albertov 5, Fysiologicky ustav, Czechoslovakia.

[3] This research was supported by a grant from the Ford Foundation and by Grant AM 10073-3 from the NIH.

[Editor's Note: Material has been omitted at this point.]

Discussion

The present data are in agreement with those of earlier workers, who showed that crude or purified SME extracts could increase the release of GH from pituitaries incubated *in vitro* (7, 8, 11). Crude extract, active *in vitro*, also evoked a depletion of GH from the pituitary when injected iv into rats, and the zone from the Sephadex fractionation which increased the release of GH *in vitro* had a similar elution volume to that which had previously been determined for GRF by *in vivo* assay (10). Thus, there is good agreement in our hands between results obtained in the living animal and with isolated pituitaries incubated *in vitro*.

To our surprise, routine screening of fractions from the Sephadex column revealed the presence of an inhibitor which reduced the release of GH from the pituitary *in vitro*. It is still too early to be certain of the physiological significance of this factor. A number of observations argue against it being a mere artifact. It was recovered in a uniform position from four consecutive Sephadex fractionations of ovine hypothalamic extract and was obtained in the same zone after fractionation of rat hypothalami. Furthermore, a dose-response relationship was observed between the dose of the inhibitor, called GH-inhibiting factor (GIF), and the degree of suppression of GH release. In other experiments (Krulich, Dhariwal and McCann, in preparation), it was determined that the GIF was separable from other releasing factors, could inhibit the response to GRF both *in vitro* and *in vivo*, and could be further purified by several additional chromatographic procedures.

If indeed the GIF has physiological significance, then its secretion might be regulated in an inverse manner to that of GRF. Situations which call forth enhanced GH release might result in increased GRF secretion and decreased release of the inhibitor and *vice versa*. The effect of crude hypothalamic extracts on GH release would then be the resultant of the GRF and GIF that they contain. Presumably, GRF is present in higher concentration than GIF in hypothalami of normal animals and this accounts for the GH-releasing activity of crude hypothalamic extracts.

References

1. Pecile, A., E. Müller, G. Falconi, and L. Martini, *Endocrinology* **77:** 241, 1965.
2. Krulich, L., A. P. S. Dhariwal, and S. M. McCann, *Proc Soc Exp Biol Med* **120:** 180, 1965.
3. Machlin, L. J., M. Horino, D. M. Kipnis, S. L. Phillips, and R. S. Gordon, *Endocrinology* **80:** 205, 1967.
4. Knobil, E., *Physiologist* **9:** 25, 1966.
5. Garcia, J. F., and I. I. Geschwind, *Nature (London)* **211:** 372, 1966.
6. Smith, G., S. Katz, A. P. S. Dhariwal, A. Bongiovanni, W. Eberlein, and S. M. McCann, *Fed Proc* **26:** 316, 1967.
7. Deuben, R. R., and J. Meites, *Endocrinology* **74:** 408, 1964.
8. Schally, A. V., S. L. Steelman, and C. Y. Bowers, *Proc Soc Exp Biol Med* **119:** 208, 1965.
9. Deuben, R. R., and J. Meites, *Proc Soc Exp Biol Med* **118:** 409, 1965.
10. Dhariwal, A. P. S., L. Krulich, S. Katz, and S. M. McCann, *Endocrinology* **77:** 932, 1965.
11. Schally, A. V., A. Kuroshima, Y. Ishida, A. Arimura, T. Saito, C. Y. Bowers, and S. L. Steelman, *Proc Soc Exp Biol Med* **122:** 821, 1966.
12. Dhariwal, A. P. S., J. Antunes-Rodrigues, L. Krulich, and S. M. McCann, *Neuroendocrinology* **1:** 341, 1965/66.
13. Krulich, L., R. W. Lackey, and A. P. S. Dhariwal, *Fed Proc* **26:** 316, 1967.
14. Krulich, L., A. P. S. Dhariwal, and S. M. McCann, Proc. 49th Mtg. Endocr. Soc., 1967, p. 87 (Abstract).
15. ———, Proc. Intn'l Symp. on GH, *Excerpta Med*, 1967, p. 32.
16. McCann, S. M., and P. Haberland, *Proc Soc Exp Biol Med* **102:** 319, 1959.
17. Greenspan, F. S., C. H. Li, M. E. Simpson, and H. M. Evans, *Endocrinology* **45:** 455, 1949.
18. Bliss, C. I., The Statistics of Bioassay, Academic Press, Inc., New York, 1962.
19. Katz, S. H., A. P. S. Dhariwal, and S. M. McCann, *Endocrinology* **81:** 333, 1967.
20. Lowry, O. H., N. J. Rosebrough, A. C. Farr, and R. J. Randall, *J Biol Chem* **193:** 265, 1951.

HYPOTHALAMIC POLYPEPTIDE THAT INHIBITS THE SECRETION OF IMMUNOREACTIVE PITUITARY GROWTH HORMONE

Paul Brazeau, Wylie Vale, Roger Burgus, Nicholas Ling, Madalyn Butcher, Jean Rivier, and Roger Guillemin

Abstract. A peptide has been isolated from ovine hypothalamus which, at 1×10^{-9}M, inhibits secretion in vitro of immunoreactive rat or human growth hormones and is similarly active in vivo in rats. Its structure is

H-Ala-Gly-Cys-Lys-Asn-Phe-Phe-Trp-Lys-Thr-Phe-Thr-Ser-Cys-OH

The synthetic replicate is biologically active.

Physiological, experimental, and clinical observations (1) have led to the concept that the hypothalamus controls and regulates the secretion of pituitary growth hormone (somatotropin). It has been generally accepted that this control would be exerted by a hypothalamic hypophysiotropic releasing factor, as is now proven to be the case for the secretion of thyrotropin (TSH) (2, 3) and the gonadotropin, luteinizing hormone (LH) (4). The nature of the postulated hypothalamic releasing factor for growth hormone, however, remains elusive, mostly due to the difficulties and ambiguities of the various assay systems used so far in attempts at its characterization [for review see (5)].

Searching to demonstrate the presence of this still hypothetical somatotropin releasing factor in the crude hypothalamic extracts used in the isolation of TRF (thyrotropin releasing factor) and LRF (luteinizing hormone releasing factor), we have regularly observed that their addition in minute doses ($\geq$ .001 of a hypothalamic fragment equivalent) to the incubation fluid of dispersed rat pituitary cells in monolayer cultures (6) significantly decreases the resting secretion of immunoreactive growth hormone (7) by the pituitary cells. This inhibition is related to the dose of hypothalamic extract added and is specific (see Table 1).

It is not produced by similar extracts of cerebellum, and the crude hypothalamic extracts that inhibit secretion of growth hormone simultaneously stimulate secretion of LH and TSH. The inhibition of growth hormone secretion could not be duplicated by addition to the assay system of [Arg⁸]-vasopressin, oxytocin, histamine, various polyamines, serotonin, catecholamines, LRF, or TRF. For operational facility, we decided to attribute this inhibitory effect on the secretion of growth hormone to a "somatotropin-release inhibiting factor" or SRIF.

Inhibition of secretion of growth hormone by crude hypothalamic preparations has been reported (8); however, the active factor possibly involved has not been characterized.

Our results on the inhibition by the hypothalamic extracts of the in vitro secretion of growth hormone by the pituitary monolayer cultures were so consistent and so easily quantitated that we decided to attempt the isolation of the postulated SRIF with the in vitro method as an assay system. Characterization of a natural inhibitory factor of hypothalamic origin was of interest in view of current efforts at designing synthetic polypeptides as antagonists of LRF (9).

The starting material was the chloroform–methanol–glacial acetic acid extract of about 500,000 sheep hypothalamic fragments (4) used in the program of characterization of the releasing factors for the gonadotropins. The extract (2 kg) had been partitioned in two systems; the LRF concentrate was subjected to ion-exchange chromatography on carboxymethyl cellulose. At that stage, a fraction with SRIF-activity was observed well separated from the LRF zone; it was further purified (10) by gel filtration (Sephadex G-25) and liquid partition chromatography (n-butanol, acetic acid, water, 4:1:5). Thin-layer chromatography and electrophoresis of the final product showed only traces of peptide impurities. The yield was 8.5 mg of a product containing 75 percent of amino acids by weight, which is approximately 2 percent of that calculated on quantitative estimates of the amount of total SRIF activity in the original extract. The low yield was not of primary concern, because the early purification stages were designed specifically for the isolation of LRF and the amount of SRIF obtained as a side fraction was considered adequate for its characterization. Samples of SRIF gave a color reaction with ninhydrin, Ehrlich reagent, but not with Pauly reagent. The biological activity was totally destroyed by hydrolysis in 6N HCl as well as by digestion with chymotrypsin. Quantitative amino acid analyses of SRIF after acid hydrolysis (11) gave the following residues: Ala, 1; Gly, 1; Thr, 2; Lys, 2; Phe, 3; Ser, 1; Cys, 2; Trp, 1; Asp, 1; NH₃, 1 (12). Amino acid analysis, after total enzymatic digestion with papain and leucine aminopeptidase, showed the same amino acid ratios except that Asp occurred as Asn.

The sequence of SRIF was determined by stepwise Edman degradation performed on the intact carboxymethylated peptide, as well as on the unresolved products of tryptic and chymotryptic digests of the peptide. The products of Edman degradation were evaluated by the subtractive method by means of amino acid analysis, determination of the successive amino terminals with [¹⁴C]dansyl chloride and mass spectrometry of 3-phenyl-2-thiohydantoin (PTH) derivatives when applicable. The primary structure of isolated ovine SRIF is

H-Ala-Gly-Cys-Lys-Asn-Phe-Phe-Trp-Lys-
|_____|
Thr-Phe-Thr-Ser-Cys-OH.

Table 1. Effects of ovine hypothalamic extracts, purified preparations, pure native and synthetic SRIF on the secretion of growth hormone by rat pituitary cells in monolayer cultures; N, number of cell culture dishes; rGH, rat growth hormone by radioimmunoassay; CMC, carboxymethyl cellulose; N.S., not significant.

Additions	Doses	N	rGH (ng/hr)	P†
Saline		4	421.7 ± 49.1	
Hypothalamic extract	0.001 fragment/ml	3	231.0 ± 13.6	<.01
Hypothalamic extract	0.01 fragment/ml	3	118.7 ± 15.8	<.01
Hypothalamic extract	0.1 fragment/ml	3	91.3 ± 9.9	<.01
CMC fraction (185–200)	20 ng/ml	3	196.3 ± 52.5	<.01
CMC fraction (185–200)	200 ng/ml	3	83.6 ± 17.1	<.01
Saline		5	354.8 ± 23.9	
Hypothalamic extract	0.002 fragment/ml	5	190.7 ± 23.4	<.01
Hypothalamic extract	0.01 fragment/ml	3	120.0 ± 22.7	<.01
Hypothalamic extract	0.05 fragment/ml	3	50.7 ± 16.4	<.01
Native ovine SRIF*	0.2 nM	3	304.0 ± 45.5	N.S.
Native ovine SRIF	1.0 nM	3	210.7 ± 17.0	<.01
Native ovine SRIF	5.0 nM	3	70.7 ± 16.8	<.01
Native ovine SRIF	25.0 nM	4	52.5 ± 8.4	<.01
Synthetic SRIF‡	0.2 nM	3	420.0 ± 23.1	N.S.
Synthetic SRIF	1.0 nM	4	205.0 ± 23.8	<.01
Synthetic SRIF	5.0 nM	3	110.0 ± 5.8	<.01
Synthetic SRIF	25.0 nM	3	100.0 ± 6.1	<.01
Synthetic SRIF	3.3 μM	3	29.3 ± 14.6	<.01

* From data obtained by a four-point assay of synthetic versus native SRIF in best fit data (interval of doses = 5), the potency ratio of synthetic SRIF to native SRIF was 0.90. † From analysis of variance and multiple comparison test of Dunnett. ‡ Concentration of native or synthetic SRIF (triacetate) based on a calculated molecular weight of 1818.

Table 2. Effects of extracts of ovine hypothalamus or cerebellum and synthetic SRIF on growth hormone in plasma in rats treated with sodium pentobarbital. Animals were anesthetized with ether; the various substances (treatments) were injected intravenously (0.2 ml); this injection was immediately followed by intravenous administration of 2.5 mg of sodium pentobarbital per 100 g of body weight (14); blood was withdrawn 15 minutes later for radioimmunoassay of rat growth hormone (rGH) (7); N, number of rats per treatment; P, as in legend for Table 1. Both experiments were designed in completely randomized blocks.

Treatment	Doses	N	rGH (ng/ml)	P
Saline		21	74.1 ± 6.3	
Hypothalamic extract	0.3 fragment	21	54.5 ± 7.8	<.05
Hypothalamic extract	1.0 fragment	21	32.1 ± 5.7	<.01
Cerebellum extract	1.0 fragment equiv.	21	73.8 ± 8.8	N.S.
Saline		10	65.6 ± 8.4	
Hypothalamic extract	1.0 fragment	10	41.2 ± 5.3	<.05
Synthetic SRIF	0.1 μg	10	70.8 ± 7.2	N.S.
Synthetic SRIF	10 μg	10	32.0 ± 7.5	<.01

The sequence -Asn-Phe-Phe-Trp-Lys- was confirmed in an acetylated, permethylated tryptic digest of SRIF by direct mass spectrometry (10).

The linear tetradecapeptide was synthesized by solid-phase methodology and purified by gel filtration in presence of 2-mercaptoethanol (10). After purification, the synthetic peptide had the biological activity of the native SRIF (Tables 1 and 2); at concentrations ≥ 1 nM, native or synthetic SRIF inhibits the secretion of growth hormone from monolayer cultures of dispersed cells of rat adenohypophysis. In one experiment, native SRIF, at a concentration of 20 nM, inhibited significantly the spontaneous secretion of growth hormone by enzymatically dispersed cells derived from the pituitary gland of a patient with confirmed active acromegaly (13). The biological results with native and synthetic SRIF do not help to resolve the question of the reduced or oxidized state of the Cys residues in the peptide when it is recognized by the pituitary receptors; both the isolation procedure and the conditions that are used in the bioassays might convert one form into the other.

With the exception of primates, no simple adequate laboratory animal model seems to exist, which would exactly duplicate in vivo what is known of the physiological regulation of the secretion of growth hormone in humans. However, we found that the crude hypothalamic extract was able to inhibit (Table 2) the elevation of the plasma of growth hormone, as determined by radioimmunoassay, induced in rats by intravenous injection of sodium pentobarbital (14). This effect is specific for the hypothalamic extract as it is not duplicated by similar extracts of sheep cerebellum. Synthetic SRIF inhibits the secretion of growth hormone in similarly prepared assay rats (Table 2).

Native or synthetic SRIF has no effect on the basal secretion of LH or FSH (follicle stimulating hormone) in vitro at concentrations at which it inhibits maximally the secretion of somatotropin.

The peptide SRIF has been isolated and characterized with the use of an in vitro assay method of considerable reliability (6); the effects observed in vivo proceed from a method the rationale of which is less clearly established. Thus a physiological role for SRIF remains to be demonstrated. Should SRIF be active in humans (15), its possible clinical significance, particularly in the treatment of acromegaly and in the management of juvenile diabetes, has not escaped our attention.

References and Notes

1. A. Pecile and E. Muller, Eds., *Growth Hormone* (Excerpta Medica, Amsterdam, 1968).
2. R. Burgus, T. F. Dunn, D. Desiderio, R. Guillemin, *C.R. Hebd. Seances Acad. Sci. Ser. D Sci. Natur. Paris* 269, 1870 (1969).
3. C. Y. Bowers, A. V. Schally, F. Enzmann, J. Bøler, K. Folkers, *Endocrinology* 86, 1143 (1970).
4. H. Matsuo, Y. Baba, R. M. G. Nair, A. Arimura, A. V. Schally, *Biochem. Biophys. Res. Commun.* 43, 1344 (1971); R. Burgus, M. Butcher, N. Ling, M. Monahan, J. Rivier, R. Fellows, M. Amoss, R. Blackwell, W. Vale, R. Guillemin, *C.R. Hebd. Seances Acad. Sci. Ser. D Sci. Natur.* (*Paris*) 273, 1611 (1971); R. Burgus, M. Butcher, M. Amoss, N. Ling, M. Monahan, J. Rivier, R. Fellows, R. Blackwell, W. Vale, R. Guillemin, *Proc. Nat. Acad. Sci. U.S.A.* 69, 278 (1972).
5. W. Vale, G. Grant, R. Guillemin, *Frontiers in Neuroendocrinology, 1973*, W. Ganong, Ed. (Oxford University Press, London, in press).
6. W. Vale, G. Grant, M. Amoss, R. Blackwell, R. Guillemin, *Endocrinology* 91, 562 (1972).
7. The radioimmunoassay for rat growth hormone is a double antibody method, with NIH-rat GH-RP-1 as reference standard; for iodination, rat GH (H III-41E) (courtesy of Dr. S. Ellis, Ames Research Center, Moffett Field, Calif.), and for antiserum, monkey antiserum to rat GH (MK 33) (courtesy of Dr. J. Lewis, Scripps Research Foundation, La Jolla, Calif.).
8. L. Krulich, A. P. S. Dhariwal, S. M. McCann, in *Growth Hormone*, A. Pecile and E. Muller, Eds. (Excerpta Medica, Amsterdam, 1968), p. 32; *Endocrinology* 83, 783 (1968); A. P. S. Dhariwal, L. Krulich, S. M. McCann, *Neuroendocrinology* 4, 282 (1969); L. Krulich and S. M. McCann, *Endocrinology* 85, 319 (1969).
9. W. Vale, G. Grant, J. Rivier, M. Monahan, M. Amoss, R. Blackwell, R. Burgus, R. Guillemin, *Science* 176, 933 (1972).
10. The methodology involved is in preparation. See also (2) and J. Rivier *et al.*, *Chimia* 26, 300 (1972).
11. T. Y. Liu and Y. H. Chang, *J. Biol. Chem.* 246, 2842 (1971).
12. Abbreviations for amino acids are Ala, alanine; Asn, asparagine; Cys, cysteine; Gly, glycine; Lys, lysine, Phe, phenylalanine; Ser, serine; Thr, threonine; Trp, tryptophan; Asp, aspartic acid.
13. Radioimmunoassay for human growth hormone, by courtesy of Drs. S. Yen and T. Siler, University of California School of Medicine, San Diego. Fragments of a human acromegalic pituitary were obtained at time of surgical hypophysectomy, courtesy of Drs. Levin, Wilson, and Aubert, University of California School of Medicine, San Francisco.
14. H. Howard and J. M. Martin, *Endocrinology* 88, 497 (1971).
15. We propose to name the peptide described here *somatostatin*, from somato(tropin), a pituitary factor affecting statural growth, and stat(in), from the Latin "to halt, to arrest" (as in hemostat and bacteriostatic). This is in keeping with the efforts of several international nomenclature committees (with which the final decision should remain) aiming at creating trivial names for biologically active polypeptides rather than maintaining the use of acronyms.
16. Research supported by contract AID/csd 2785 from A.I.D., Ford Foundation, Rockefeller Foundation, and Edna McConnell Clark Foundation and a Canadian Medical Research Council postdoctoral fellowship to P.B.

Effects of Somatostatin on the Secretion of Thyrotropin and Prolactin

WYLIE VALE, CATHERINE RIVIER, PAUL BRAZEAU, AND ROGER GUILLEMIN

The Salk Institute for Biological Studies, Neuroendocrinology Laboratory, La Jolla, California

ABSTRACT. Somatostatin, a tetradecapeptide isolated from ovine hypothalamic extracts on the basis of its ability to inhibit the spontaneous secretion of growth hormone (GH) by pituitary cell cultures, has been found to inhibit the stimulated secretion of thyrotropin (TSH) mediated by TRF (pGlu-His-Pro-NH$_2$), 10 × [K$^+$], or theophylline *in vitro*, while having no effect on the secretion of luteinizing hormone (LH) due to LRF. The spontaneous release of PRL *in vitro* is also inhibited by somatostatin but to a lesser extent than is the spontaneous secretion of GH. *In vivo*, the TRF-triggered secretion of TSH but not of PRL is suppressed by somatostatin in the estrogen–progesterone-pretreated male rat. The injection of TRF leads to a greater rise in both plasma TSH and PRL in estrogen–progesterone-pretreated male rats than in untreated male rats. Somatostatin acts rapidly but reversibly to inhibit the secretion of TSH due to TRF in a dose-dependent manner. Thyroid hormones and somatostatin exhibit summation in their inhibition of TSH secretion *in vivo* and *in vitro*. These data indicate the potential for somatostatin, along with thyroid hormones and TRF, to play a physiological role in the regulation of TSH secretion. (*Endocrinology* 95: 968, 1974)

RECENTLY our laboratory reported the isolation, characterization and synthesis (1–3) of a peptide purified from ovine hypothalami which inhibits the secretion of radioimmunoassayable somatotropin (GH) by the adenohypophysis. This somatotropin release inhibiting factor (SRIF) was termed somatostatin. Somatostatin was identified throughout its purification by its ability to inhibit the spontaneous secretion of GH by cultures of enzymatically dissociated rat anterior pituitary cells (3). Somatostatin also inhibits the stimulated GH secretion mediated by dibutyryl 3′, 5′-cyclic AMP or theophylline *in vitro* (4). Subsequently, somatostatin was shown to inhibit "resting" or "stimulated" GH secretion in rats (5,6), dogs (7), baboons (8) and humans (9).

In preliminary communications we have reported that somatostatin can also inhibit the secretion of thyrotropin (TSH) and, in some circumstances, prolactin (PRL) (10,11). Although the existence and partial purification of a growth hormone release inhibiting activity in the hypothalamus had been noted by Krulich et al. (12) and others (13,14), no reports until the above preliminary communication (10) had described the presence of TSH release inhibiting activity in extracts of mammalian hypothalami; Peter has suggested (15) that in the goldfish the hypothalamus has an inhibitory effect on the secretion of TSH mediated by a hypothalamic TSH release inhibiting factor.

The following report presents evidence that somatostatin inhibits the secretion of TSH stimulated *in vitro* by various agents: TSH releasing factor (TRF), pGlu-His-Pro-NH$_2$, high medium potassium and theophylline. The *in vitro* spontaneous release of PRL is also decreased by somatostatin. *In vivo*, the TRF-mediated secretion of TSH but not of PRL is inhibited by somatostatin. We will furthermore describe experiments investigating the possible similarities of action between somatostatin and other inhibitors of TSH secretion, the thyroid hormones.

[*Editor's Note:* Material has been omitted at this point, including figures 1 through 6 and tables 1 through 6.]

potent inhibitor of TSH secretion *in vivo* and *in vitro*. Our original observations (10,11) of the effects of somatostatin on the secretion of TSH have now been confirmed in other laboratories with baboons (8) and human subjects (23).

In vitro, as little as 1 nM somatostatin (Fig. 7) decreases the TSH response to 10 nM TRF; *in vivo*, 1 µg somatostatin inhibits the TSH release due to 13-120 ng TRF (Fig. 4). Concentrations of somatostatin required for TSH release inhibiting activity *in vitro* are therefore in the range of those required for the inhibition of spontaneous GH release (11) and, in addition, are similar to the doses required for the activity of the hypothalamic releasing hormones TRF and LRF (apparent affinity constants of ca.3 and 0.5 nM, respectively (3)).

In vivo, TRF and LRF are effective in stimulating the secretion of the appropriate hormones in the rat at doses 10 to 1000 times less than the amounts of somatostatin that have been administered to evince inhibition of TSH and GH (5,6) secretion in the same species. The most likely explanation for this discrepancy in the minimal effective doses as seen *in vivo* is that the releasing hormones need only increase the secretion rate of a pituitary hormone for a

Discussion

The results presented here have demonstrated that somatostatin, which was purified on the basis of its ability to inhibit the secretion of growth hormone by rat anterior pituitary cell cultures, is also a

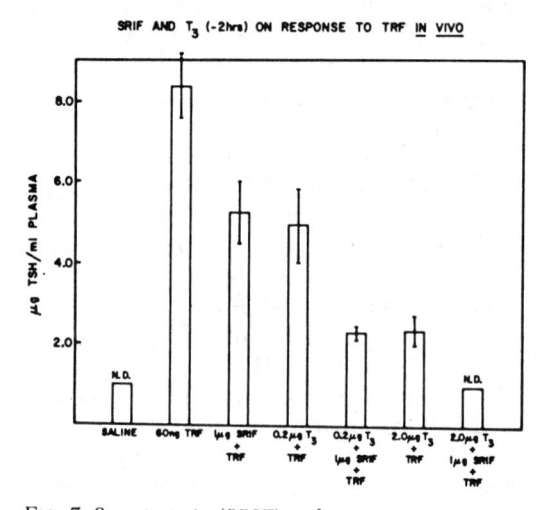

FIG. 7. Somatostatin (SRIF) and pretreatment (−2 hr) with triiodothyronine (T_3) on the TRF-mediated elevation in plasma TSH levels 5 min after injection in the estrogen–progesterone-primed rat.

short time in order to increase its plasma levels. An inhibitor of secretion must be present in an effective concentration throughout much of the period during which suppression is desired. As shown by Table 5, somatostatin is rapidly cleared from its site of action, since 20 µg of somatostatin is active when administered iv simultaneously with TRF but is not effective when given 5 or 20 min before TRF. It is therefore probable that high levels of somatostatin must be administered *in vivo* in order to maintain effective levels of the inhibitor throughout the period that TRF is present. Since blood radioactivity is sampled in the mouse bioassay 2 hr after the injection of TRF and/or somatostatin, the secretion of TSH as monitored takes place over a longer period of time in the mouse TRF bioassay than in the rat bioimmunoassay where blood is taken 5 min after injections. Perhaps the difference in time over which the secretion of TSH is followed explains the difference in the sensitivity of the two methods to somatostatin; alternatively, a species related difference in sensitivity is possible. The relative insensitivity of the mouse bioassay to somatostatin might reveal the reason that much higher levels of TRF are estimated in crude hypothalamic extracts with the mouse bioassay than with the rat bioimmunoassay (17).

Patterns of the specificity of action of somatostatin are evidenced by its inability to inhibit the secretion of LH due to LRF; more interestingly, the *in vivo* secretion of prolactin which is stimulated by TRF in the estrogen–progesterone-pretreated rat is not inhibited by somatostatin. Since we have presented earlier data showing that the TRF receptors on PRL-secreting cells and TSH-secreting cells are similar (17,24), these results suggest that somatostatin does not inhibit the TRF-mediated secretion of TSH by competing for binding to TRF receptors. This is further supported by the noncompetitive nature of the *in vitro* inhibition of TRF by somatostatin (Table 1A) and by the observation that somatostatin can suppress the spontaneous secretion of TSH in long-term experiments where TRF is presumably not involved and furthermore, can block the secretion of TSH stimulated by high potassium and theophylline. The *in vivo* reversibility of the somatostatin block by large doses of TRF possibly reflects the longer time of action of TRF at the higher doses; in other words, following iv administration, 120 ng TRF might remain in the circulation at effective levels longer than does 1 µg somatostatin. Thus, although the inhibition kinetics are not of the competitive type, the dynamics of action and rapid clearance of the two neurohormones allow fine modulation of TSH secretion.

No effect of somatostatin on the basal secretion of TSH *in vitro* is observed in short-term (<4 hr) experiments. However, in the 3-day experiment (Fig. 3), somatostatin inhibited the basal release of TSH by the pituitary cells in culture. The long-term administration of TRF to cultured pituitary cells increases the total TSH (fluids plus intracellular) in the cultures as we had reported earlier (3). Somatostatin is able to inhibit the increase in total TSH due to TRF. One interpretation of these data is that TRF enhances the rate of synthesis of TSH and that somatostatin suppresses the rate of synthesis of TSH. It is possible that the influences of both TRF and somatostatin on the synthesis of TSH are secondary to their effects on secretion.

The observation that pretreatment with sex steroids increases the secretion of TSH due to TRF in the rat is not surprising since similar results have been obtained in humans (25). Estrogens have been found to increase the responses of the PRL (17,26), GH (27) and gonadotropin-secreting (28) pituitary cells to various stimuli.

Although somatostatin does not inhibit the secretion of PRL stimulated by TRF *in vivo*, we usually observe an inhibition of PRL secretion by somatostatin *in vitro* (Table 3). This effect is seen often with pituitary cells from normal or estrogen–progesterone-treated rats and invariably with pituitary cells from castrated donor rats. It has been reported earlier that the ability of the rat anterior pituitary to secrete PRL in response to TRF is modified by the presence or absence of thyroid hormones (24) or steroids (25). It would therefore appear that the secretion of PRL can be influenced by a number of factors whose interrelations are not fully defined at the moment.

The *in vitro* influence of somatostatin on the secretion rate of PRL is considerably less than on the secretion of GH. Since this effect on PRL has not been seen in the intact rat, its significance is open to question, but we had anticipated that one might be rewarded by looking closely at the effects of somatostatin on the secretion of PRL in other species and under various pathological conditions. Indeed, somatostatin has been found (23) to lower plasma PRL levels in some acromegalic patients but not in normal subjects, an observation reminiscent of the effects of TRF (29) and LRF (30) on the secretion of GH in acromegalics.

All of the characterized hypothalamic hormones have been found to have multiple actions on the anterior pituitary: LRF releases both LH and FSH; TRF stimulates the secretion of TSH, PRL and under some conditions, GH (31). Somatostatin inhibits the secretion of GH, TSH and PRL as a function of the experimental situations. It would appear that there is a nonexclusive distribution of hypothalamic hormone receptors between the several pituitary cell types and that a variety of pathological and experimental circumstances (including the levels of peripheral hormones) can influence the functionality of those receptors. Whether these multiple activities are phylogenetic vestiges or represent important mechanisms for the synchronization of endocrine events remains to be defined. In view of the now unfolding extra-pituitary effects of the hypothalamic hypophysiotropic hormones on the nervous system (32,33,34), and endocrine pancreas (8,23) these questions should command even more attention in the future.

While the relationships between TRF, somatostatin, sex steroids and thyroid hormones on one hand and the secretion of TSH, GH and PRL on the other are obviously in need of clarification, a hypothesis can be suggested relating TRF, somatostatin and thyroid hormones to the regulation of the secretion of TSH.

Thyroid hormones have long been known to be feedback inhibitors of the secretion of TSH (35,36 for review). Later experiments have indicated that T_3 and T_4 can act at the pituitary level *in vivo* (37,38) and *in vitro* (39) to inhibit the release of TSH due to TRF. It is therefore possible that TRF controls the "setting" of the concentration at which thyroxine inhibits the secretion of TSH (40,41). The demonstration (37) of the functionally competitive relationship between thyroxine and TRF as they influence the secretion of TSH is consistent with this hypothesis. However, thyroid hormones and TRF do not directly compete for binding to the same receptor, as evidenced by the inhibitory effect of thyroxine on the secretion of TSH stimulated by elevating the potassium concentration of the medium (42). Experiments (21,22) with inhibitors of RNA and protein synthesis led further to the hypothesis that thyroid hormones induce in thyrotrophs a polypeptide or protein that mediates their suppression of TSH secretion. In contrast, the effects of somatostatin are not blocked by cycloheximide (Table 7). Furthermore, the time course of action of thyroid hormones and somatostatin differs. Somatostatin acts immediately to inhibit the response to TRF and is rapidly reversed when cleared from the pituitary; on the other hand, thyroid hormones have a longer latent period and greater persistence of action.

The observation (Figs. 6 and 7) that somatostatin and thyroid hormones exhibit pharmacological summation *in vivo* and *in vitro* are consistent with the suggestion that the ultimate steps in the mechanisms of action of those hormones might be common. Thus, the experimental evidence reported here raises the possibility that the secretion of TSH is under acute positive control by TRF and negative control chronically by thyroid hormones and acutely by somatostatin, with all three elements modulating TSH secretion in a concentration and time dependent manner.

Acknowledgments

The authors wish to thank Dr. J. Rivier for the synthesis of the peptides used in this study and C. Otto, A. Nussey, E. Tucker, K. Setbacken, V. Page, J. White and A. MacNiel for their excellent technical assistance. Research was supported by AID csd 2785 to R. Guillemin, Canadian Medical Research Council Fellowship to P. Brazeau and Edna McConnell Clark, Rockefeller and Ford Foundation Grants for the Salk Institute, and NIH AM 16707-01 to W. Vale.

References

1. Brazeau, P., W. Vale, R. Burgus, N. Ling, M. Butcher, J. Rivier, and R. Guillemin, Science 179: 77, 1973.
2. Rivier, J., P. Brazeau, W. Vale, N. Ling, R. Burgus, C. Gilon, J. Yardley, and R. Guillemin, C R Acad Sci (Paris) [D] 276: 2737, 1973.
3. Vale, W., G. Grant, M. Amoss, R. Blackwell, and R. Guillemin, Endocrinology 91: 562, 1972.
4. ———, P. Brazeau, G. Grant, A. Nussey, R. Burgus, J. Rivier, N. Ling, and R. Guillemin, C R Acad Sci (Paris) [D] 275: 2913, 1972.
5. Brazeau, P., J. Rivier, W. Vale, and R. Guillemin, Endocrinology 94: 184, 1974.
6. Martin, J., Endocrinology 94: 497, 1974.
7. Lovinger, R., M. Connors, A. Boryzcka, S. L. Kaplan, and M. M. Grumbach, Endocrinology 93: A-82, 1973.
8. Koerker, D. J., W. Ruch, E. Chickedel, J. Palmer, C. J. Goodner, J. Ensinck, and C. C. Gale, Science 184: 482, 1974.
9. Siler, T. M., G. Vandenberg, S. S. C. Yen, P. Brazeau, W. Vale, and R. Guillemin, J Clin Endocrinol Metab 37: 632, 1973.
10. Vale, W., P. Brazeau, C. Rivier, J. Rivier, G. Grant, R. Burgus, and R. Guillemin, Fed Proc 32: 211, 1973.
11. ———, ———, ———, ———, ———, ———, and ———, Endocrinology 93: A-139, 1973.
12. Krulich, L., A. P. S. Dhariwal, and S. M. McCann, In Pecile, A., and Muller, E. (eds.), Growth Hormone, Excerpta Medica, Amsterdam, 1968, p. 32.
13. ———, P. Illner, C. P. Fawcett, M. Quijada, and S. M. McCann, In Pecile, A., and E. Muller (eds.), Growth Hormone, Excerpta Medica, Amsterdam, 1972, p. 306.
14. Knobil, E., V. Meyer, and A. V. Schally, In Pecile, A., and E. Muller (eds.), Growth Hormone, Excerpta Medica, Amsterdam, 1968, p. 226.
15. Peter, R. E., Gen Comp Endocrinol 14: 334, 1970.
16. Vale, W., and G. Grant, In O'Malley, B. W., and J. G. Hardman (eds.), "Hormones and Cyclic Nucleotides", Methods in Enzymology, Academic Press, New York (In press).
17. Rivier, C. and W. Vale, Endocrinology 95: 50, 1974.
18. Ramirez, V. D., and S. M. McCann, Endocrinology 75: 206, 1964.
19. Vale, W., R. Burgus, T. F. Dunn, and R. Guillemin, Hormones 2: 193, 1971.
20. Sakiz, E., and R. Guillemin, Proc Soc Exp Biol Med 115: 856, 1964.
21. Vale, W., R. Burgus, and R. Guillemin, Neuroendocrinology 3: 34, 1968.
22. Bowers, C. Y., K. L. Lee, and A. V. Schally, Endocrinology 82: 303, 1968.
23. Yen, S. S. C., T. Siler, G. DeVane, J. Rivier, W. Vale, P. Brazeau, and R. Guillemin, Advances in Human Growth Hormone Research, Raiti, S.(ed.), DHEW, p. 159, 1973.
24. Vale, W., R. Blackwell, G. Grant, and R. Guillemin, Endocrinology 93: 26, 1973.
25. Sanchez-Franco, F., G. L. Cacicedo, A. Martin-Zurro, and F. Escobar del Ray, J Clin Endocrinol Metab 37: 736, 1973.
26. Valverde-R, C., V. Chieffo, and S. Reichlin, Endocrinology 91: 982, 1972.
27. Malacara, J. M., C. Valverde-R, S. Reichlin, and J. Bollinger, Endocrinology 91: 1189, 1972.
28. Arimura, A., and A. V. Schally, Proc Soc Exp Biol Med 136: 290, 1971.
29. Saito, S., K. Abe, H. Yoshida, T. Kaneko, E. Nakamura, N. Shimizu, and N. Yanaihara, Endocrinol Jap 18: 101, 1971.
30. Rubin, A. L., S. E. Levin, R. I. Bernstein, J. B. Tyrrell, C. Naocco, and H. P. Forsham, J Clin Endocrinol Metab 37: 160, 1973.
31. Carlson, H., and I. Mariz, Endocrinology 93: A-186, 1973.
32. Plotnikoff, N. P., A. J. Prange, G. R. Breese, M. S. Anderson, I. C. Wilson, Science 178: 417, 1972.
33. Moss, R. L., and S. M. McCann, Science 181: 177, 1973.
34. Segal, D. S., and A. J. Mandell, In Prange, A. J. Jr. (ed.), Thyroid Axis, Drugs and Behavior, Raven Press, 1973.
35. Hoskins, R. G., J Clin Endocrinol 9: 1429, 1949.
36. Reichlin, S., In Martini, L., and W. F. Ganong (eds.), Neuroendocrinology, VI, Academic Press, New York, 1966, p. 445.
37. Vale, W., R. Burgus, and R. Guillemin, Proc Soc Exp Biol Med 125: 210, 1967.
38. Schally, A. V., C. Y. Bowers, T. W. Redding, and J. F. Barrett, Biochem Biophys Res Commun 25: 165, 1966.
39. Guillemin, R., E. Yamazaki, D. A. Gard, M. Jutisz, and E. Sakiz, Endocrinology 73: 564, 1963.
40. VonEuler, C., and B. Holmgren, J Physiol (Lond) 131: 125, 1956.
41. Reichlin, S., Endocrinology 66: 327, 1960.
42. Vale, W., and R. Guillemin, Experientia 23: 855, 1967.

The Regional Distribution of Somatostatin in the Rat Brain

M. BROWNSTEIN,[†] A. ARIMURA,[††] H. SATO,[††] A. V. SCHALLY,[††] AND J. S. KIZER[†]

[†] *Laboratory of Clinical Science, National Institute of Mental Health, Bethesda, Maryland 20014; and* [††] *Endocrine and Polypeptide Laboratories, Veterans Administration Hospital and Department of Medicine, Tulane University Medical Center, New Orleans, Louisiana 70140*

THE secretion of growth hormone (GH) by the anterior pituitary appears to be regulated by both releasing and inhibitory factors which are secreted into the portal capillaries of the median eminence. Massive hypothalamic lesions made in brains of weanling animals cause growth retardation which may be attributable to a decrease in the resting rate of GH release (1–8). The secretion of GH has been shown to be depressed following stalk transection, pituitary transplantation, or hypothalamic lesions (9–11). Thus, it has been postulated that the hypothalamus normally stimulates the cells of the anterior pituitary which synthesize and release GH. This tonic stimulation is believed to be mediated by a GH-releasing factor (GH-RF) or hormone (GH-RH).

In the rat, stress results in the acute inhibition of GH secretion. This phenomenon has been postulated to be due to the elaboration of an inhibitory factor (12). Recently, Guillemin and his coworkers have isolated from ovine hypothalami, characterized, and synthesized a peptide which inhibits the release of immunoreactive GH *in vivo* and *in vitro* (13–15). This peptide has been named somatostatin, GH release inhibiting factor or hormone. We have recently generated antisera to synthetic somatostatin in rabbits and developed a sensitive and specific radioimmunoassay for this tetradecapeptide (16,17). Using this assay, we have determined the localization of somatostatin within the central nervous system of the rat and studied its distribution among the nuclei of the hypothalamus.

Materials and Methods

Female Osborne-Mendel (NIH strain) rats weighing 200 g were housed under diurnal lighting conditions (light: 6 AM to 6 PM; dark: 6 PM to 6 AM) and were given food and water *ad lib*. All animals were killed by decapitation between 8:00 to 9:00 AM.

Dissection of the brain. Initially, the concentration of somatostatin was measured in several large regions of the brain. Samples of these regions were prepared as follows: The *olfactory bulbs* were removed from the brain, and then a cut was made through the brain in the frontal plane at the level of the caudal end of the optic chiasm. With the aid of a plexiglass template second and third cuts were made parallel to the first one exactly 3 mm rostral and caudal to it respectively.* Thus, two slices of brain were

---

* In order to make this template, a hole, the shape of the dorsal surface of the brain, is cut in a block of plexiglass. The hole is deep enough so that the ventral surface of the brain is lower than the top surface of the block when the brain is set into it. Narrow grooves, just wide enough to accommodate double-edged razor blades, are cut in the plexiglass. These must extend as deep as the bottom of the hole. The grooves are cut perpendicular to the long axis of the brain and are spaced 3mm from one another. The brain is

---

Received November 18, 1974.

Please direct requests for reprints to: M. J. Brownstein, M.D., Laboratory of Clinical Science/NIMH, Building 10, Room 2D-47, Bethesda, Maryland 20014.

obtained which were 3 mm thick. The brain which remained rostral to the most anterior cut made up part of the sample of *cortex*. It contained part of the striatum. The portion of brain caudal to the most posterior cut was divided into samples of *cerebellum, mesencephalon,* and *brainstem* (18).

The more rostral 3 mm slice of brain was dissected into samples of *septum* and *preoptic area, striatum,* and *cortex*. The sample of septum and preoptic area also contained the anterior portion of the hypothalamus. It was limited laterally by vertical lines passing through the lateral ventricles, dorsally by the corpus callosum, and ventrally by the base of the brain. The sample of striatum was removed from the slice by making a cut which followed the contours of the corpus callosum and the anterior commissure. The striatum having been removed, the cortex was added to the sample of cortex obtained earlier.

The more caudal 3 mm slice of brain was divided into samples of *hypothalamus, thalamus,* and *cortex*. The hypothalamic sample extended from the base of the brain to the top of the third ventricle dorsally, and as far as the amygdala laterally. The thalamus was cut from the slice using the hippocampus and the internal capsule as landmarks. The cortex was added to the portions dissected earlier. The samples were immediately frozen on dry ice, weighed, homogenized in 10 volumes of ice cold 2N acetic acid, and centrifuged. The supernatants were lyophilized.

Since the entire brain was preserved in the course of the above dissection, the contribution of each individual region to the total amount of somatostatin in the brain could be determined. In order to define more precisely the localization of somatostatin within the various regions of the brain, a microdissection procedure was used. The brains were frozen and serial, coronal sections 300 μm in thickness were cut in a cryostat at -10 C. Samples were cut from the frozen sections with a Graefe knife or punched from them with small stainless steel needles according to the method of Palkovits (19). The dissections of nuclei of the hypothalamus (20,

positioned in the hole with its ventral surface uppermost, such that the rear of the optic chiasm is beneath one of the grooves. Then razor blades are placed in this groove as well as the ones immediately in front of and behind it.

21), brainstem (22) and limbic system (23) have been described in detail elsewhere. For determination of somatostatin in the relatively larger areas cut from the frozen slices (e.g., the amygdala, mamillary body, and substrantia nigra) tissue fragments from two rats were pooled and homogenized in microhomogenizers (Micrometric Instrument Company) in 200 μl of ice cold 2N acetic acid. For measurement of somatostatin in the hypothalamic nuclei, tissue fragments from six rats were pooled and homogenized in 200 μl of 2N acetic acid. After homogenization, 5 μl of each homogenate were removed for determination of protein (24) using bovine serum albumin as the standard. The homogenates were then centrifuged and the supernatants removed and lyophilized.

Assay of somatostatin. Somatostatin was determined by radioimmunoassay (RIA) as described elsewhere (16,17). Rabbit anti-somatostatin serum (No. 103) was used at a final dilution of 1:4900. Synthetic Tyr^1-somatostatin, iodinated with ^{125}I, served as the labeled hormone. The standard was synthetic cyclic somatostatin prepared by Dr. Coy. An excellent dose-response curve was obtained in a range from 4 to 512 pg somatostatin/tube in this RIA system (Fig. 1). There was no interference by other hypothalamic or pituitary hormones including TRH and LH-RH (16–17). The lyophilized samples were dissolved in 5–10 ml (for large tissue extracts) or 0.5–1 ml (for extracts of hypothalamic nuclei) of 0.1% gelatin/0.01M phosphate buffer/0.15M NaCl/0.025M EDTA, pH 7.4 and 20 or 100 μl of these solutions were assayed for somatostatin.

Results

The concentration of somatostatin in the nine major regions of the brain appear in Table 1. Not unexpectedly, the concentration of somatostatin is considerably higher in the hypothalamus than it is elsewhere, but somatostatin is not confined to the hypothalamus. The samples of septum and preoptic area, midbrain, brainstem, thalamus, and cortex all contained considerable amounts of somatostatin. While the concentrations of somatostatin in these regions were only about 1/3 to 1/10 of that found in the hypothalamus, the total

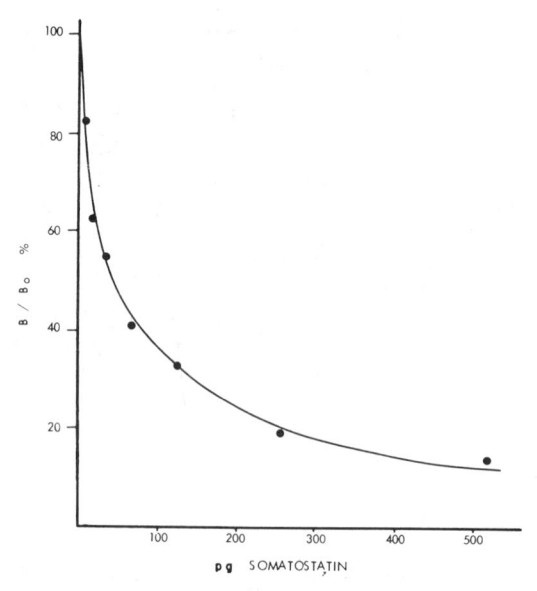

FIG. 1. Dose response curve of RIA for somatostatin. B and Bo represent bound radioactivity in the presence or absence of unlabeled hormone, respectively. Labelled hormone was [^{125}I]Tyr^1-somatostatin. Unlabelled hormone was cyclic somatostatin. Bound and free hormone were separated by dextran-coated charcoal. Rabbit antiserum against somatostatin, #103, was diluted 1:4900; 38% of total radioactivity was bound to the antibody in the absence of unlabeled hormone.

amount of somatostatin found in them was quite large. Thus, the hypothalamus only contains 28% of the somatostatin found in the brain. The cortex contains 22%, the brainstem 11%, the midbrain 7%, the thalamus 12%, and the septum and preoptic area 18%.

When selected areas of the above regions were removed from 300 μm sections and assayed, it was found that somatostatin was unevenly distributed within them (Table 2). For example, the preoptic area contains considerably more somatostatin than the septum, and the amygdala is richer in somatostatin than are the hippocampus and parietal cortex. The central grey is richer in somatostatin than the interpeduncular nucleus and the substantia nigra.

The distribution of somatostatin among the nuclei of the hypothalamus also proved to be markedly heterogenous (Table 3). As might have been expected, the concentration of somatostatin in the median eminence was very high; 7 times greater than that of the arcuate nucleus, which had a higher concentration of somatostatin than any other hypothalamic nucleus. Unlike luteinizing hormone releasing hormone (21), somatostatin was detected in all of the hypothalamic nuclei. The arcuate, periventricular, ventral premamillary and ventromedial nuclei had the highest concentrations. The median eminence which weighs about 0.28 mg (28 μg protein) contains 8.7 ng somatostatin, approximately 20% of the amount which was measured in our 18.5 mg hypothalamic sample (Table 1).

Discussion

Our results show that somatostatin is scattered among several hypothalamic nuclei and that it is present in extra-hypothalamic sites. Figure 2 shows the distribution of somatostatin in the hypothalamus. It is found in higher concentrations in regions adjacent to the third ventricle than areas located more laterally. In general, it is present in greater amounts caudally than rostrally.

Like luteinizing hormone releasing hormone (LH-RH), somatostatin is found in highest concentrations in the median eminence and arcuate nucleus. But unlike LH-RH, somatostatin does not seem to be

TABLE 1. Regional distribution of somatostatin (SRIF) in the rat brain

Region	Weight (mg) ± SEM	SRIF (ng/mg wet weight) ± SEM	ng/region
Olfactory bulb	51.9 ± 1.0	0.02 ± 0.01	1.0
Septum and preoptic area	38.6 ± 4.0	0.64 ± 0.04	24.7
Hypothalamus	18.5 ± 0.3	2.12 ± 0.08	39.3
Thalamus	116.4 ± 4.9	0.15 ± 0.01	17.5
Midbrain	158.5 ± 12.0	0.06 ± 0.01	9.5
Brain stem	195.7 ± 13.0	0.05 ± 0.01	9.8
Cerebellum	226.7 ± 7.6	0.02 ± 0.003	4.5
Striatum	64.8 ± 1.6	0.05 ± 0.004	3.2
Cortex	1,000 ± 12.6	0.03 ± 0.002	30.0
		Total	139.4

The brain was dissected as described in the text and the somatostatin content of each region was determined. The means and standard errors of the mean (SEM) of 3 separate determinations are given.

TABLE 2. Somatostatin content of selected brain areas

	ng/mg protein ± SEM
Cortical areas	
Amygdala	3.9 ± 0.4
Parietal cortex	2.4 ± 0.3
Hippocampus	1.1 ± 0.2
Brainstem-mesencephalun	
Substantia nigra	0.9 ± 0.1
Interpeduncular nucleus	1.0 ± 0.4
Central grey	3.3 ± 0.4
Dorsal raphe	1.1 ± 0.1
Diencephalon	
Habenula	1.3 ± 0.1
Mamillary body	2.7 ± 0.6
Pineal gland	0.5 ± 0.1
Olfactory tubercle	6.3 ± 0.9
Septum	2.1 ± 0.3
Preoptic area	8.4 – 1.3

The brain was frozen and serially sectioned and specific areas of the brainstem and limbic system were cut from the sections with a Graefe knife or punched from the sections with stainless steel needles. Means and standard errors (SEM) of 4 separate determinations are presented.

produced solely in the arcuate nucleus. As was postulated for thyrotropin releasing hormone (TRH) (25), somatostatin may be synthesized in cell bodies present in several hypothalamic nuclei, reaching neuronal terminals in the median eminence (26) by axoplasmic flow. In view of its widespread distribution throughout the brain, it is possible that somatostatin may function as a neurotransmitter in areas of the brain remote from the median eminence and as a release inhibitory hormone when it is secreted into the pituitary portal circulation.

The distribution of somatostatin (27) has recently been studied by means of a bioassay method (28). Extracts of hypothalamus and of other areas of brain inhibit the secretion of growth hormone by pituitary monolayers. Somatostatin-like activity has been found in extracts of discrete hypothalamic nuclei in a distribution similar to that described in the present manuscript. There is, however, one important difference between the results obtained by bioassay and immunoassay: Somatostatin-like activity is not detectable in the ventromedial nucleus (VMN) by bioassay. This suggests that there may be as much or more growth hormone releasing activity in the ventromedial nucleus as there is growth hormone inhibitory activity. This is compatible with the observations that lesions of the VMN cause a decrease in plasma growth hormone levels (8,29) and that electrical stimulation of the VMN causes a prompt increase in plasma growth hormone levels (30–34). Krulich et al. (12) have also concluded that somatostatin-releasing factor may primarily be produced in the VMN because hypothalamic slices which contain the VMN appear to be especially rich in releasing activity.

The distribution of somatostatin—measured by radioimmunoassay or by bioassay—summarized above differs from that reported by Hökfelt and his colleagues (35). Hökfelt used an immunohistochemical method for localizing SRIF. He employed the same antiserum which we used, but was able to detect SRIF only in axons of the ventromedial nucleus and median eminence. Since our radioim-

TABLE 3. Distribution of somatostatin among nuclei of the hypothalamus

	ng/mg protein ± SEM
Medial preoptic nucleus	10.4 ± 2.5
Periventricular nucleus	23.7 ± 9.0
Suprachiasmatic nucleus	8.0 ± 0.6
Supraoptic nucleus	3.2 ± 0.6
Anterior hypothalamic nucleus	8.6 ± 1.5
Lateral anterior nucleus	4.9 ± 1.1
Parventricular nucleus	4.4 ± 1.8
Arcuate nucleus	44.6 ± 6.1
Ventromedial nucleus	14.6 ± 2.1
Dorsomedial nucleus	5.4 ± 2.1
Perifornical nucleus	3.8 ± 0.7
Lateral posterior nucleus	3.5 ± 0.7
Ventral premamillary nucleus	17.3 ± 4.4
Dorsal premamillary nucleus	4.3 ± 0.7
Posterior hypothalamic nucleus	3.8 ± 0.8
Median eminence	309.1 ± 60.8

Means and standard errors (SEM) of 6 *separate* determinations are presented.

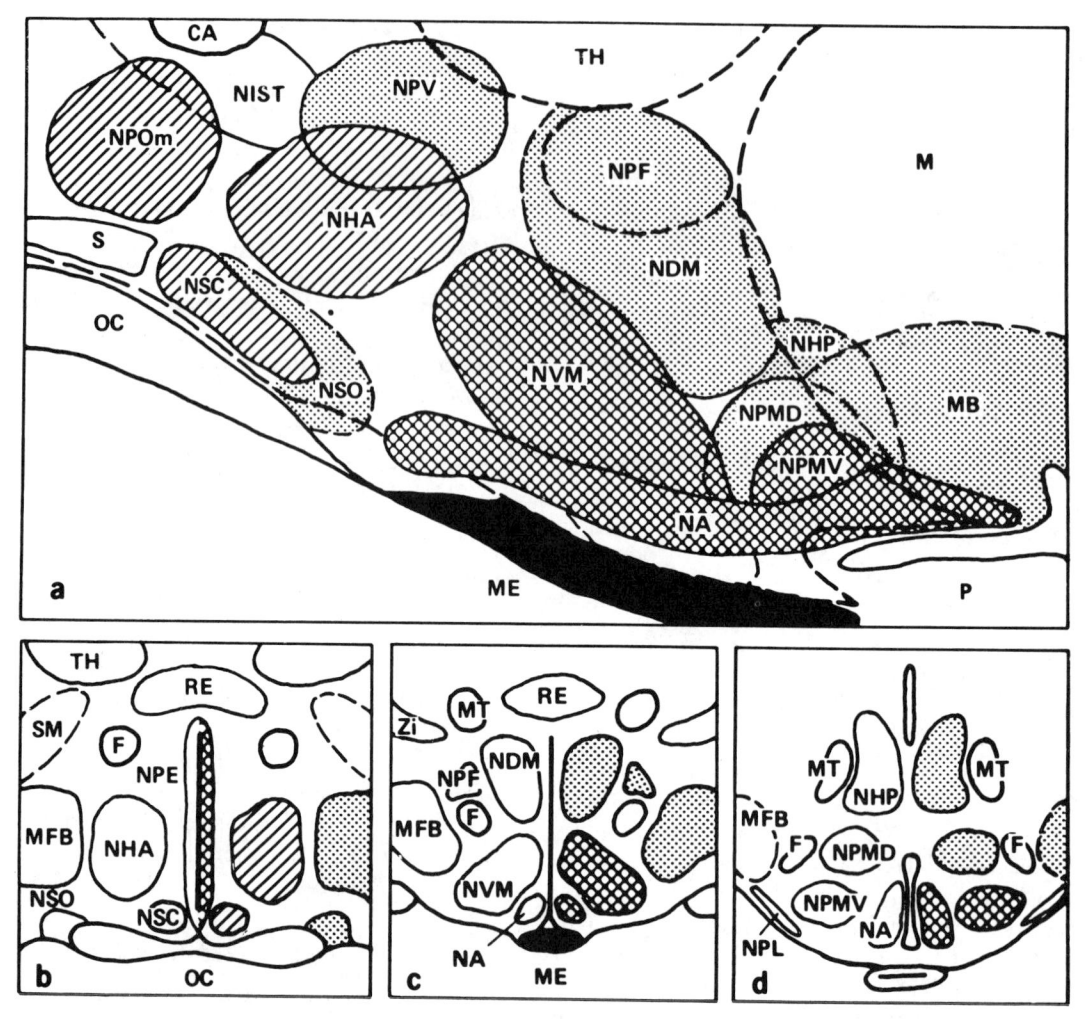

FIG. 2. Localization of somatostatin in nuclei of the hypothalamus. Drawing (a) is of a parasagittal section through this area of the brain. Drawings (b), (c), and (d) are of frontal sections through the anterior hypothalamus, the tuberal region, and the premamillary region, respectively. Relative concentrations of somatostatin are denoted as follows: ■ > ▨ > ▨ > ▣. Abbreviations: CA, anterior comissure; F, fornix; M, mesencephalon; MB, mamillary body; MT, mamillothalamic tract; ME, median eminence; MFB, medial forebrain bundle; NA, arcuate nucleus; NDM, dorsomedial nucleus; NHA, anterior hypothalamic nucleus; NHP, posterior hypothalamic nucleus; NIST, nucleus interstialis striae terminalis; NPE, periventricular nucleus; NPF, perifornical nucleus; NPL, prelateral mamillary nucleus; NPMD, dorsal premamillary nucleus, NPMV, ventral premamillary nucleus; NPOm, medial preoptic nucleus; NPV, paraventricular nucleus; NSC, suprachiasmatic nucleus; NSO, supraoptic nucleus; NVM, ventromedial nucleus; OC, optic chiasm; P, pituitary; RE, nucleus reuniens thalami; S, preoptic suprachiasmatic nucleus; SM, stria medullaris; TH, thalamus; ZI, zona incerta.

munoassay appears to be quite specific for SRIF, it is unlikely that the material which we have measured outside of the ventromedial nucleus and median eminence is another molecule which cross-reacts with the antiserum. Moreover, if this were the case, Hökfelt should have visualized the second molecular species in his study because he also used antisomatostatin serum No. 103. The most likely explanation for the discrepancy between our results and those of Hökfelt is that we are able to detect somatostatin in areas where its concentration is relatively low by means of pooling tissue obtained from several animals. It also seems that the cell bodies which manufacture releasing hormones and release inhibitory hormones can rarely be visualized. The reason for this is not known.

It is unlikely that the SRIF which we have found in our samples of tissue from the arcuate nucleus is there because of contamination by tissue from the adjacent median eminence. This contamination would not occur in the course of sectioning the brains, and care is always taken to remove the median eminence *before* the sample of arcuate nucleus is punched from the section.

Techniques based on the combination of microassay and microdissection have proven to be useful adjuncts to histochemical methods for the mapping of putative neurotransmitters and releasing hormones in the central nervous system of the rat. The widespread distribution of TRH (25), SRIF and prolactin release inhibiting activity (27) suggests a much broader role for peptidergic neurones in the brain than had been suspected. The interrelationship between peptidergic neurones and those which use other transmitters remains to be determined.

References

1. Endröczi, E., S. Kovács, and K. Lissák., *Endokrinologie* **33**: 271, 1956.
2. Kennedy, G. C., *Endocrinology* **16**: 9, 1957.
3. Hinton, G. C., and J. A. F. Stevenson, *Fed Proc* **18**: 69, 1959.
4. ———, and ———, *Can J Biochem Physiol* **40**: 1239, 1962.
5. Reichlin, S., *J Lab Ann Med* **54**: 937, 1959.
6. ———, *Endocrinology* **66**: 340, 1960.
7. ———, *Endocrinology* **67**: 760, 1960.
8. ———, *Endocrinology* **69**: 225, 1961.
9. Malacara, J. M., C. Valverde-R., S. Reichlin, and J. Bollinger, *Endocrinology* **91**: 1189, 1972.
10. Frohman, L. A., J. W. Maran, and A. P. S. Dhariwal, *Endocrinology* **88**: 1483, 1971.
11. Stachura, M. E., A. P. S. Dhariwal, and L. A. Frohman, *Endocrinology* **91**: 1071, 1972.
12. Krulich, L., P. Illner, C. P. Fawcett, M. Quijada, and S. M. McCann. In Pecile, A., and E. E. Müller (eds.),Growth and Growth Hormone, ICS 244, Excerpta Medica, Amsterdam, 1972, p. 306.
13. Vale, W., P. Brazeau, G. Grant, A. Nussey, R. Burgus, J. Rivier, N. Ling, and R. Guillemin, *C R Acad Sci (Paris)* **275**: 2913, 1972.
14. Brazeau, P., W. Vale, R. Burgus, N. Ling, M. Butcher, J. Rivier, and R. Guillemin, *Science* **179**: 77, 1973.
15. Rivier, J., P. Brazeau, W. Vale, N. Ling, R. Burgus, C. Gilon, J. Yardley, and R. Guillemin, *C R Acad Sci (Paris)* **276**: 666, 1973.
16. Arimura, A., H. Sato, and D. H. Coy, Program, 56th Meeting of the Endocrine Society, Abstract No. 196, p. A-153, 1974.
17. ———, ———, ———, and A. V. Schally, *Proc Soc Exp Biol Med* **148**: 784, 1975.
18. Glowinski, J., and L. L. Iverson, *J Neurochem* **13**: 655, 1966.
19. Palkovits, M., *Brain Res* **59**: 449, 1973.
20. ———, M. Brownstein, J. M. Saavedra, and J. Axelrod, *Brain Res* **77**: 137, 1974.
21. ———, A. Arimura, M. Brownstein, A. V. Schally, and J. M. Saavedra, *Endocrinology* **96**: 554, 1974.
22. ———, M. Brownstein, and J. M. Saavedra, *Brain Res* **80**: 237, 1974.
23. ———, J. M. Saavedra, R. M. Kobayashi, and M. Brownstein, *Brain Res* **79**: 443, 1974.
24. Lowry, O. H., N. Y. Rosenbrough, A. L. Farr, and R. J. Randall, *J Biol Chem* **193**: 265, 1951.
25. Brownstein, M., M. Palkovits, J. M. Saavedra, R. M. Bassiri, and R. D. Utiger, *Science* **185**: 267, 1974.
26. Pelletier, G., F. Labrie, A. Arimura, and A. V. Schally, *Am J Anat* **140**: 445, 1974.
27. Vale, W., C. Rivier, M. Palkovits, J. M. Saavedra, and M. Brownstein, Program of 56th Meeting of the Endocrine Society, Abstract No. 146, p. A-128, 1974.
28. ———, G. Grant, M. Amoss, R. Blackwell, and R. Guillemin, *Endocrinology* **91**: 562, 1972.
29. Frohman, L. A., and L. L. Bernardis, *Endocrinology*, **82**: 1125, 1968.
30. ———, L. L. Bernardis, and K. J. Kant, *Science* **162**: 530, 1968.
31. Bernardis, L. L., and L. A. Frohman, *Neuroendocrinology* **7**: 193, 1971.
32. Martin, J. B., *Endocrinology* **91**: 107, 1972.
33. ———, P. Mead, and J. A. Kontoz, *Endocrinology* **92**: 1352, 1973.
34. ———, *Endocrinology* **94**: 497, 1974.
35. Hökfelt, T., S. Efendic, O. Johansson, R. Luft, and A. Arimura, *Brain Res* **80**: 165, 1974.

Part VI
HYPOTHALAMIC-HYPOPHYSIAL CONTROL OF PROLACTIN SECRETION

Editor's Comments on Papers 46 Through 49

46 EVERETT
Luteotrophic Function of Autografts of the Rat Hypophysis

47 RATNER and MEITES
Depletion of Prolactin-Inhibiting Activity of Rat Hypothalamus by Estradiol or Suckling Stimulus

48 GROSVENOR, McCANN, and NALLAR
Inhibition of Nursing-Induced and Stress-Induced Fall in Pituitary Prolactin Concentration in Lactating Rats by Injection of Acid Extracts of Bovine Hypothalamus

49 JACOBS et al.
Increased Serum Prolactin after Administration of Synthetic Thyrotropin Releasing Hormone (TRH) in Man

Everett (Paper 46) demonstrated in female rats that removal of the hypophysis shortly after ovulation and transplanting it under the renal capsule maintained (actually favored) functional corpus lutea. The hypophysial luteotropic factor in rats was known at that time to be the lactogenic hormone; thus, he suggested that the results of his data indicated that removal of the hypophysis from its normal relationship with the hypothalamus actually results in increased hypophyseal secretion of the lactogenic hormone (prolactin). He also demonstrated that liberation of prolactin (PRL) from the transplanted hypophysis occurs independently of estrogen pretreatment. Deslin had previously shown that renal capsule grafts of adenohypophyses evoked corpus lutea hypertrophy and modification of the vagina, comparable to that seen in pregnancy, when the rats were treated with estrogen. Deslin's interpretation of his results was that estrogen caused luteotropin (PRL) secretion by a direct action on the transplanted hypophysial tissue. Everett's study showed that the effect was not due to a direct effect of estrogen. He further observed continuous secretory function by the corpus lutea up to ninety days after transplanatation of the hypophysis. Thus, Everett was the first to show that PRL secretion is tonically inhibited by the hypothalamus.

Ratner and Meites (Paper 47) studied the effects of suckling, estradiol, epinephrine, acetylcholine, and electrical stimulation of the uterine cervix on the content of PIF in the hypothalamus of rats. The PIF activity was determined by biological assay of extracted hypothalamus, tested by two hours of incubation with rat hypophysis and the media subsequently assayed for PRL. Suckling, reserpine, and estradiol completely depleted the hypothalamus of PIF activity. This study demonstrated that these factors that increase PRL release do so by decreasing levels of PIF in the hypothalamus, presumably by decreasing synthesis of PIF. Studies from the same laboratory demonstrated that a homogenate or acid extract of rat hypothalamus acts directly on the rat adenohypophysis in vitro to inhibit PRL synthesis and release. This group coined the term *prolactin inhibitory factor* (PIF) since the hypothalamic extract inhibited both synthesis and release of PRL.

Grosvenor et al. (Paper 48) demonstrated that PIF activity present in acid extracts of bovine stalk–median eminence inhibited the suckling-induced and stress-related fall in PRL content in vivo in lactating rats. Treatment with extracts of bovine cerebral cortex or ovine PRL did not inhibit this response. They concluded that the data provided in vivo evidence for the existence of a hypothalamic inhibitor factor in the normal regulation of PRL release and this PIF decreases in response to stress or nursing. They further suggested that PIF is always present, and probably is stored in the hypothalamus, and that the hypothalamic response to the suckling and stress stimulus is one of temporary inhibition of the tonic release of PIF. They believed that the pronounced effect of stress on PRL release makes it imperative that much care be taken to minimize stress in studies concerned with regulation of PRL secretion. They also suggested the possibility that a prolactin-stimulating factor is also present in the hypothalamus.

Barraclough and Sawyer (Paper 22) noted that animals treated with reserpine or chlorpromazine display an interruption of their estrus and menstrual cycles and that ovaries of rats treated with these agents contain numerous corpus lutea similar in size and appearance to those observed during pregnancy. They also noted that galactorrhea frequently occurs in female mammals and humans receiving these drugs. They performed a study to determine whether the administration of these drugs produces pseudopregnancy by causing the secretion of luteotrophic hormone (PRL). The results indicated that the pseudopregnant condition produced in rats was due to the increased secretion of PRL. They postulated that these drugs increase luteotrophic hormone release by blocking the hypothalamic control over hypophysial release of this hormone. This was the first description of what was later termed the *galactorrhea-amenorrhea syndrome* being produced by antidopaminergic drugs that interfere with hypothalamic release of a prolactin release-inhibitor factor (PIF).

In 1971, Jacobs (Paper 49) demonstrated that TRH is a potent and rapidly acting releaser of PRL in normal man, with mean peak responses occurring at approximately fifteen minutes after an intravenous bolus of TRH. These authors postulated, partly on the basis of prior in vitro work, that TRH stimulates PRL release by exerting a direct effect on the hypophysis, rather than via a hypothalamic effect mediated by inhibition of PIF release.

46

Copyright © 1954 by J. B. Lippincott Company

Reprinted from *Endocrinology* 54:685-690 (1954)

LUTEOTROPHIC FUNCTION OF AUTOGRAFTS OF THE RAT HYPOPHYSIS[1]

JOHN W. EVERETT

Department of Anatomy, Duke University School of Medicine, Durham, North Carolina

WESTMAN and Jacobsohn (1938) in experiments with hypophyseal stalk-sections in rats, reported certain results that have been difficult to explain. Adult, cyclic females were operated on during estrus or proestrus by the authors' usual technique. This included the placing of a barrier of metal foil between the cut end of the stalk and the hypophyseal capsule (Jacobsohn, personal communication). Although the intended purpose of the barrier was to prevent regeneration of nerve fibers, regeneration of the hypophyseal portal veins must have been equally impossible. Control animals were totally hypophysectomized. In all cases the cervix uteri was electrically stimulated 2 to 5 hours *after operation*. The uteri were traumatized 5 or 6 days later and were subsequently examined for deciduomata. Whereas the 7 completely hypophysectomized animals were negative, the 5 stalk-sectioned rats were positive. With the stalk having been cut before the time of cervical stimulation, how could the latter have induced pseudopregnancy, if this involves a reflex that is analogous to the ovulation reflex of the rabbit? It is important to note that Westman and Jacobsohn did not include control experiments in which the stalks were cut and cervical stimulation was omitted.

Recently Desclin (1950) described experiments in which he transplanted anterior hypophyses of estrogenized adult female rats to the kidney, obtaining luteotrophic function of the grafts in the absence of any fragments of gland remaining in the original site. In this instance the test for corpus luteum function was vaginal mucification in the presence of amounts of estrogen sufficient to cause vaginal cornification in the hypophysectomized controls. Desclin's interpretation is that estrogen can cause luteotrophin secretion by direct action on the hypophyseal tissue; that this does not require integrity of the connection of the hypophysis with the hypothalamus. No control experiments were reported that would test the possible luteotrophic activity of grafted hypophyses in the absence of estrogen.

Received for publication November 18, 1953.

[1] This investigation was supported in part by a grant from the Research Council of Duke University.

The present investigation demonstrates that anterior hypophyses, removed from female rats shortly after ovulation and transplanted to the renal capsule, will maintain fully functional corpora lutea without any stimulus other than may have resulted from the operation itself.

MATERIALS AND METHODS

Thirty adult, cyclic, virgin rats of the Vanderbilt strain were employed in these experiments, ranging in age from 5 to 11 months. Vaginal smear histories were recorded for several weeks preceding operation. The time of ovulation in the current cycle was judged on the basis of regularity of the preceding cycles (Everett, 1948; Everett, Sawyer and Markee, 1949; Everett and Sawyer, 1949). All operations were performed on the day after presumptive ovulation, when the vaginal smear registered full cornification.

Hypophysectomy was accomplished by the parapharyngeal route under ether anesthesia. To minimize fluid in the respiratory passages and resulting obstruction of the tracheal cannula,[2] atropine sulfate (10 mg./kg. body weight, in physiological saline)[3] was injected subcutaneously about 10 minutes before induction of anesthesia. The hypophysis was removed by suction and was recovered by a trap in the vacuum line.

In most of the transplantation experiments surgical approach to the left kidney was performed at the very outset, the wound then being temporarily closed until hypophysectomy had been accomplished. The pars distalis, usually in 2 pieces, was separated from the posterior lobe and inserted into a pocket inside the renal capsule. Pressure of the perirenal fat served to hold the graft in place as the body wall was being repaired. In 2 cases transplantation of pars distalis was made to a fascial pocket postero-lateral to the left common carotid artery.

Four days after transplantation or simple hypophysectomy the uterus was traumatized at laparotomy (ether anesthesia). Two silk threads were looped through short segments of the left uterus and tied along the antimesometrial border.

Eight days after the initial operation, hence 4 days after uterine traumatization, the uteri were examined for gross evidence of deciduomata. The degree of response was estimated on a scale of four. Portions of the traumatized uterine segments and at least one ovary were fixed in Zenker's fluid for histological examination. The cranium was opened, the brain was removed and a portion of the cranial floor including the pituitary capsule was placed in Heidenhain's Susa fixative for 24 hours. Decalcification was completed in 5% trichloracetic acid for 48 to 72 hours, after which washing and dehydration were accomplished in successive changes of 95% alcohol and dioxane. Serial sections were then prepared and rigorously searched for remnants of the hypophysis.

---

[2] The tracheal cannula that proved most satisfactory is a 10 cm. length of polyethylene tubing (1.57×2.08 mm. inside and outside diameters, resp., Clay-Adams #PE205). The tube is beveled at the tip to aid its passage through the glottis by way of the oral cavity and pharynx. A retractable soft wire core maintains a slight curve of the beveled end of the tube during its introduction, and is then removed. A stiff rubber washer, placed along the tube about 4 cm. from the tip is caught by the upper incisor teeth to prevent accidental retraction during manipulation of the trachea and pharynx.

[3] This amount of atropine is far below the minimal subcutaneous dose (230 mg./kg.) effective in blockade of the ovulatory stimulation of the rat hypophysis (Everett and Sawyer, 1953).

RESULTS AND DISCUSSION

The result are summarized in Table 1. The definitive control and experimental groups (I and II) comprise animals in which complete removal of pars distalis had been accomplished. The inclusion of additional groups in which hypophysectomy had been incomplete requires explanation. Inadequate vacuum during the early stages of the investigation resulted in a surprisingly large number of such cases. Where extensive fragments of retained pars distalis were found in the control series the data are included because the results bear on the question at issue (group V). The least amount found in this group (in the negative case) was a single fragment measuring approximately $1.0 \times 0.5 \times 0.2$ mm. Groups III and IV retained considerably less. In control group III the largest amount was a single piece approximately $0.55 \times 0.5 \times 0.1$ mm. One other rat had almost as much, while the other four had much less. Group IV was purposely limited to grafted animals in every one of which the aggregate of retained bits was obviously far less than the largest amount in group III.

Inspection of the table will disclose that every hypophysectomized animal that bore a graft of pars distalis developed a strong deciduoma reaction in the traumatized uteri. Among the controls deciduomata were absent in group I in which hypophysectomy had been complete, as well as in group III in which minute fragments of anterior lobe remained *in situ*. Retention of a large fragment, however, was nearly always sufficient in itself to produce deciduomata that were often of maximal size (group V).

The corpora lutea of all the animals that developed deciduomata were distinctly larger than in the negative cases, resembling those of normal pseudopregnancy histologically. On the other hand, examination of serial sections of the ovaries discloses no evident difference between grafted animals and controls with respect to status of follicles and interstitial tissue. No healthy follicles are found beyond the stage of incipient antrum formation. In this respect the ovarian picture is decidely at variance with that of

TABLE 1. DECIDUOMA FORMATION IN FEMALE RATS BEARING AUTOGRAFTS OF ANTERIOR HYPOPHYSIS

Group no.	Hypophysectomy	Grafted to:	No. of rats	Deciduoma reaction ++	+++	++++	Total pos.	Total neg.
I	Complete	—	3				0	3
II	Complete	Renal capsule	6		1	5	6	0
III	Nearly complete	—	6				0	6
IV	Nearly complete	Renal capsule	6		2	4	6	0
		Neck	2		1	1	2	0
V	Extensive fragment left	—	7	2	1	3	6	1

normal pseudopregnancy, where prominent vesicular follicles are common. It is also significant that wide spread wheel-cell formation appears in the interstitial tissue of both the grafted and the control animals. Thus, neither the grafts (groups II and IV) nor the retained fragments of anterior lobe (group V) had been secreting effective amounts of either FSH or LH. They had been releasing sufficient luteotrophin, however, to maintain corpus luteum function.

The grafts were uniformly well vascularized, as attested in the fresh tissue by their normal pink color. In the histological sections the sinusoids are seen to be well-developed; the parenchyma remains in good condition save in the interiors of the grafts, where it has been replaced by connective tissue. Characteristically, healthy parenchyma extends inward from all surfaces to a depth of some 0.1–0.2 mm., while the dimensions of the connective tissue core vary with form of the graft. The inner regions must have been severely damaged before circulation became reestablished.

It must be assumed that for some ill-defined period of time after transplantation hormones already present were passed into circulation by absorption from necrotic tissue. In fact, the question arises whether maintenance of corpora lutea throughout the 8-day period may have been produced by such absorption rather than by actual secretion of luteotrophin. Several considerations, however, favor the latter alternative. According to current views, the hypophyseal luteotrophic factor in rats is the lactogenic hormone (Evans et al., 1941; Tobin, 1942; Nelson and Pichette, 1943; Everett, 1944; Gaarenstroom and de Jongh, 1946; Desclin, 1948; Mayer, 1951). In substitution experiments the required amounts of lactogen for maintaining pseudopregnancy are on the order of 15 to 20 I.U. injected subcutaneously once daily. According to Reece and Turner (1937) the average lactogen content of group of estrous rat hypophyses was 4.8 bird units per gland, equivalent to approximately 0.2 I.U. (1 Reece-Turner unit = ca. 0.045 I.U.— Meites et al., 1941). One must admit, of course, that minute amounts released gradually and continuously may be far more effective than a large amount injected once daily. Yet the maturity of the connective tissue in the internal portion of the grafts indicates that deterioration of parenchyma and its removal had been precipitous rather than gradual. Such would be expected *a priori*. Thus it seems almost certain that corpus luteum function in the grafted animals reflected actual luteotrophin secretion.

Conclusive evidence is furnished by certain additional experiments that will be fully described in a subsequent publication. These are long-term experiments that demonstrate corpus luteum secretory function for 33, 60 and even 90 days after transplantation of pars distalis to the renal capsule.

There is no evidence of the formation of additional corpora lutea. Follicular apparatus and interstitial tissue remain atrophic.

It should be emphasized that in none of the experiments just mentioned or those listed in Table 1 was there any special stimulation administered that was designed to cause pseudopregnancy. It seems that the mere fact of removal of the gland from its normal relation with the hypothalamus favors luteotrophin secretion at the expense of the other gonadotrophic factors.

In this connection it is significant that pseudopregnancy was obtained in most of the control animals (group V) in which a large fragment of anterior lobe remained in place. These experiments are analogous to the stalk-sectioned series of Westman and Jacobsohn (*loc. cit.*). There now seems little doubt that the additional factor of cervical stimulation in their animals was superfluous. The fact of stalk-section itself was apparently the cause of pseudopregnancy.

Some readers may insist that irritation of the hypophysis during either the act of cutting the stalk or the act of transplantation is sufficient to account for this luteotrophic function. This hardly seems likely in view of the great length of time during which the new activity can be maintained. To this writer it seems the better choice to regard the effect as a release phenomenon. It is interesting that Greep and Jones (1950), considering possible explanations of the production of pseudopregnancy in rats by estrogen treatment, suggested that the fundamental action of estrogen here may be suppression of FSH and LH secretion, after which luetotrophin secretion "proceeds apace."

Desclin's interpretation of his results, to the effect that estrogen invoked luteotrophin secretion by direct action on the grafted hypophyses, does not now appear to be correct. The estrogen was superfluous. Nevertheless, the present experiments amply confirm his original observation of the fact that the rat hypophysis, although isolated from the central nervous system by transplantation to the kidney, can yet secrete luteotrophic hormone. The new information is that secretion of this particular hormone is actually favored by such isolation. In addition the present results emphasize sharply the physiological distinction in this species between the two gonadotrophic hormones FSH and LH, on the one hand, and the luteotrophic factor, on the other.

SUMMARY

Adult virgin female rats were hypophysectomized on the day following ovulation. In the experimental animals the anterior hypophysis was autotransplanted to the renal capsule (12 cases) or the vicinity of the common carotid artery (2 cases). Control animals were simply hypophysectomized.

The uteri of all rats were traumatized 4 day later and autopsy was performed on the eighth day.

None of the 9 control rats in which hypophysectomy had been either complete or nearly complete formed deciduomata. However, good deciduomata were formed in 6 grafted animals that had been completely hypophysectomized and 8 in which hypophysectomy had been nearly complete. In addition, 6 of 7 partially hypophysectomized, non-grafted animals that retained large fragments of the gland gave significant deciduoma reactions.

The results indicate that removal of the gland from its normal relationship with the hypothalamus, or even local interference with such relationship, not only allows luteotrophin secretion to take place, but actually favors this activity.

REFERENCES

DESCLIN, L.: *Compt rend. Soc. biol.* **142**: 1436. 1948.
DESCLIN, L.: *Ann. d'endocrinol.* **11**: 656. 1950.
EVANS, H. M.; M. E. SIMPSON, W. R. LYONS AND K. TURPEINEN: *Endocrinology* **28**: 933. 1941.
EVERETT, J. W.: *Endocrinology* **35**: 507. 1944.
EVERETT, J. W.: *Endocrinology* **43**: 389. 1948.
EVERETT, J. W. AND C. H. SAWYER: *Endocrinology* **45**: 581. 1949.
EVERETT, J. W. AND C. H. SAWYER: *Endocrinology* **52**: 83. 1953.
EVERETT, J. W., C. H. SAWYER AND J. E. MARKEE: *Endocrinology* **44**: 234. 1949.
GAARENSTROOM, J. H. AND S. E. DE JONGH: Contribution to the Knowledge of the Influences of Gonadotropic and Sex Hormones on the Gonads of Rats. Elsevier Publ. Co., New York. 1946.
GREEP, R. O. AND I. C. JONES: *Recent Progr. Hormone Res.* **5**: 197. 1950.
MAYER, G.: *Arch. sc. physiol.* **5**: 247. 1951.
MEITES, J., A. J. BERGMAN AND C. W. TURNER: *Endocrinology* **28**: 707. 1941.
NELSON, W. O. AND J. W. PICHETTE: *Fed. Proc.* **2**: 36. 1943.
REECE, R. P. AND C. W. TURNER: *Mo. Agri. Exper. Sta. Res. Bull.* No. 266. 1937.
TOBIN, C. E.: *Endocrinology* **31**: 197. 1942.
WESTMAN, A. AND D. JACOBSOHN: *Acta path. microbiol. Scandinav.* **15**: 445. 1938.

Depletion of Prolactin-Inhibiting Activity of Rat Hypothalamus by Estradiol or Suckling Stimulus[1]

ALBERT RATNER AND JOSEPH MEITES[2]

Michigan State University, Department of Physiology, East Lansing, Michigan

ABSTRACT. Previous studies from this laboratory have shown that the hypothalamus contains a factor(s) which inhibits prolactin synthesis and release *in vitro*. The present experiments were undertaken to determine whether certain prolactin-releasing agents acted by depressing hypothalamic production of "prolactin-inhibiting factor" (PIF). Anterior pituitary incubated in a Dubnoff shaker at 37 C for 2 hr in a medium containing hypothalamic extract from rats injected with estradiol, or from suckled postpartum rats, released 114 and 133% more prolactin, respectively, than similar pituitaries incubated with hypothalamic extract from control cycling rats. Hypothalamic extract from the estradiol-treated or suckled rats had no significant effect on prolactin release by incubated anterior pituitary, whereas hypothalamic extract from control cycling rats inhibited prolactin release by some 50%. These results indicate that estradiol and suckling can deplete the hypothalamus of PIF, thus removing hypothalamic inhibition to pituitary prolactin release. (*Endocrinology* 75: 377, 1964)

MANY studies have demonstrated that the central nervous system (CNS), in particular the hypothalamus, exerts an inhibitory effect on prolactin secretion. Placement of appropriate lesions in the hypothalamus, transection of the pituitary stalk, transplantation of the anterior pituitary to noncranial sites, administration of various CNS depressant drugs and culture of the anterior pituitary *in vitro* result in a marked decrease in secretion of all anterior pituitary hormones except prolactin (1). Prolactin secretion following removal of hypothalamic connections is increased, as indicated *in vivo* by prolonged maintenance of the corpora lutea in rats and mice, and induction of mammary growth and lactation in these and other species. Under *in vitro* conditions, the rat pituitary can release many times more prolactin per day than is present in the pituitary *in situ* (2, 3). These observations suggested that the hypothalamus produces a factor(s) which reaches the anterior pituitary through the hypothalamic-hypophysial portal system and inhibits prolactin secretion. Talwalker, Ratner and Meites (4) recently demonstrated that a homogenate or acid extract of rat hypothalamus acts directly on rat anterior pituitary *in vitro* to inhibit prolactin synthesis and release. Rat cerebral cortical extract had no effect. Since the hypothalamic extract inhibited both synthesis and release of prolactin, the active agent was tentatively named "prolactin-inhibiting factor" (PIF). Pasteels (5) has similarly reported that rat hypothalamus inhibits pituitary prolactin release *in vitro*.

Received February 20, 1964.

This work was supported in part by grants from the NIH (AM 4784-04) and the Michigan Cancer Foundation.

[1] Published with the approval of the Michigan Agricultural Experiment Station as journal article no. 3327.

[2] An oral report of these results was presented by the junior author at the Symposium on Regulation of the Secretion of Gonadotrophins, Fed. of Am. Soc. for Exper. Biology, April 18, 1963, Atlantic City, N. J.

Our laboratory has demonstrated that many agents, including hormones, drugs, certain environmental stimuli and stresses can increase prolactin release and initiate mammary secretion in rats or rabbits (1). We suggested that some of these factors may act by suppressing hypothalamic inhibition of prolactin release. With the demonstration of the existence of a prolactin-inhibiting factor, studies were undertaken to determine whether certain of the prolactin-releasing agents could act by depressing hypothalamic production of PIF. Two natural agents which have been shown to be particularly potent for inducing pituitary prolactin release *in vivo* are estrogen and the suckling stimulus. These agents can initiate lactation in a variety of species, and suckling has an important role in postpartum maintenance of lactation (6). Our present study demonstrates that estradiol and suckling can completely deplete the rat hypothalamus of PIF.

Materials and Methods

Animals. Mature female rats of the Wistar strain (Wilson and Son, Acton, Indiana) were used in all experiments. They were housed in a temperature-controlled room at 75 ± 1 F and fed Wayne Lab Blox pellets *ad lib*. White King squabs, 5–8 weeks old, were used for prolactin assays.

Incubations. After decapitation, the posterior lobe was removed and discarded, and the anterior pituitary was hemisected. One half was placed in a 25 ml Erlenmeyer flask (control) containing 2 ml of medium, and the other half was placed into a similar flask (experimental) containing 2 ml of medium. The equivalent of 3 anterior pituitaries was placed into each flask. Hypothalamic extract was placed in some of the flasks as shown in the tables. All incubations were carried out at pH 7.4 in a Dubnoff metabolic shaker (60 cycles/min) under constant gassing with humidified $96\% \; O_2$-$5\% \; CO_2$, at 37 C for 2 hr.

Preparation of Hypothalamic Extracts and Medium. Hypothalamic extract was prepared from (a) suckled rats which were constantly with their litters until killed on day 12–18 postpartum and (b) rats injected subcutaneously daily with 50 µg estradiol benzoate in 0.1 ml corn oil for 10 days. Each hypothalamus, including the median eminence, was removed and placed in cold 0.1N HCl (10 hypothalami/ml), homogenized and centrifuged at $20,000 \times g$ for 30 min at 4 C. The supernatant was added to protein-free medium 199 (Difco Laboratories, Detroit, Michigan) and the pH was adjusted to 7.4 by addition of $5.6\% \; NaHCO_3$ solution. The final volume was made up so that each ml of medium contained extract equivalent to 3 rat hypothalami. Control hypothalamic extract was prepared in the same manner from cycling rats. The hypothalamic tissue from the control and experimental animals was removed and extracted at the same time.

Prolactin Assay and Statistical Treatment. After incubation the medium was assayed for prolactin in 5- to 8-week-old White King squabs by the intradermal method (7). The medium from each flask pair was assayed in 4 birds, or the medium from 2 flask pairs was pooled and assayed in 8 birds. The medium from the control flask was injected over one side of the crop sac and the medium from the experimental flask was injected over the other side. This permitted each bird to serve as its own control and provided a direct comparison between the 2 samples. The prolactin responses in each bird were rated by the method of Reece and Turner (7), and these responses were converted to International Units by using a standard dose-response curve established in the same breed of pigeons with NIH prolactin (3). The results from the assays of the control and experimental medium in each experiment were analyzed by the *t* test for paired experiments (8). The percentage difference in prolactin content between the control and experimental medium was determined as follows:

$$\% \; \text{Difference} = \frac{\text{Experimental} - \text{Control}}{\text{Control}} \times 100.$$

It should be pointed out that the prolactin assay results from different experiments are not comparable, since the amounts of prolactin released into the medium by pituitary tissue from different rats vary greatly from one experiment to another. The only valid

TABLE 1. Effect of hypothalamic extract (HE) from estradiol-injected rats on pituitary prolactin release *in vitro*

Experiment No.	No. of flask pairs	No. of assays	No. of pigeons	Average prolactin released into medium IU/100 mg AP* Control	Experimental	Average % difference	p† C vs. E
HE from control cycling rats vs. HE from estradiol-treated rats								
1	5	3	19	1.3	3.3	+153	.01
2	4	2	13	1.5	2.6	+ 73	.05
3	4	2	15	2.5	5.4	+116	.01
No HE vs. HE from estradiol-treated rats								
4	4	2	15	3.7	3.8	+ 3	NS‡
5	4	2	16	1.1	1.3	+ 18	NS
6	4	2	14	2.4	2.3	− 4	NS
No HE vs. HE from control cycling rats								
7	4	2	14	2.6	1.2	− 54	.01

* Anterior pituitary.
† Computed using the *t* test for paired experiments.
‡ Not significant.

comparisons that can be made are between the amounts of prolactin released by 2 anterior pituitary halves from the same rat pituitary, assayed in the same pigeon.

Results

1. *Effect of Hypothalamic Extract from Estradiol-Treated Rats on Pituitary Prolactin Release* in Vitro (Table 1). Medium containing hypothalamic extract from estradiol-treated rats was added to the experimental flask and an equivalent amount of hypothalamic extract from control cycling rats was added to the corresponding control flask. A total of three separate experiments were carried out, and 2 to 6 flask pairs were incubated per experiment. It can be seen (Experiments 1, 2, 3) that anterior pituitary halves incubated with hypothalamic extract from estradiol-treated rats released an average of 114% more prolactin into the medium than anterior pituitary halves incubated with hypothalamic extract from control cycling rats.

In a second series of experiments, hypothalamic extract from estradiol-treated rats was added to each experimental flask, but no hypothalamic extract was added to the corresponding control flask. No significant difference was observed in the amount of prolactin released by the anterior pituitary tissue incubated with hypothalamic extract from estradiol-treated rats as compared to pituitary incubated without hypothalamic extract (Experiments 4, 5, 6), showing that the hypothalamic extract had lost its ability to inhibit prolactin release. When anterior pituitary was incubated with hypothalamic extract from control cycling rats (Experiment 7), 54% less prolactin was released into the medium than by the corresponding control pituitary incubated in the absence of hypothalamic extract. This corresponds to a 54 to 72% reduction in pituitary prolactin release after incubation with hypothalamic extract from cycling rats reported by Talwalker *et al.* (4).

2. *Effect of Hypothalamic Extract from Suckled Rats on Pituitary Prolactin Release* in Vitro (Table 2). Anterior pituitary incubated with hypothalamic ex-

TABLE 2. Effect of hypothalamic extract (HE) from suckled rats on pituitary prolactin release *in vitro*

Experiment No.	No. of flask pairs	No. of assays	No. of pigeons	Average prolactin released into medium IU/100 mg AP* Control	Experimental	Average % difference	p† C vs. E
			HE from control cycling rats vs. *HE from suckled rats*				
1	6	3	22	1.1	2.6	+136	.01
2	3	3	13	0.8	2.2	+175	.01
3	4	2	14	1.7	3.2	+ 88	.01
			No HE vs. *HE from suckled rats*				
4	4	2	11	1.6	1.5	− 6	NS‡
5	4	2	14	1.1	1.2	+ 9	NS
6	4	2	13	1.6	1.3	− 19	NS
			No HE vs. *HE from control cycling rats*				
7	4	2	15	3.0	1.6	− 47	.05

* Anterior pituitary.
† Computed using the t test for paired experiments.
‡ Not significant.

tract from suckled rats released an average of 133% more prolactin into the medium than anterior pituitary incubated with hypothalamic extract from control cycling rats (Experiments 1, 2, 3). No significant difference was observed in the amount of prolactin released by pituitary incubated with hypothalamic extract from suckled rats when compared to the corresponding pituitary incubated without hypothalamic extract (Experiments 4, 5, 6), indicating that suckling had removed hypothalamic PIF. When anterior pituitary was incubated with hypothalamic extract from control cycling rats (Experiment 7), 47% less prolactin was released into the medium than by the corresponding control pituitary incubated in the absence of hypothalamic extract.

Discussion

The present study indicates that estradiol and the suckling stimulus can suppress hypothalamic inhibition of prolactin secretion. Hypothalamic extract from estradiol-treated or suckled rats had no capacity to inhibit prolactin release by incubated rat anterior pituitary tissue, whereas hypothalamic extract from control cycling rats inhibited release of prolactin by the anterior pituitary by 47 to 54%. These results indicate, therefore, that estradiol or the suckling stimulus can completely deplete the rat hypothalamus of PIF. Depletion of PIF is attributed to reduced PIF synthesis rather than to increased release, since an increase in PIF release should have resulted in inhibition of pituitary prolactin release. On the contrary, estrogen administration or the suckling stimulus induces increased prolactin release and initiates lactation (6).

Acid extracts of the hypothalamus apparently contain the follicle-stimulating, luteinizing, thyrotropic, corticotropic and somatotropic releasing factors, as well as the prolactin-inhibiting factor (4). Changes in hypothalamic content of three of these neurohumors in response to changes in circulating hormone titers have recently been reported. Vernikos-Dannellis (9) observed an increase in corticotropin-releasing activity of rat hypothalamic extract after stress, and

Kobayashi et al. (10) reported an increase in gonadotropin-releasing activity of rat hypothalamus after ovariectomy. Deuben and Meites (unpublished) recently noted that thyroxine increased hypothalamic growth hormone releasing activity in the rat. These observations support the concept that release of anterior pituitary hormones can be altered by stimulating or depressing production of hypothalamic neurohumors which control release of pituitary hormones. This does not rule out other possible modes of action, such as a direct effect by some hormones or drugs on the anterior pituitary itself.

Nicoll and Meites (11) reported that estradiol incorporated into a tissue culture medium can act directly on the anterior pituitary to increase prolactin release. We have also found that anterior pituitaries from rats injected with estradiol released significantly more prolactin upon incubation than pituitaries from untreated rats (13). Michael (12) reported that some systemically administered radioactive hexestrol collects in the hypothalamus, and it is possible that some of the estradiol injected into our rats entered the hypothalamus. If the estradiol remained in the hypothalamic acid extract, it could have acted directly on the incubated pituitary. However, a preliminary observation in which rat pituitary was incubated with estradiol for two hours suggests that no significant stimulation of prolactin release occurred during this brief period.

Kanematsu and Sawyer (14) made localized implants of estrogen into the hypothalamus and anterior pituitary of rabbits, and found that estrogen acted directly on the pituitary to stimulate prolactin release. Implants in the hypothalamus apparently promoted storage of prolactin in the pituitary without release. In rats, however, Ramirez et al. (15) found that estrogen implants into the hypothalamus promoted prolactin release. Estrogen injected in vivo elicits an increase in prolactin content of the pituitary and blood, and promotes mammary growth and lactation (16, 17). It is apparent, therefore, that in the rat estrogen may elicit prolactin release either by a direct action on the pituitary or on the hypothalamus, or by acting on both tissues.

Suckling results in a reflex discharge of prolactin and promotes mammary development and lactation (16). Since suckling stimulates the nerve endings in the nipples (18), it is reasonable to assume that its action is mediated through a neural circuit ending in the hypothalamus. It has been suggested that oxytocin, which is reflexly discharged by the suckling stimulus, may be responsible for inducing prolactin release from the anterior pituitary (19). However, most of the recent evidence from in vivo and in vitro experiments does not support this concept (1, 20, 21). It is evident from our present study that suckling promotes pituitary prolactin release by removing hypothalamic inhibition.

There is considerable evidence that, while estrogen and the suckling stimulus can promote prolactin release, they can inhibit release of FSH and LH by the pituitary (1). Thus, transplantation of the anterior pituitary (22), placement of appropriate hypothalamic lesions (23, 24) or implantation of estrogen into the hypothalamus (15) promote prolactin release but inhibit FSH-LH release. It has been suggested that the hypothalamic factor which stimulates release of LH may be the same factor which inhibits prolactin release (22, 24). Preliminary assays of several purified preparations of hypothalamic LH releasing factor recently sent to us by Dr. A. V.

Schally indicate that they do not contain PIF activity (unpublished observations).

Reserpine and chlorpromazine are effective in promoting prolactin release, as indicated by their ability to elicit mammary growth and lactation in a variety of species and to induce pseudopregnancy in rats (1, 25). Recently we found that reserpine, like estradiol and the suckling stimulus, can deplete the rat hypothalamus of PIF (unpublished observations). Danon et al. (26) also observed that perphenazine (a chlorpromazine derivative) acted similarly to suppress hypothalamic inhibition of pituitary prolactin release. Kanematsu and Sawyer (27) reported that reserpine implanted directly into the hypothalamus of rabbits evoked prolactin release, whereas similar implants into the anterior pituitary had no effect.

The present and related experiments suggest that environmental factors, drugs and hormones may influence anterior pituitary hormone secretion by increasing or decreasing the production of neurohumoral factors in the hypothalamus which regulate the secretion of anterior pituitary hormones. Current investigations in our laboratory are intended to determine whether agents other than estradiol, suckling or reserpine can similarly alter hypothalamic content of PIF.

References

1. Meites, J., C. S. Nicoll, and L. K. Talwalker, In Nalbandov, A. V. (ed.), Advances in Neuroendocrinology, Univ. of Illinois Press, Urbana, 1963, p. 238.
2. Meites, J., R. H. Kahn, and C. S. Nicoll, Proc Soc Exp Biol Med 108: 440, 1961.
3. Nicoll, C. S., and J. Meites, Endocrinology 72: 544, 1963.
4. Talwalker, P. K., A. Ratner, and J. Meites, Amer J Physiol 205: 213, 1963.
5. Pasteels, J. L., C R Soc Biol (Paris) 254: 2664, 1962.
6. Meites, J., In Cole, H. H., and P. T. Cupps (eds.), Reproduction in Domestic Animals, Academic Press, New York, 1959, vol. 1, p. 539.
7. Reece, R. P., and C. W. Turner, Res Bull Mo Agr Exp Sta 266: 8, 1937.
8. Batson, H. C., An Introduction to Statistics in the Medical Sciences, Burgess Publishing, Minneapolis, 1961, p. 16.
9. Vernikos-Dannellis, J., In Program 45th Ann. Meeting, Endocrine Soc., Atlantic City, 1963, p. 28 (Abstract).
10. Kobayashi, T., T. Kobayashi, T. Kigawa, M. Mizuno, and Y. Amenomori, Endocr Jap 10: 16, 1963.
11. Nicoll, C. S., and J. Meites, Endocrinology 70: 272, 1962.
12. Michael, R. P., Excerpta Med, Proc. of the Internat. Union of Physiological Sciences, vol. 1, part 2, 1962, p. 650.
13. Ratner, A., P. K. Talwalker, and J. Meites Proc Soc Exp Biol Med 112: 12, 1963.
14. Kanematsu, S., and C. H. Sawyer, Endocrinology 72: 243, 1963.
15. Ramirez, V. D., R. M. Abrams, and S. M. McCann, Fed Proc 22: 2063, 1963 (Abstract).
16. Meites, J., In Kon, S. K., and A. T. Cowie (eds.), Milk: The Mammary Gland and Its Secretion, Academic Press, London, 1961, p. 321.
17. Wolthuis, O. L., Acta Endocr (Kobenhavn) 43: 137, 1963.
18. Eayrs, J. T., and R. M. Baddeley, J Anat 90: 161, 1956.
19. Benson, G. K., and S. J. Folley, J Endocr 16: 189, 1957.
20. Meites, J., and T. F. Hopkins, J Endocr 22: 207, 1961.
21. Nicoll, C. S., and J. Meites, Endocrinology 70: 927, 1962.
22. Everett, J. W., Endocrinology 58: 786, 1956.
23. McCann, S. M., and H. M. Friedman, Endocrinology 67: 597, 1960.
24. Haun, C. K., and C. H. Sawyer, Endocrinology 67: 270, 1960.
25. Meites, J., In Guillemin, R. (ed.), Proc. First International Pharmacological Meeting, Pergamon Press, Oxford, 1963, vol. 1, p. 151.
26. Danon, A., S. Dikstein, and F. G. Sulman, Proc Soc Exp Biol Med 114: 366, 1963.
27. Kanematsu, S., and C. H. Sawyer, Proc Soc Exp Biol Med 113: 967, 1963.

Inhibition of Nursing-Induced and Stress-Induced Fall in Pituitary Prolactin Concentration in Lactating Rats by Injection of Acid Extracts of Bovine Hypothalamus

CLARK E. GROSVENOR[1], S. M. McCANN, AND R. NALLAR[2]

Department of Physiology and Biophysics, University of Tennessee, Memphis, Tennessee, and Department of Physiology, University of Pennsylvania, Philadelphia, Pennsylvania

ABSTRACT. The concentration of prolactin in the anterior pituitary glands of lactating rats killed with either ether or Nembutal after 10½ hr of isolation from their litters averaged .073 IU/mg (prenursed level). Thirty min of nursing, laparotomy with bleeding from the inferior vena cava during 5 min of ether anesthesia, and the stress of cervical stunning followed by decapitation, each reduced the pituitary prolactin concentration significantly below the prenursed level. Nembutal prevented the fall of prolactin concentration which resulted from laparotomy and bleeding. Nursing, followed by ether anesthesia and the stress of laparotomy and bleeding, did not lower pituitary prolactin content more than nursing alone. Injections of acid extracts of bovine stalk-median-eminence (1 SME/rat) inhibited the fall in prolactin concentration which followed the combined stimuli of nursing and stress. Treatment with extracts of bovine cerebral cortex, or with ovine prolactin (12 mg), did not. These results provide *in vivo* evidence for the existence of a hypothalamic inhibitory factor in the normal regulation of prolactin release in response to nursing or stress. (*Endocrinology* **76**: 883, 1965)

SEVERAL studies have indicated that the hypothalamus possesses a factor(s) which normally inhibits prolactin release from the adenohypophysis. Transplantation of the anterior pituitary, transection of the pituitary stalk, and placement of hypothalamic lesions result in increased prolactin secretion, as manifested by induction and maintenance of milk secretion and preservation of corpora lutea in the rat (1). In *in vitro* studies utilizing organ cultures of rat anterior pituitary glands, the amount of prolactin released into the medium is reduced significantly by the addition of homogenates and acid extracts of rat hypothalamus (2–4). However, neither the effectiveness *in vivo* of a prolactin inhibiting factor(s) nor the physiologic role of such a factor in the normal regulation of prolactin release in an *in vivo* system have heretofore been demonstrated.

In the initial part of the studies being reported, we found that acid extracts of bovine hypothalamus could completely inhibit the normal fall in pituitary prolactin concentration caused by nursing (5–8). Early in the course of these experiments it was realized that two of the procedures we were using, *viz.*, laparotomy with bleeding in rats anesthetized with ether and cervical stunning prior to decapitation, each resulted in a fall in pituitary prolactin concentration similar to that which follows nursing. Our investigations, therefore, were extended to include the stress-induced discharge of prolactin in the lactating rat and to

Received September 14, 1964.
Supported by USPHS Grants A-3637 and AM-01236-08.
[1] Career Research Development Awardee of the USPHS.
[2] Supported by Consejo Nacional de Investigaciones Cientificas y Technicas (Argentina).

demonstrate that hypothalamic extracts could also prevent this type of prolactin release. Part of the results has appeared in abstract form (9).

Materials and Methods

Adult primiparous rats of the Sprague Dawley-Rolfsmeyer strain were used. The litter of each rat was reduced to 8 young on day 2 and 6 young on day 4. Each mother and her litter were weighed daily. On postpartum day 14 the young were removed from the cages. Ten and one-half hr later, groups of 9–11 mothers (prenursed groups) were killed by one of the following methods: a) placing them in small ether-saturated containers; b) injecting 40 mg Nembutal subcutaneously and, after the onset of deep anesthesia, injecting 25–90 mg more Nembutal intraperitoneally; c) stunning by a sharp blow to the cervical region, followed quickly by decapitation. Two additional groups of mothers were deeply anesthetized with ether (11 rats) or with 4.5 mg/100 g Nembutal (10 rats), then laparotomized and bled (4–5 ml) from the inferior vena cava. Five min later, each rat in these 2 groups was killed by injecting Nembutal directly into the inferior vena cava. The litters of the remaining rats were returned after 10 hr of separation, and the mothers were permitted to nurse 30 min (postnursed groups).

Extracts were made by grinding hypothalamic or cortical fragments (which had been frozen following their collection) in 0.1N HCl. Prior to injection the extracts were buffered with phosphate buffer (pH 6.8), neutralized with 0.1N NaOH and centrifuged. The supernatant was injected intraperitoneally into groups of mothers 1–2 min prior to replacement of young at a dose equivalent to 1 bovine SME (or cortical tissue equivalent weight)/rat and in a volume of .2–.4 ml saline. Saline (.2 ml) was injected intraperitoneally 1–2 min prior to replacement of young in the controls. Ovine prolactin (6 mg) (NIH P-S5, assaying 17 IU/mg) was injected subcutaneously into one group of mothers 1 hr, and again 10 min, prior to replacement of young. At the end of the 30-min nursing period, all groups of mothers but one were laparotomized, bled from the inferior vena cava under ether anesthesia and killed with ether or iv Nembutal. The remaining group was killed with ether immediately after nursing. All young were killed at the same time and their stomachs were examined for the presence of milk.

The anterior pituitary lobe of each mother was immediately removed, weighed and frozen. Those of each group were pooled, homogenized in saline and assayed for prolactin using a modification (10) of the intradermal pigeon crop-sac method (11). A 4-point assay was conducted for each group, utilizing 6 or 7 female pigeons (5–7 yr old) per point, $i.e.$, 24 or 28 pigeons/assay. The 2 dose levels of standard ovine prolactin (NIH Lot S-10209, assaying 15 IU/mg) were 12 μg and 3 μg/pigeon, and the higher dose of the pituitary homogenate was 4$\times$ that of the lower dose. One side of the pigeon's crop sac was routinely used, since preliminary assays revealed no significant differences between the responses of the right and left sides. Replicate assays were performed for some of the groups. Standard tests for validity, parallelism and precision were done for each assay on the bases of the combined standard deviations of all responses and the combined slope for all parallel responses (12). The results of replicate assays or assays of separate groups of pituitaries obtained from the same experimental group were combined by the method of Sheps and Moore (13). Differences between groups were judged significant if the level of statistical probability was 5% or less.

Calculation of pituitary prolactin concentration of the separate groups from a single combined dose-response curve to standard prolactin was eschewed, since one of us (CEG) found that the slope of the crop-sac responses to the same doses of standard prolactin (12 and 3 μg/pigeon) varied from 1.14 to 2.58 in 48 individual 4-point assays (including the 21 assays in the present study). Only 1 of the 48 assays, however, was invalid because of lack of parallelism between the slopes of the response to the 2 doses of the standard and the 2 doses of the pituitary homogenate.

Results

The anterior pituitary concentration of prolactin of lactating rats after a 10½ hour period of isolation from their litters (prenursed level) averaged .073 IU/mg pituitary in both rats killed with ether and those killed with Nembutal (Table

TABLE 1. Effect of nursing, method of killing and stress [laparotomy with bleeding (4–5 ml) from inferior vena cava applied for 5 min after onset of anesthesia] upon prolactin concentration in anterior pituitary glands of lactating rats

Treatment	No. of rats	Method of killing	Relative potency (IU/mg)	95% Limits	Index of assay precision (lambda)	Mean relative potency (IU/mg)	95% Limits
Prenursed	10	Ether	.069	.042–.117	.290		
			.083	.054–.126	.229		
	10	Ether	.071	.048–.105	.216	.073	.057–.095
Prenursed: laparotomy and bleeding	11	Ether	.035	.026–.050	.190	.035	.026–.050
Postnursed	9	Ether	.047	.033–.068	.199	.039	.029–.053
			.032	.021–.050*	.211		
Postnursed: laparotomy and bleeding	10	Ether	.036	.023–.057	.251		
			.033	.021–.053	.225		
	12	Ether	.041	.024–.068*	.259	.038	.029–.048
Prenursed	9	Nembutal	.074	.044–.126	.297	.073	.053–.102
			.072	.048–.108	.224		
Prenursed: laparotomy and bleeding	10	Nembutal	.066	.047–.093	.189	.067	.051–.089
			.068	.039–.117	.289		
Prenursed	9	Stun and Decapitation	.047	.030–.071	.226	.049	.036–.066
			.051	.033–.083	.256		

* Six pigeons for each assay point, *i.e.*, 24 pigeons/assay. All other assays utilized 7 pigeons for each assay point.

1). Death generally occurred in three to four minutes following placement of rats in small ether-saturated containers. Generally they would slump and become unconscious after a few respirations. Subcutaneously administered Nembutal quickly produced unconsciousness, though death from Nembutal overdosage did not occur until 40 to 105 minutes after the initial injection. The pituitary prolactin concentration of rats killed by stunning from a blow to the cervical region followed quickly by decapitation averaged only .049 IU/mg. This concentration was significantly less than that in the pituitary gland of rats killed with ether or Nembutal (Table 1).

Thirty minutes of nursing (postnursed level) and the combined stress of laparotomy and bleeding from the inferior vena cava resulted in average pituitary prolactin concentrations of .039 and .035 IU/mg, respectively, values significantly less than the prenursed level (Table 1). The combination of these stimuli (nursing followed by ether anesthesia, laparotomy and bleeding) did not lower pituitary prolactin concentration further. Laparotomy with bleeding performed under Nembutal anesthesia resulted in a prolactin concentration of .067 IU/mg, which was not significantly different from that of the Nembutal-killed prenursed rat (.073 IU/mg).

Injections of bovine SME extract prevented the fall in prolactin concentration in response to the combined stimuli of nursing and stress (Table 2), whereas, in

TABLE 2. Effect of acid extracts of bovine stalk median eminence (SME), bovine cerebral cortex and ovine prolactin upon stress-induced and nursing-induced discharge of prolactin in the lactating rat

Treatment	No. of rats	Relative potency (IU/mg)	95% Limits	Index of assay precision (lambda)	Mean relative potency (IU/mg)	95% Limits
Prenursed	10	.069	.042–.117	.290		
		.083	.054–.126	.229	.073*	.057–.095
	10	.071	.048–.105	.216		
Postnursed:† saline		.036	.023–.057	.251		
	10	.033	.021–.053	.225	.038*	.029–.048
	12	.041	.024–.068‡	.259		
Postnursed:† bovine cortical extract (1 SME wt equivalent /rat)	10	.047	.032–.071	.206	.046	.036–.057
	8	.045	.030–.069	.211		
Postnursed:† bovine SME extract (1 SME/rat)	8	.084	.051–.141	.287		
		.086	.056–.132	.243	.111	.084–.146
	9	.137	.084–.221	.220		
Postnursed:† prolactin	10	.032	.015–.066†	.381	.032	.015–.066

* Same data as in Table 1.

† Laparotomized and bled (4–5 ml) from the inferior vena cava under ether anesthesia immediately after nursing and prior to death.

‡ Six pigeons for each assay point, *i.e.*, 24 pigeons/assay. All other assays utilized 7 pigeons for each assay point.

two separate trials, in rats treated with equivalent by weight doses of bovine cortical extract, the combined stimuli to prolactin release resulted in pituitary concentrations averaging .046 IU/mg. These concentrations of prolactin were not significantly different from the saline-injected nursed control concentration of .038 IU/mg, but were significantly less than the prenursed level of .073 IU/mg.

Injections of a total of 12 mg prolactin during the hour before nursing and subsequent laparotomy and bleeding did not significantly impair the fall in pituitary prolactin concentration in response to the combined stimuli (.032 vs. .038 IU/mg). None of the injections produced any visible alterations in nursing or maternal behavior. All mothers gathered up their young when they were replaced in the cage and quickly commenced nursing. The stomachs of all young were distended with milk.

Discussion

Our finding that 30 minutes of nursing leads to a significant reduction in pituitary prolactin concentration in lactating rats previously deprived of their pups for ten hours agrees with other reports (6–8). Morphologic confirmation of the influence of nursing in releasing prolactin in the rat recently has been obtained by Pasteels (14). He found, using light microscopy, that the prolactin cells of anterior pituitary glands of lactating rats became engorged with granules when the mothers were separated from their litters for ten hours. Thirty minutes of nursing caused a disappearance of the granules from the cells but did not affect the size or number of the prolactin cells. The prolactin granules almost completely disappeared following nursing on post-partum day 6. Less depletion occurred following nursing on post-partum day 14, and on day 21 only small depletion of granules was observed. We had previously observed that the prolactin content of rats on post-partum day 21 was not reduced appreciably by 30 minutes of nursing (7).

Pasteels (14) also observed, using electronmicroscopy, that the excretion of prolactin granules occurred at the pole of the cell into the perisinusoidal spaces. The granules quickly lost their individuality once they were excreted. Smith found (R. E. Smith, personal communication), using electronmicroscopic techniques, that a short period of nursing following a period of non-nursing in rats results in quick extrusion of prolactin granules into the pericapillary and intracellular spaces of the pituitary gland. The granules continue to be extruded for about one hour after the cessation of nursing. Denamur (R. Denamur, personal communication) recently observed a significant reduction in the prolactin concentration in the pituitary of the lactating goat following nursing, which suggests that discharge of prolactin in response to the nursing stimulus is not limited to the rat.

Nicoll et al. (15) have shown that various noxious stimuli known to release ACTH, e.g., cold, heat, restraint and formalin injections, all induced varying degrees of mammary secretion in estrogen-primed, nonlactating rats, suggesting that release of prolactin as well as ACTH had occurred. In the present study, stress was found to be as effective as nursing in discharging prolactin. The fall in pituitary prolactin concentration occurred within five minutes in rats stressed by laparotomy and bleeding under ether anesthesia, whereas that following stunning and decapitation apparently occurred within a few seconds. In the latter instance, even if some stress was generated as a result of positioning the animal prior to stunning, the duration of stress was less than a minute.

The effect of stress upon prolactin release renders it apparent that considerable care must be exercised to ensure a minimum of stress in studies concerned with the regulation of prolactin secretion or in studies in which the presence of elevated levels of prolactin in the circulation might be desirable. Particular care should be exercised in the handling of the animal prior to killing and in the method of killing employed. No differences in prolactin concentration were apparent between rats killed with ether and Nembutal, suggesting that at least ether is not a potent stimulus for prolactin discharge, although it is for ACTH (16, 17). Since Nembutal actually prevented the reduction in pituitary prolactin concentration which resulted from the stress of laparotomy with bleeding from the inferior vena cava, and, in the same dosage (4.5 mg/100 g), prevents the nursing-induced discharge of prolactin (18), it seems unlikely that Nembutal itself causes prolactin release.

Nursing and the laparotomy with bleeding stress lowered pituitary prolactin concentration to the same extent. However, the two stimuli were no more effective in combination than either one alone. This suggests either that each stimulus effected maximal prolactin discharge or that the pituitary or the neural prolactin-releasing mechanism was somehow refractory to the second stimulus. The prolactin assay method can easily detect .007 IU/mg pituitary, so it is unlikely that the result was the consequence of working at the lower limits of sensitivity of the assay.

The concept has developed, since the early work of Desclin (19) and Everett (20, 21), that the hypothalamus chronically holds prolactin discharge in check. This is now thought to be by means of an inhibitor substance(s) which is manufactured in the hypothalamus and which presumably passes to the pituitary via the hypophysial portal system (22). Pasteels (2) showed that the addition of hypothalamic extracts or explants to anterior pituitary tissue in organ cultures decreased the quantity of prolactin released into the medium. This was demonstrated independently by Talwalker *et al.* (3) and confirmed by Danon *et al.* (4). Talwalker *et al.* (3) demonstrated further that no prolactin inhibition occurred when any one of the then recognized hypothalamic neurohumors was added to the organ culture. Gala and Reece (23) reported, however, that co-cultures of rat anterior pituitary and rat hypothalamic fragments did not result in a significant decrease in prolactin production. They noted that hypothalamic tissue viability was not maintained throughout the three-day culture period.

We have now inhibited, *in vivo*, the release of prolactin resulting from nursing and stress by injecting acid extracts of bovine hypothalamus, but not by injecting bovine cerebral cortical extract. Our data not only support the *in vitro* evidence that a "prolactin-inhibiting" factor(s) can be extracted from the hypothalamus; they suggest that this factor may have a physiological role in the normal regulation of secretion and/or the discharge of prolactin. The pituitary prolactin concentration following injections of bovine SME extracts were significantly higher in one group of nine rats than in the prenursed controls. This result, in all probability, was due to chance. It is possible, however, that this level more closely represents the true prenursed concentration of prolactin and that the prenursed levels which we observed in control animals actually represented a partial discharge of prolactin resulting from stimuli of unknown origin. The assumption is made that the SME extracts inhibited prolactin discharge resulting from all stimuli for the duration of the experiment. Another possibility which we believe to be less likely is that a "prolactin-stimulating" factor also resides in bovine hypothalamic tissue which promotes the rapid synthesis of prolactin.

Ratner and Meites (24), using an *in vitro* system, failed to find any "prolactin-inhibiting" activity in hypothalami obtained from suckled rats. They concluded that suckling depleted the hypothalamus of "prolactin-inhibiting" factor. We have recently shown, however (unpublished data), that acid extracts of as little as one third whole rat hypothalamus obtained either from prenursed, postnursed, or stressed lactating rats, are able to inhibit nursing or stress-induced discharge of prolactin in the lactating rat. These observations plus those of the present investigation indicate that the hypothalamic "prolactin-inhibiting" factor(s) is remarkably potent and long lasting in its effect.

We have also examined the possibility that prolactin itself may feed back to inhibit further discharge of prolactin. Injection of a large amount of ovine prolactin prior to nursing and stress, however, failed to influence the normal fall in prolactin concentration produced by these stimuli.

Acknowledgment

The author wishes to thank Mrs. Betty Martin and Miss Dorothy Schaefgen for their capable assistance.

References

1. Meites, J., C. S. Nicoll, and P. K. Talwalker, *In* Nalbandov, A. V. (ed.), Advances in Neuroendocrinology, University of Illinois Press, Urbana, 1963, chapt. 8.
2. Pasteels, J. L., *C R Acad Sci (Paris)* **253**: 3074, 1961.
3. Talwalker, P. K., A. Ratner, and J. Meites, *Amer J Physiol* **205**: 213, 1963.
4. Danon, A., S. Dikstein, and F. G. Sulman, *Proc Soc Exp Biol Med* **114**: 366, 1963.
5. Reece, R. P., and C. W. Turner, *Proc Soc Exp Biol Med* **35**: 621, 1937.
6. Grosvenor, C. E., and C. W. Turner, *Proc Soc Exp Biol Med* **96**: 723, 1957.
7. ———, *Endocrinology* **63**: 535, 1958.
8. Moon, R. C., and C. W. Turner, *Proc Soc Exp Biol Med* **101**: 332, 1959.
9. Grosvenor, C. E., S. M. McCann, and R. Nallar, Program, Endocrine Society, 1964, p. 96.
10. Grosvenor, C. E., and C. W. Turner, *Endocrinology* **63**: 530, 1958.
11. Lyons, W. R., and E. Page, *Proc Soc Exp Biol Med* **32**: 1049, 1935.
12. Bliss, C. I., The Statistics of Bioassay, Academic Press, New York, 1952.
13. Sheps, M. C., and E. A. Moore, *J Pharmacol Exp Ther* **128**: 99, 1960.
14. Pasteels, J. L., *Arch Biol (Liege)* **74**: 439, 1963.
15. Nicoll, C. S., P. K. Talwalker, and J. Meites, *Amer J Physiol* **198**: 1103, 1960.
16. Biegelman, P. M., M. A. Slusher, G. G. Slater, and S. Roberts, *Proc Soc Exp Biol Med* **93**: 608, 1956.
17. Matsuda, K., C. Duyck, J. W. Kendal, and M. A. Greer, *Endocrinology* **74**: 981, 1964.
18. Grosvenor, C. E., and C. W. Turner, *Proc Soc Exp Biol Med* **97**: 463, 1958.
19. Dresclin, L., *Ann Endocr (Paris)* **11**: 656, 1950.
20. Everett, J. W., *Endocrinology* **54**: 685, 1954.
21. ———, *Ibid.*, **58**: 786, 1956.
22. Nikitovitch-Winer, M., and J. W. Everett, *Endocrinology* **62**: 522, 1958.
23. Gala, R. R., and R. P. Reece, *Proc Soc Exp Biol Med* **115**: 1030, 1964.
24. Ratner, A., and J. Meites, *Endocrinology* **75**: 377, 1964.

Copyright © 1971 by J. B. Lippincott Company

Reprinted from *J. Clin. Endocrinol. Metab.* 33:996-998 (1971)

INCREASED SERUM PROLACTIN AFTER ADMINISTRATION OF SYNTHETIC THYROTROPIN RELEASING HORMONE (TRH) IN MAN[1]

Laurence S. Jacobs, Peter J. Snyder, John F. Wilber, Robert D. Utiger, and William H. Daughaday, Endocrine Divisions, Departments of Medicine, Washington University School of Medicine, Northwestern University School of Medicine, and The University of Pennsylvania School of Medicine.

The ability of two synthetic hypothalamic releasing hormones to stimulate secretion of adenohypophysial hormones has been established (1-3). The luteinizing hormone releasing hormone (LRH) stimulates the secretion of both LH and FSH (3). Administration of thyrotropin releasing hormone (TRH) to human subjects (1,2) has caused elevations only of serum thyrotropin (TSH) levels; no consistent changes in serum levels of luteinizing hormone (LH), follicle stimulating hormone (FSH), growth hormone (GH), or cortisol were observed, and monotropic specificity of TRH action was assumed (1).

Recently, Tashjian et al. (4) have demonstrated stimulation of prolactin release by TRH from cloned rat pituitary tumor cells *in vitro*. An inconsistent stimulatory effect of TRH on prolactin secretion from bovine anterior pituitary *in vitro* has also been reported (5). The recent development of radioimmunoassay methods for the measurement of human prolactin (6,7) has made it feasible to examine human prolactin levels following the administration of synthetic TRH in man. In accord with the *in vitro* observations on normal and tumorous animal adenohypophyses, we report here the striking stimulatory effect of TRH on serum prolactin levels in man.

[1]Submitted July 27, 1971

MATERIALS AND METHODS

Ten normal volunteers (three females, seven males) were given TRH[2] after an overnight fast while hospitalized. After placement of an indwelling scalp vein needle 100 to 800 micrograms of synthetic TRH were given as a bolus injection in 10 cc. saline at zero time, and blood was collected frequently thereafter. Human prolactin (HPr) was measured by a mixed heterologous radioimmunoassay system employing ^{125}I-labelled porcine prolactin tracer and a guinea pig anti-ovine prolactin antiserum. Results are expressed as microliter equivalents per ml. of a prolactin-rich human plasma. On the basis of biological assay each microliter equivalent represents about 2 nanograms of human prolactin, assuming equal biologic potency of human and ovine prolactin. This radioimmunoassay is sufficiently sensitive to detect fasting prolactin levels in about 50% of normal adult human beings. No significant cross reaction has been observed with any pituitary hormone tested, including GH, LH, TSH or the placental peptides, human chorionic gonadotropin (HCG) or human chorionic somatomammotropin (HCS). Full methodologic details of

[2]Gift of Michael S. Anderson, M.D., Abbott Laboratories, Chicago, Illinois

this assay will be given elsewhere (manuscript in preparation).

RESULTS

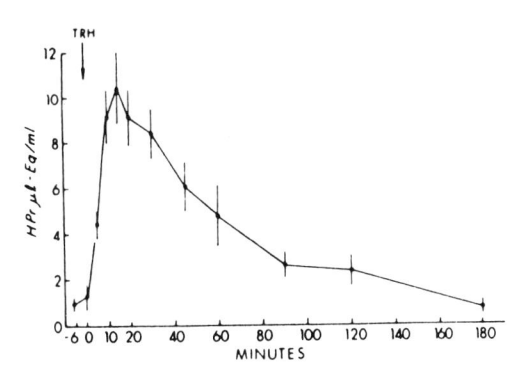

Fig. 1. Mean (± S.E.) prolactin levels before and after TRH injection in 10 normal volunteers. Each microliter-equivalent equals approximately 2 ng. of human prolactin (see text).

Figure 1 shows the mean (± S.E.) HPr responses to TRH in the 10 normal subjects. A striking and consistent elevation in HPr levels was seen 5 minutes after intravenous TRH. The peak values occurred at 15 to 20 minutes and thereafter serum HPr fell slowly toward baseline. Neither the peak responses nor the individual HPr patterns (Figure 2) appeared to differ after varying doses of TRH ranging from 100 to 800 micrograms. All 10 sets of infusion data, therefore, were treated as one group for statistical and graphic analysis. This observation suggests that the minimum effective dose for stimulation of prolactin release is probably less than 100 μg, although more experience at low dosage levels will be required to substantiate this impression. All subjects had normal (i.e. greater than 2-fold) increases in serum TSH levels (2) following TRH.

Two lines of evidence suggest that the rise in radioimmunoassayable HPr demonstrated in these studies is not an artifact produced by elevations of circulating TSH or TRH levels. First, HPr levels were only slightly increased in subjects with primary hypothyroidism (2.99 ± 0.44 vs. 1.75 ± 0.25 in normal adults, $p < .01$). These patients had invariably elevated TSH levels (Table 1).

TABLE 1. HPr and H-TSH Levels in Patients with Primary Hypothyroidism.

Patient	HPr μl-Eq/ml	H-TSH μU/ml
1	2.3	> 100
2	2.0	> 100
3	5.8	300
4	2.0	67
5	3.4	54
6	4.1	255
7	4.0	223
8	2.3	114
9	3.1	258
10	< 0.9	63

Further, we have observed patients (to be reported separately) with thyroid and pituitary disease who showed minimal, if any, HPr responses to TRH despite post-injection circulating TRH levels presumably not different from those of the normal volunteers. Second, the addition of as much as 500 μU TSH to individual HPr assay tubes failed to alter either the HPr standard curve or the assay results on specimens with known HPr levels from prior assays.

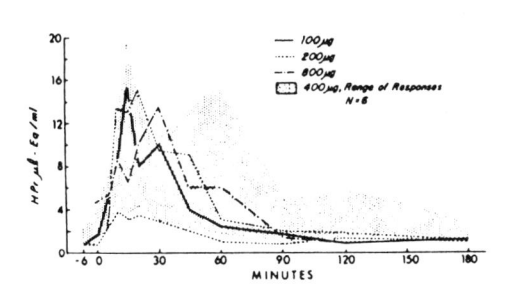

Fig. 2. Range of HPr levels observed after administration of various doses of TRH.

DISCUSSION

The present studies demonstrate that the ability of TRH to stimulate prolactin release is not limited to rat pituitary tumor cells or bovine pituitary pieces in vitro, but extends to normal man in vivo. Although the physiologic significance of these observations is unclear at this time, the fact that TRH stimulation of prolactin release is preserved in vitro on isolated pituitary cells suggests that the findings reported here may be the result of a direct pituitary action of the infused TRH, rather than a hypothalamic effect via inhibition of prolactin inhibiting factor (PIF).

Our finding of near normal levels of prolactin in chronic hypothyroidism suggests that chronic hypersecretion of TRH in this condition may not sustain substantially increased prolactin secretion. Alternatively, TRH may not be involved in the TSH hypersecretion in this condition.

Since both Nicoll et al. (8), and Valverde and Chieffo (9) have identified prolactin-releasing activity (PRF) in the hypothalamic tissue of a variety of species, it is possible that TRH may be identical with or structurally similar to PRF. Evidence bearing on this possibility must await further purification of PRF.

REFERENCES

1. Fleischer, N., R. Burgus, W. Vale, T. Dunn, and R. Guillemin, J. Clin. Endocrinol. Metab. 31:109, 1970.

2. Anderson, M. S., C. Y. Bowers, A. J. Kastin, D. S. Schalch, A. V. Schally, R. D. Utiger, P. J. Snyder, J. F. Wilber, and A. J. Wise, Clin. Res. 19:366, 1971 (Abstract).

3. Kastin, A. J., A. V. Schally, D. S. Schalch, S. G. Korenman, C. Gual, and E. Perez Pasten, J. Clin. Invest. 50:53a, June 1971 (Abstract).

4. Tashjian, A. H., Jr., N. J. Barowsky, and D. K. Jensen, Biochem. Biophys. Res. Comm. 43:516, 1971.

5. LaBella, F. S., and S. R. Vivian, Endocrinology 88:787, 1971.

6. Guyda, H., H. Friesen, and P. Hwang, J. Clin. Endocrinol. Metab. 32:120, 1971.

7. Bryant, G. D., T. M. Siler, L. L. Morgenstern, B. Webster, and F. C. Greenwood, Second International Symposium on Growth Hormone, ICS #236, p. 5 (Abstract), May 1971.

8. Nicoll, C. S., R. P. Fiorindo, C. T. McKennee, and J. A. Parsons, in Hypophysiotropic Hormones of the Hypothalamus, ed. J. Meites, pp. 115-144, 1970.

9. Valverde-R, C., and V. Chieffo, Presented at the 53rd Annual Meeting of The Endocrine Society, June 25, 1971. Program, Abstract #83, p. A-84, 1971.

Research supported in part by USPHS Grants AM 05105, AM 10699, AM 05071, AM 14997, T01 AM 05649, R01 AM 14039, FR-SO, 5F03 AM 48051.

Laurence S. Jacobs is a Special Research Fellow of the NIAMD, NIH.

Editor's Comments
on Papers 50 Through 53

50 LU and MEITES
    Inhibition by L-Dopa and Monoamine Oxidase Inhibitors of Pituitary Prolactin Release; Stimulation by Methyldopa and d-Amphetamine

51 MacLEOD and LEHMEYER
    Excerpts from *Studies on the Mechanism of the Dopamine-Mediated Inhibition of Prolactin Secretion*

52 SOWERS et al.
    Effect of Dexamethasone on Prolactin and TSH Responses to TRH and Metoclopramide in Man

53 RIVIER et al.
    Stimulation in vivo *of the Secretion of Prolactin and Growth Hormone by β-Endorphin*

Lu and Meites in 1971 (Paper 50) demonstrated that administration of L-dopa and monoamine oxidase inhibitors impede PRL release in rats; administration of methyldopa, which inhibits dopa decarboxylase and reduces synthesis of dopamine and norepinephrine, increases PRL release. They suggested that drugs reducing hypothalamic catecholamine activity increase PRL release, and those increasing catecholamine decrease PRL secretion from the adenohypophysis. They also noted that catecholamine-altering drugs could be acting directly at the hypophysial level. When they assayed hypothalami from rats treated with L-dopa and monoamine oxidase inhibitors, PIF activity was found to be proportional to suppression of PRL release. These findings demonstrated that L-dopa and monoamine oxidase inhibitors result in increased PIF hypothalamic activity, which, in turn, depresses adenohypophyseal release of PRL.

MacLeod and Lehmeyer (Paper 51) showed that PRL release could be inhibited by co-incubation of cultured hypophyses with dopamine. They further demonstrated that direct inhibition of PRL release from adenohypophysial cells can be prevented by pretreating animals from which the hypophysis has been obtained or by pre-incubating or co-incubating the hypophysis with dopamine-blocking drugs. Thus, there is very good evidence for dopamine receptors on PRL secreting cells and for dopamine to act directly at the hypophysis to inhibit PRL secretion in very low concentration (5×10^{-7} mol/l). It is interesting that psychotrophic drugs such as chlorpromazine, noted by Barraclough and Sawyer (Paper 22) to interfere with normal menstrual cycles and produce the galactorrhea associated with hyperprolactinemia, act centrally as inhibitors of dopamine synthesis or dopamine receptor blocking agents which interfere with generation of PIF at the hypothalamic level and also exert direct inhibitory effects on dopamine receptors of the adenohypophysial prolactin secreting cells.

Sowers et al. (Paper 52) demonstrated that acute administration of high doses of glucocorticoids inhibit PRL secretion. These investigators showed that administration of 8 mg of dexamethasone daily for five days significantly reduced baseline PRL and TSH levels and blunted the PRL and TSH response to TRH. A similar inhibitory effect was observed in the PRL response to metoclopramide, a central dopamine antagonist that Sowers et al. (1976) previously showed to be a very potent releaser of PRL, probably exerting its effects at both the hypothalamic and hypophysial levels. Sowers et al. (1979) have also shown that high dose glucocorticoid administration blunts the LH and FSH responses to LH-RH and clomiphene citrate. The data from this laboratory indicate that glucocorticoids suppress PRL, as well as TSH, LH, and FSH, release by exerting suppressive effects at both the hypothalamic and hypophysial levels.

Rivier et al. (Paper 53) demonstrated that morphine sulfate (MS) and the opiate peptide β-endorphin, the C-terminal fragment of β-lipotropin (β-LPH (61-91)), stimulate PRL and GH release when injected intravenously or intracisternally in rats. The in-vivo stimulatory effects of β-endorphin on PRL secretion was reversed by the opiate antagonist naloxone. On a molecular basis, β-endorphin was found to be at least twenty times more potent than MS. The observation of no in-vitro effects of morphine and β-endorphin on PRL and GH secretion by cultured rat hypophysial cells was interpreted as indicating that they have a CNS site of action. These investigators have found that other pharmacological stimuli of PRL secretion, including TRH, neurotensin, substance P, and histamine, are not affected by concomitant naloxone administration, indicating that the stimulatory activity of most PRL-releasing agents does not involve an opiate receptor-dependent mechanism. Thus, the significance of opiate-like peptide in the physiological control of PRL and GH secretion remains to be elucidated; however, the results of this study further indicate similarity in the biological activity of MS and the neurotropic brain peptides related to β-endorphin. The PRL- and GH-releasing effects of β-endorphin demonstrated in this study suggest the possibility of autoregulation at the hypophysial level. Lipotropin secretion by the hypophysis, with or without conversion to endorphin, could modulate the secretion of PRL and GH. Thus a number of factors exert control either at the hypothalamic or directly at the hypophysial level on PRL secretion. Whether all of these factors modulate PRL release through common pathways remains to be elucidated.

REFERENCES

McCallum, R. W., J. R. Sowers, J. M. Hershman, and R. A. L. Sturdevant. 1976. Metoclopramide Stimulates Prolactin Secretion in Man. *J. Clin. Endocrinol. Metabol.* **44**:1148.

Sowers, J. R., R. M. McCallum, J. M. Hershman, and H. E. Carlson. 1976. Comparison of Metoclopramide with Other Dynamic Tests of Prolactin Secretion. *J. Clin. Endocrinol. Metab.* **43**:856.

Sowers, J. R., and J. Fayez. 1979. Effect of Dexamethasone on Gonadotropin Responsiveness to Luteinizing Hormone-Releasing Hormone and Clomiphene in Women with Secondary Amenorrhea. *Am. J. Obstet. Gynecol.* **134**:325.

INHIBITION BY L-DOPA AND MONOAMINE OXIDASE INHIBITORS OF PITUITARY PROLACTIN RELEASE; STIMULATION BY METHYLDOPA AND d-AMPHETAMINE

Kuew-Hsiung Lu and J. Meites[1]

Department of Physiology, Michigan State University, East Lansing, Michigan 48823

[1] This investigation was aided in part by NIH Research Grants AM 4784 and CA 10771.

Numerous studies have indicated that hypothalamic catecholamines (CA) influence secretion of several anterior pituitary (AP) hormones, including prolactin. An adrenergic tonus is believed to inhibit prolactin release, and a reduction in hypothalamic CA's to promote prolactin release (1, 2). Recently we reported that a single intracarotid injection of dopamine, epinephrine, but not norepinephrine, evoked small but significant decreases in AP prolactin levels but no significant changes in serum prolactin levels (3). On the other hand, a single injection of reserpine, chlorpromazine, α-methyl-*para*-tyrosine or α-methyl-*meta*-tyrosine, all known to depress hypothalamic CA's (2, 3), produced a rapid increase in serum prolactin concentration and, with the exception of α-methyl-*meta*-tyrosine, a decrease in AP prolactin concentration.

Inasmuch as dopamine, epinephrine, and norepinephrine do not readily pass through the blood–brain barrier (4, 5), the present study was undertaken to determine whether other drugs known to enter the brain and increase CA levels could depress serum prolactin values. The drugs used included L-dopa, the immediate precursor of dopamine; 3 monoamine oxidate inhibitors (pargyline, Lilly-15641, and iproniazid) that depress normal metabolism of epinephrine and norepinephrine and therefore increase brain catecholamine levels; methyldopa, which inhibits dopa decarboxylase and reduces synthesis of dopamine and norepinephrine; and *d*-amphetamine, a sympatheticomimetic drug.

Materials and Methods. Animals. Mature 4- to 5-month-old female Sprague-Dawley rats (Spartan Research Animals, Haslett, Mich.), weighing 225–255 g each, were used in all experiments. The rats were housed in a temperature-controlled (25±1°) and artificially illuminated (lights on at 5:00 a.m., off at 7:00 p.m.) animal room, and maintained on Wayne Lab Blox pellets and water *ad libitum*. Two complete estrous cycles of 4 to 5 days duration were followed on all female rats before they were injected with one of the drugs at 10 a.m. on the day of proestrus. Since the main objective of these experiments was to determine whether some of the drugs could depress serum prolactin levels, proestrous rats with relatively high serum prolactin levels were used. The experiments were terminated 2 hr (12 a.m.) after each injection.

Drugs. The rats were injected intraperitoneally once with one of the following drugs:[2] L-dopa, methyldopa, pargyline hydrochloride, iproniazid phosphate, *d*-amphetamine sulfate, and Lilly-15641. All drugs except L-dopa and methyldopa were dissolved directly in neutral phosphate buffer saline. The L-dopa and methyldopa were each dissolved in a warm solution of 0.5 N HCl to which 0.5 N NaOH was added to bring the pH to 2.8. Two control groups were injected once with saline or pH 2.8 solution. The doses of drugs used represents the total amount given per rat, and similar doses were shown by us and other investigators to be effective in rats (1, 8, 9).

---

[2] We are indebted to Dr. S. L. Steelman, Merck Institute for Therapeutic Research, Rahway, N.J., for supplying L-dopa and methyldopa; Dr. R. W. Fuller, Lilly Research Labs., Eli Lilly and Co., Indianapolis, Ind., for Lilly-15641 and *d*-amphetamine; Dr. K. E. Moore, Pharmacology Dept., Michigan State University, for pargyline; and Hoffmann-La Roche Inc., Nutley, N.J., for iproniazid phosphate.

TABLE I. Effects of a Single Intraperitoneal Injection of Drugs on Serum and Pituitary Prolactin Concentrations.

Treatment (7 rats/group) per rat	Serum prolactin (ng/ml) Pre-treatment	30 min	1 hr	2 hr	AP prolactin conc (μg/mg of AP)
pH 2.8 solution, 0.3 ml (controls)	158.6 ± 16.4[a]	143.6 ± 12.0	146.4 ± 10.3	130.1 ± 9.7	10.34 ± 0.19
L-dopa, 12 mg	174.1 ± 12.7	85.1 ± 3.2[c]	90.1 ± 8.8[c]	66.7 ± 4.1[c]	12.08 ± 0.79[b]
Methyldopa, 80 mg	204.3 ± 21.8	955.3 ± 85.3[c]	1319.1 ± 171.5[c]	984.1 ± 188.1[c]	8.19 ± 0.28[c]
Saline, 0.5 ml (controls)	169.6 ± 10.1	193.1 ± 26.7	192.9 ± 24.6	181.9 ± 11.6	9.32 ± 0.29
Pargyline, 15 mg	187.4 ± 15.5	112.7 ± 7.0[c]	107.1 ± 10.9[c]	100.0 ± 11.1[c]	9.35 ± 0.37
Pargyline, 15 mg + L-dopa, 12 mg	149.6 ± 13.3	66.7 ± 3.0[c]	63.7 ± 6.0[c]	70.1 ± 5.4[c]	10.63 ± 0.11
Lilly-15641, 8 mg	208.0 ± 28.9	208.6 ± 32.9	173.1 ± 25.2	126.0 ± 21.7[b]	11.63 ± 0.44[c]
Iproniazid, 40 mg	195.6 ± 25.5	182.6 ± 40.0	168.7 ± 38.1	89.4 ± 13.8[c]	8.89 ± 0.37
d-Amphetamine, 1.2 mg	142.9 ± 6.7	568.3 ± 126.1[c]	1056.1 ± 211.4[c]	956.1 ± 245.1[c]	5.88 ± 0.32[c]

[a] Mean ± standard error of mean.
[b] Significantly different from controls: $p < 0.05$; [c] $p < 0.01$.

Collection of sera and AP's for assay. Individual blood samples (0.6 or 0.7 ml) were collected by cardiac puncture under light ether anesthesia at 0, 0.5, 1, and 2 hr following each treatment. This method of blood collection was previously shown not to alter normal serum prolactin values in rats (6). A pretreatment blood sample was taken from each animal prior to drug injection for comparison with subsequent blood samples. The animals were decapitated by guillotine after the last blood samples were collected. The AP's were removed immediately, weighed on a Mettler balance, and homogenized in neutral phosphate buffer saline with a ultrasonic cell disruptor. Blood samples were first stirred gently and then placed in a refrigerator at 4° for 24 hr to separate the serum. The sera and AP homogenates were kept in a freezer at −20° until assayed for prolactin.

Prolactin assay. Prolactin activity in individual serum samples and AP homogenates were assayed by radioimmunoassay (7). Each sample was assayed at two dilutions, averaged, and expressed in terms of a purified rat prolactin reference standard (NIAMD-Rat-Prolactin-RP-1) obtained from NIH, Rat Pituitary Hormone Program, Bethesda, Md. Sample means and standard error of means were calculated for each experimental group. Student's "t" test was used to determine significance of differences in serum prolactin values between pretreatment and posttreatment samples, and also for differences in AP prolactin concentrations between groups.

Results. Table I shows that a single intraperitoneal injection of saline or pH 2.8 solution (controls) had no effect on subsequent serum prolactin levels. Administration of L-dopa reduced serum prolactin about 50% by 30 min or 1 hr after injection as compared to pretreatment values. By 2 hr after injection serum prolactin values were reduced about 60% and AP prolactin concentration was significantly increased. Pargyline produced smaller reductions in serum prolactin and no significant change in AP prolactin concentration. When both L-dopa and pargyline were given together, there were greater decreases in serum prolactin values than when either drug was given alone. The combination produced no significant change in AP prolactin concentration. Lilly-15641 or iproniazid produced no effect on serum prolactin by 30 min or 1 hr after injection, but elicited about a 40–50% reduction by 2 hr after injection. Lilly-15641 but not iproniazid significantly increased AP concentration of prolactin.

A single injection of amphetamine increased serum prolactin over pretreatment values about 4-fold by 30 min, about 7-fold by 1 hr and about 6-fold by 2 hr after injection. This drug reduced AP prolactin concentration by about 44%. An injection of methyldopa increased serum prolactin over pretreatment levels about 5-fold by 30 min, about 6-fold by 1 hr, and about 5-fold by 2 hr after injection. This drug significantly reduced AP prolactin concentration.

Discussion. These results demonstrate that a single injection of L-dopa, the precursor of dopamine, produced a rapid decrease in serum prolactin and an increase in AP prolactin concentration. The ability of L-dopa to raise brain CA levels (2, 4, 5) is believed to be responsible for the decrease in prolactin release. Rapid reductions in serum prolactin were also observed shortly after L-dopa injection by Wedig and Gay (8) and Schneider and Midgley (9), but the latter noted an increase in serum prolactin by 26 to 100 min after injection. We did not observe any increase in serum prolactin levels even by 2 hr after injecting L-dopa, and have recently confirmed this in another experiment with several doses of L-dopa (unpublished).

The monoamine oxidase inhibitors, pargyline, Lilly-15641 and, iproniazid, all reduced serum prolactin levels significantly, presumably by interfering with the metabolism of CA's (5) and thereby increasing their concentration in the hypothalamus. Pargyline was the most effective of the 3 monoamine oxidase inhibitors used for decreasing serum prolactin concentration, and when given together with L-dopa, the reduction in serum prolactin was greater than when either drug was given alone, presumably because synthesis of CA was enhanced and metabolism of CA was reduced. We previously reported that iproniazid inhibited mammary growth and lactation (10), and depressed mammary tumor growth in rats (11), although no significant change in serum prolactin was found. Since blood samples were collected from these animals about 24 hr after the last injection of iproniazid, it is possible that any decrease which may have occurred earlier was missed.

The large increase in serum prolactin and significant fall in pituitary prolactin produced by injection of methyldopa is probably due to a reduction in brain CA's, since this drug interferes with synthesis of dopamine and norepinephrine (1, 4). The action of amphetamine is more difficult to understand, although it has been observed that amphetamine induces a brief liberation of norepinephrine from adrenergic terminals and that it may inhibit monoamine oxidase activity (4, 5). Amphetamine also blocks dopamine reuptake by nerve endings (Fuller, personal communication), which would block synthesis of norepinephrine. Further work will be necessary to elucidate the stimulating action of amphetamine on prolactin release.

In general, the results reported here are in agreement with the concept that an adrenergic tonus in the hypothalamus inhibits prolactin release (1, 2). Recent work by Kamberi *et al.* (12) has shown that an injection of dopamine into the 3rd ventricle of rats increases PIF activity in the hypothalamo-pituitary portal blood and decreases serum concentration of prolactin. The present study demonstrates that several drugs known to enhance brain CA activity produce a decrease in AP prolactin release. Drugs that reduce hypothalamic CA activity, including methyldopa, reserpine, and chlorpromazine, increase prolactin release. Possible direct effects of these drugs on the AP can not be excluded, although CA have been reported to produce equivocal effects on AP prolactin release *in vitro* (13).

Summary. A single intraperitoneal injection of L-dopa, the precursor of dopamine, into female rats significantly reduced serum prolactin concentration at 30 min, 1 hr, and 2 hr after injection compared to pretreatment levels or control rats not given this drug. A single injection of each of 3 monoamine oxidase inhibitors, pargyline, iproniazid or Lilly-15641, also significantly decreased serum prolactin below pretreatment values. Injection of L-dopa and pargyline together was more effective than either alone in lowering serum prolactin. Each of the above drugs is believed to reduce pituitary prolactin release because it increases catecholamine activity in the hypothalamus. By contrast, a single injection of methyldopa, which inhibits catecholamine synthesis, increased serum prolactin many fold over pretreatment levels. A single injection of *d*-amphetamine, a sympatheticomimetic drug, also greatly increased serum prolactin concentration.

Addendum

The hypothalami of the rats treated with saline (controls), iproniazid, pargyline, L-dopa or pargyline and L-dopa together, were assayed for PIF activity by our standard *in vitro* procedure. All drugs increased hypothalamic PIF activity and the combination of pargyline and L-dopa was more effective than either alone. These observations suggest that the increase in hypothalamic catecholamines produced by these drugs results in increased hypothalamic PIF activity, and this in turn depresses prolactin release by the pituitary.

---

1. Coppóla, J. A., J. Reprod. Fert., Suppl. **4**, 35 (1968).
2. Fuxe, K., and Hokfelt, T., *in* "Frontiers in Neuroendocrinology, 1969" (W. F. Ganong, and L. Martini, eds.), p. 47. Oxford Univ. Press, London/New York (1969).
3. Lu, K. H., Amenomori, Y., Chen, C. L., and Meites, J., Endocrinology **87**, 667 (1970).
4. Innes, I. R., and Nickerson, M., *in* "The Pharmacological Basis of Therapeutics" (L. S. Goodman and A. Gilman, eds.), p. 50. Macmillan Co., New York (1970).
5. Koelle, G. B., *in* "The Pharmacological Basis of Therapeutics" (L. S. Goodman, and A. Gilman, eds.), pp. 422–432. Macmillan Co., New York (1970).
6. Wuttke, W., and Meites, J., Proc. Soc. Exp. Biol. Med. **135**, 648 (1970).
7. Niswender, G. D., Chen, C. L., Midgley, A. R., Jr., Meites, J., and Ellis, S., Proc. Soc. Exp. Biol. Med. **130**, 793 (1969).
8. Wedig, J., and Gay, V. L., Abstr. Pap. Soc. Study Reprod. 3rd Annu. Meet., 1970, 13.
9. Schneider, H. P. G., and Midgley, A. R., Jr., Abstr. Pap., Soc. Study Reprod., 3rd Ann. Meet., 1970, 12.
10. Mizuno, H., Talwalker, P. K., and Meites, J., Proc. Soc. Exp. Biol. Med. **115**, 604 (1964).
11. Nagasawa, H., and Meites, J., Proc. Soc. Exp. Biol. Med. **135**, 469 (1970).
12. Kamberi, I. A., Mical, R. S., and Porter, J. C., Fed. Proc., Fed. Amer. Soc. Exp. Biol. **29**, 378 (1970).
13. Koch, Y., Lu, K. H., and Meites, J., Endocrinology **87**, 673 (1970).

Received Jan. 12, 1971. P.S.E.B.M., 1971, Vol. 137.

ERRATUM

Page 480, line 28 in the left-hand column should read: "mine, 3 monoamine oxidase inhibitors (par-"

Studies on the Mechanism of the Dopamine-Mediated Inhibition of Prolactin Secretion[1]

ROBERT M. MACLEOD,[2] AND JOYCE E. LEHMEYER

Department of Internal Medicine, University of Virginia School of Medicine, Charlottesville, Virginia 22901

ABSTRACT. A study of the *in vitro* effect of dopamine on the release of newly synthesized prolactin is reported. Pituitary glands of female rats were incubated with 4,5-^{3}H-leucine and the radioactive prolactin present in the pituitary gland and that released into the incubation medium were measured. Incubation with 5×10^{-7}M dopamine caused an 85% decrease in prolactin release. Prior injection of the rats with perphenazine or haloperidol rendered the pituitary gland refractory to the *in vitro* inhibitory effect of dopamine. Although *in vitro* perphenazine and haloperidol had little or no effect on release of prolactin, 5×10^{-9}M of these drugs directly blocked the *in vitro* action of dopamine on prolactin release. Phentolamine, an α-blocking agent, was partially able to block the inhibitory effect of dopamine. Propranolol, however, was not effective. Apomorphine, an agent known to mimic the effects of dopamine, caused a significant decrease in the amount of radioactive and radioimmunoassayable prolactin released into the incubation medium. This *in vitro* effect of apomorphine was blocked by the *in vitro* presence of perphenazine. Apomorphine did not block the effect of dopamine. 3×10^{-9}M ergocryptine caused a complete inhibition of prolactin release but the effect of this drug, which binds to α-adrenergic receptors, was completely blocked by the *in vitro* presence of perphenazine or haloperidol. The results of this study demonstrate that agents known to stimulate α-adrenergic or dopaminergic receptors cause an inhibition in prolactin release. Since hypothalamic catecholamines, including dopamine, have an important role in the control of prolactin secretion and because these catecholamines can directly inhibit the *in vitro* secretion of prolactin by the pituitary, consideration has been given to the hypothesis that dopamine is the physiological inhibitor of prolactin secretion that acts directly on the pituitary gland by stimulating specific receptors. (*Endocrinology* **94**: 1077, 1974)

THE *in vivo* secretion of prolactin by the anterior pituitary gland is normally inhibited by the hypothalamus. When the pituitary gland is transplanted to organs remote from the hypothalamus, when it is incubated *in vitro*, or when lesions are placed in the median eminence region of the hypothalamus, the pituitary gland secrets large amounts of prolactin (1). The role that hypothalamic catecholamines play in the process of prolactin release has received considerable attention recently, and it has been clearly demonstrated that catecholamines can directly inhibit the *in vitro* secretion of prolactin (2,3). We have shown that treatment of rats with reserpine or perphenazine stimulates prolactin synthesis (4). In the present study we demonstrate that several α-adrenergic blocking agents antagonize the inhibitory *in vitro* action of dopamine on prolactin secretion and hypothesize that the hypothalamic catecholamines have an important physiological function in controlling prolactin release by a direct action on the pituitary gland.

Received August 2, 1973.

[1] This investigation was supported by USPHS Research Grant CA-07535 from the National Cancer Institute. A preliminary report of this work was presented at the Annual Meeting of the Endocrine Society, Chicago, Illinois, June 1973.

[2] Portions of this investigation were conducted while RMM was a recipient of a Research Career Development Award CA-07665 from the National Cancer Institute.

[Editor's Note: Material has been omitted at this point.]

Discussion

The suggestion that hypothalamic catecholamines influence the release of pituitary hormones followed the observations of Sawyer *et al.* (13) that adrenergic drugs caused ovulation whereas antiadrenergic drugs blocked ovulation in rabbits and rats. The high concentration of dopamine in the median eminence region first observed by Fuxe (14) provided support for the concept that the monaminergic tubero-infundibular neural system could be responsible for the direct control of prolactin secretion proposed by Van Maanen and Smelik (15). To date, however, there is no evidence that brain catecholamines are released and transported by the portal blood vessels. Nevertheless, agents which deplete the stores of hypothalamic catecholamines or block their synthesis induce prolactin secretion and its subsequent effects (2, 16–19). The injection of other drugs such as chlorpromazine or pimozide also significantly increase serum prolactin levels (1,9). Injection of the metabolic precursor of the brain catecholamines, L-dopa, causes a decrease in serum prolactin (7,12). Similarly, apomorphine treatment blocks the suckling-induced rise in serum prolactin (9). These studies provide evidence that prolactin secretion is greatly influenced by hypothalamic catecholamines. The mechanism, however, through which the catecholamines act has not been agreed upon.

The argument that hypothalamic catecholamines increase PIF which subsequently decreases prolactin secretin received support from the finding of Kamberi et al. (24) that direct perfusion of the pituitary gland with catecholamines was without effect on serum prolactin whereas intraventricular injection caused a decrease in its concentration. The data presented herein do not agree with those of Kamberi et al. Our data show that the inhibitory effect of dopamine on newly synthesized prolactin is much greater than on total secreted prolactin. In this respect our data are in agreement with those of Swearingen (25,26) who demonstrated that prolactin secretion *in vitro* is heterogeneous and that agents which inhibit prolactin secretion have a selective inhibitory effect on the fast turnover component.

Few studies involving the *in vitro* effect of perphenazine on pituitary function have appeared. Danon, Ben-David and Sulman (8,20,21) presented evidence that injection of rats with perphenazine or incubation of hypothalami and pituitary glands with the drug produced an increase in prolactin secretion by the pituitary gland. They suggested that perphenazine caused prolactin secretion by blocking the release of prolactin-inhibiting factor (PIF) from the hypothalamus although they never measured PIF activity. Their experimental data, in our opinion, are insufficient to support their conclusions.

Haloperidol is a known competitive antag-

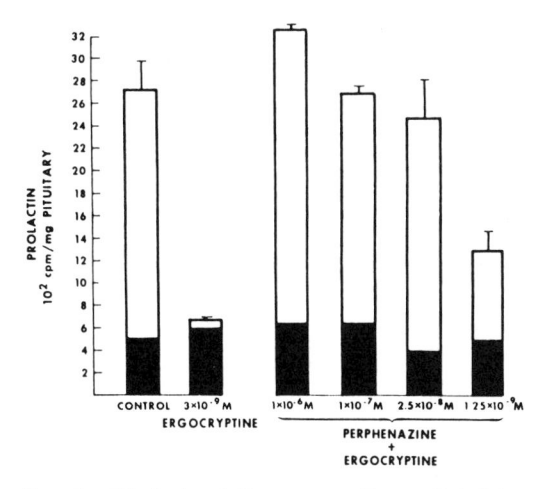

FIG. 9. Blockade of the ergocryptine-mediated inhibition of prolactin release by perphenazine. 3×10^{-9}M ergocryptine was incubated alone and in the presence of varying concentrations of perphenazine in flasks containing 4 hemipituitary glands. Three flasks per group.

onist of catecholamines and blocks neurotransmission in dopaminergic receptors (22). When this drug was administered to rats, Dickerman et al. (23) observed a prompt increase in serum prolactin. They attributed this increase to a haloperidol-mediated decrease in hypothalamic PIF.

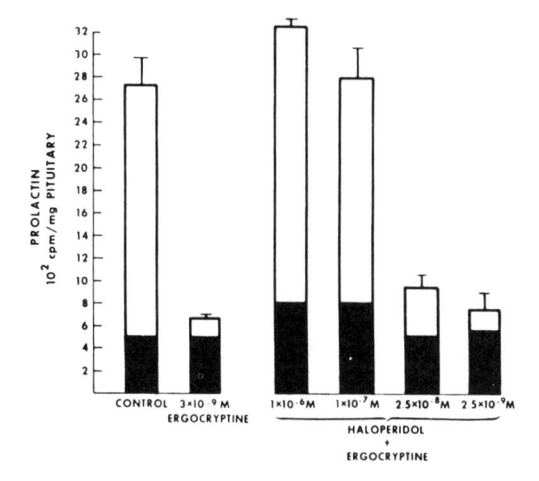

FIG. 10. Blockade of the ergocryptine-mediated inhibition of prolactin release by haloperidol. 3×10^{-9}M ergocryptine was incubated alone and in the presence of varying concentrations of haloperidol in flasks containing 4 hemipituitary glands. Three flasks per group.

Although the experimental data presented here utilizing the *in vivo* administration of pharmacological agents are in agreement with data obtained by others, the present *in vitro* use of these agents necessitates that we interpret our results in a different manner. Studies by MacLeod (2) and Birge *et al.* (3) demonstrated that catecholamines can act directly on the pituitary gland to decrease prolactin secretion *in vitro*. The present results confirm earlier work and provide evidence for the concept that dopamine is a physiological regulator of prolactin secretion and that it acts directly upon the pituitary gland.

Perphenazine and haloperidol have certain conformational similarities to dopamine and both drugs stimulate prolactin secretion following their injection. Since the biochemical action of these drugs in other tissues is to block catecholamine action at their receptor site, it can be reasoned that the drugs increase prolactin production by altering the function of catecholamines in the pituitary gland or in the hypothalamus. Evidence for the former possibility has been presented in that we have shown that pituitary glands from perphenazine and haloperidol-treated rats are refractory to the inhibitory action of dopamine on prolactin secretion. Furthermore, incubating pituitary glands *in vitro* with perphenazine or haloperidol completely inhibits the effect of dopamine. In addition to these drugs, the conventional α-adrenergic blocking agent, phentolamine, will partially block the action of dopamine at the pituitary level.

The data presented here demonstrate that in addition to dopamine, pharmacological agents such as apomorphine and ergocryptine, which bind to "dopaminergic" or "α-adrenergic" receptors, inhibit the *in vitro* secretion of newly synthesized prolactin, further suggesting the presence of these receptors in the pituitary. This inhibition is blocked by co-incubation of the tissue with perphenazine or haloperidol, suggesting that one of the *in vivo* effects of these tranquilizing drugs is to block the activity of hypothalamic catecholamines. Since the α-adrenergic or dopaminergic blocking agents are active at such low concentrations, it may be that their action is at or near the control point regulating prolactin secretion. These data are consistent with the concept that prolactin cells in the pituitary gland have dopaminergic or α-adrenergic receptors which when stimulated inhibit the secretion of prolactin. Preliminary evidence suggests that C^{14}-dopamine is capable of binding to pituitary gland receptor sites.

Acknowledgment

The authors gratefully acknowledge the excellent technical assistance of Mr. Ronald C. Pace.

References

1. Meites, J., and J. A. Clemens, *Vitam Horm* **30:** 165, 1972.
2. MacLeod, R. M., *Endocrinology* **85:** 916, 1969.
3. Birge, C. A., L. S. Jacobs, C. T. Hammer, and W. H. Daughaday, *Endocrinology* **86:** 120, 1970.
4. MacLeod, R. M., E. H. Fontham, and J. E. Lehmeyer, *Neuroendocrinology* **6:** 283, 1970.
7. Turkington, R. W., *J Clin Endocrinol Metab* **34:** 306, 1972.
9. Smalstig, E. B., B. D. Sawyer, M. E. Roush, and J. A. Clemens, *Fed Proc* **32:** 521, 1973.
12. Lu, K. H., and J. Meites, *Proc Soc Exp Biol Med* **137:** 480, 1971.
13. Sawyer, C. H., J. E. Markee, and B. F. Townsed, *Endocrinology* **44:** 18, 1949.
14. Fuxe, K., Z. Zellforsch, *Mikrosk Anat* **61:** 710, 1964.
15. VanMaanen, J. H., and P. G. Smelik, *Neuroendocrinology* **3:** 177, 1968.
16. Kanematsu, S., J. Hilliard, and C. H. Sawyer, *Acta Endocrinol* **44:** 467, 1963.
17. Lu, K. H., Y. Amenomori, C. L. Cheng, and J. Meites, *Endocrinology* **87:** 667, 1970.
18. Donoso, A. O., W. Bishop, C. P. Fawcett, L. Krulich, and S. M. McCann, *Endocrinology* **89:** 774, 1971.
19. Turkington, R. W., *Arch Intern Med* **130:** 349, 1972.
22. Anden, N. E., A. Dahlstrom, K. Fuxe, and T. Hokfelt, *Acta Physiol Scand.* **68:** 419, 1966.
23. Dickerman, S., J. Clark, E. Dickerman, and J. Meites, *Neuroendocrinology* **9:** 332, 1972.
24. Kamberi, I. A., R. S. Mical, and J. C. Porter, *Endocrinology* **88:** 1012, 1971.

Effect of Dexamethasone on Prolactin and TSH Responses to TRH and Metoclopramide in Man

JAMES R. SOWERS, HAROLD E. CARLSON, NACHMAN BRAUTBAR, AND JEROME M. HERSHMAN

Endocrine Section, Medical and Research Services, Veterans Administration Wadsworth Hospital Center and Department of Medicine, University of California, Los Angeles, California

THERE IS considerable evidence that the suppressive effects of glucocorticoids at the hypothalamic-pituitary level are not entirely specific to the adrenocorticotropic axis. Previous studies have shown that both the prolactin (PRL) and the growth hormone (GH) responses to insulin-induced hypoglycemia in man and stress-induced PRL release in rats can be suppressed by prior administration of dexamethasone (1–3); the normal nocturnal elevation of plasma PRL is absent in Cushing's disease (4). Other studies in rats and man have demonstrated that dexamethasone suppresses baseline thyrotropin (TSH) levels and that a rebound phenomenon occurs when the medication is withdrawn (5,6). Administration of glucocorticoids also eliminates the normal periodicity of TSH secretion (6). There are conflicting reports on the effects of glucocorticoids on the TSH and PRL responses to thyrotropin releasing hormone (TRH). In patients with Cushing's syndrome, normal TRH-induced TSH (7,8) responses have been observed. Woolf *et al.* reported that neither acute nor chronic administration of glucocorticoids affected the basal concentration of TSH or the TSH response to TRH (9). Haigler *et al.* observed no significant blunting of the TSH response to TRH in 4 hypothyroid patients given 8 mg of dexamethasone for two days (10). In contrast, Otsuki *et al.* (11) observed a blunted TSH response to TRH in patients on high doses of glucocorticoids and in patients with Cushing's syndrome. Physiological concentrations of cortisol decrease synthesis of PRL in rat pituitary tumor cell cultures (12). Dussault *et al.* reported that administration of 2 mg of dexamethasone daily for 3 days suppressed baseline serum levels of TSH and PRL and blunted the TSH but not the PRL response to TRH in 13 normal subjects (13).

To determine the effects of short term administration of high doses of glucocorticoids on TSH and PRL secretion and the site of this effect in man, we administered 8 mg of dexamethasone daily for 5 days and studied baseline serum TSH and PRL and their responses to TRH and metoclopramide. Metoclopramide is a dopamine antagonist that appears to increase PRL release by blocking dopamine-mediated hypothalamic inhibition of prolactin-secretion (14,15).

Supported by VA Research Program 3590 and USPHS Research Grant HD-7181.

Reprint requests to: Jerome M. Hershman, M.D., VA Wadsworth Hospital Center, Wilshire and Sawtelle Boulevards, Los Angeles, California 90073.

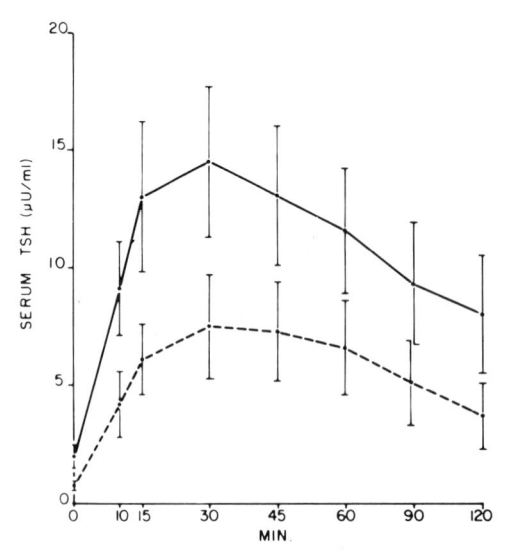

FIG. 1. Mean serum TSH responses to TRH (given at 0 time) in 9 normal men before (solid line) and after (broken line) dexamethasone administration; vertical bars show SEM.

Materials and Methods

Nine normal male volunteers (ages 29–55) were fasted overnight and given an iv bolus of 500 μg of TRH at 0800 h before and after receiving dexamethasone 2 mg orally every 6 h for 5 days. Baseline samples of blood (−15 and 0 min) were drawn through an indwelling 19-gauge needle and further blood samples were obtained at 10, 15, 30, 45, 60, 90 and 120 min after injection of TRH. Seven normal male volunteers (ages 35–58) were fasted overnight and an indwelling 19-gauge needle was placed in an antecubital vein at 0800 h. The 7 men were given 10 mg of metoclopramide orally before and after receiving dexamethasone 8 mg daily for 5 days. Baseline samples of blood were drawn (−15 and 0 min) and further blood samples were obtained at 30, 45, 60, 90, 120 and 150 min after ingestion of metoclopramide. Serum PRL was measured by minor modification of the homologous radioimmunoassay described by Sinha et al. (16); the mean basal serum PRL was 5.7 ± 3 (SD) in a large group of normal male controls. Serum TSH was measured by the double antibody method described by Pekary et al. (17); the mean basal TSH in normal controls was 1.5 ± 1.0 (SD) μU/ml. Serum triiodothyronine (T_3) and thyroxine (T_4) were determined by modifications of the double antibody radioimmunoassays described by Chopra et al. (18,19); the normal mean basal serum T_3 was 148 ± 32 ng/dl and the normal mean basal serum T_4 was 7.9 ± 1.5 μg/dl. All hormone determinations were done in the same assay to eliminate inter-assay variation. Statistical comparisons of serum hormone concentrations before and after dexamethasone administration were made using Student's paired t test.

Results

As shown in Fig. 1, dexamethasone administration reduced the mean baseline TSH ($P < 0.005$). The mean serum TSH response to TRH in the 9 men before taking dexamethasone was greater ($P < 0.005$) at all sampling times from 10 min to 120 min after TRH administration than the response after dexamethasone administration (Fig. 1). As shown in Fig. 2, dexamethasone administration reduced the mean baseline serum PRL ($P < 0.005$). The mean serum PRL

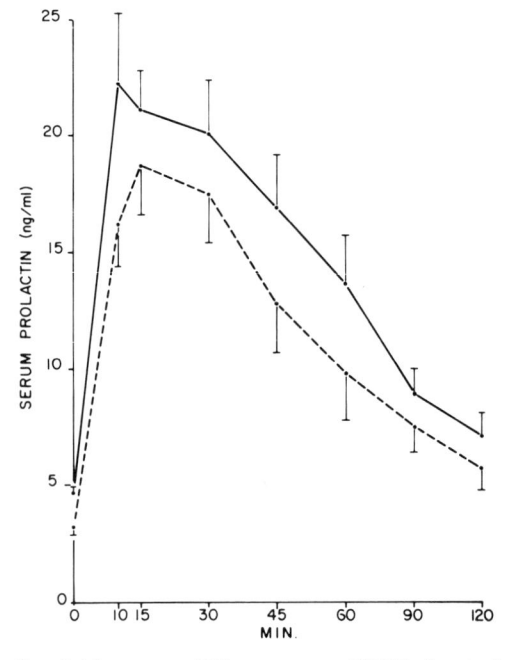

FIG. 2. Mean serum PRL responses to TRH in 9 normal men before (solid line) and after (broken line) dexamethasone administration; vertical bars show SEM.

response prior to taking dexamethasone in the 9 men was greater ($P < 0.05$) at sampling times from 10 through 60 min after TRH administration (Fig. 2). As shown in Fig. 3, dexamethasone administration reduced the mean baseline serum T_3 ($P < 0.005$). Figure 3 shows that the mean serum T_3 response to TRH of these 9 men prior to their taking dexamethasone was greater ($P < 0.005$) at all sampling times from 10 through 120 min and the mean serum T_4 response was greater at the 90 and 120 min sampling times. The peak and maximum increment of PRL, TSH, T_3 and T_4 following TRH was greater ($P < 0.005$) before dexamethasone than after dexamethasone.

The mean serum PRL response in the 7 men receiving metoclopramide was greater ($P < 0.005$) at all sampling times from 30 through 150 min when the metoclopramide was given prior to dexamethasone administration (Fig. 4). The peak and max ΔPRL response to metoclopramide was greater ($P < 0.005$) prior to administration of dexamethasone than after receiving dexamethasone.

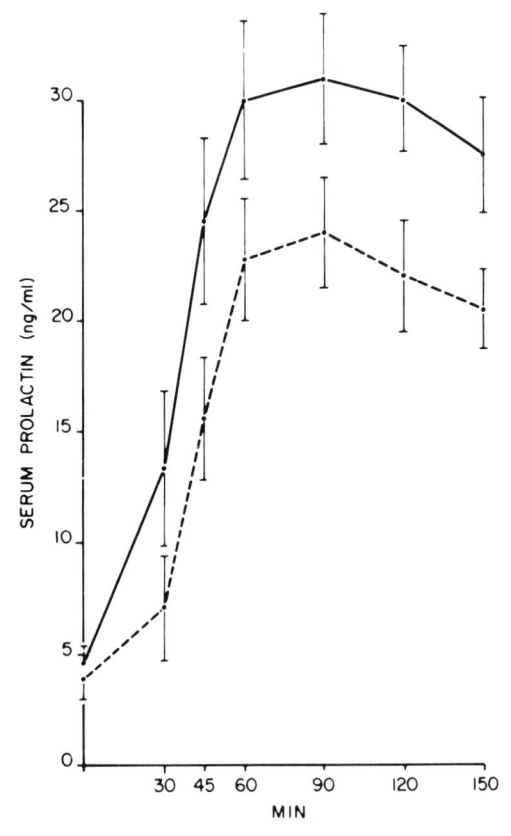

FIG. 4. Mean serum PRL responses to metoclopramide (given at 0 time) in 7 normal men before (solid line) and after (broken line) dexamethasone administration; vertical bars show SEM.

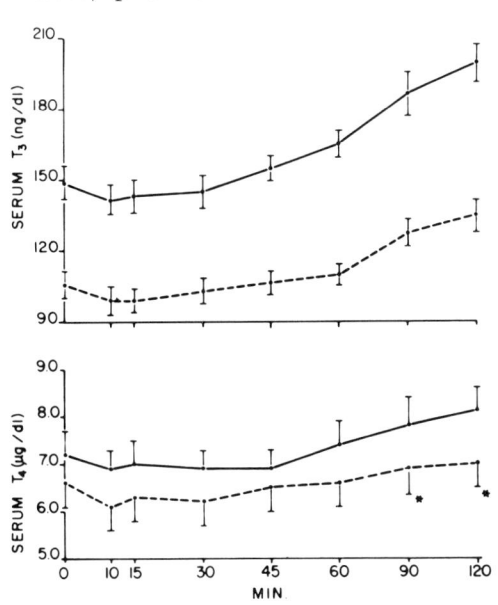

FIG. 3. Mean serum T_3 and T_4 responses to TRH in 9 normal men before (solid line) and after (broken line) dexamethasone administration; vertical bars show SEM;* denotes significant difference between the T_4 response at these times.

Discussion

This study clearly shows that short-term high dose glucocorticoid administration decreases baseline serum levels of PRL, TSH and T_3. Our results confirm the findings of other investigators that glucocorticoids suppress basal TSH secretion (5,6,13). Our finding that glucocorticoids suppress baseline serum PRL is in agreement with previous reports of glucocorticoids suppressing PRL secretion *in vitro* (12) and baseline PRL levels in normal man (1,13). The present observation that pharmacological doses of glucocorticoids lead to a reduction in basal circulating T_3 without significantly affecting the serum T_4 levels are similar to the findings of other investigators (20,21) in euthyroid subjects which suggest that glucocorticoids may, in part, reduce circulating levels of serum T_3 by interfering with the peripheral conversion of T_4 to T_3. This concept is further supported by the work of Chopra et al. who showed that short-term administration of pharmacological doses of dexamethasone resulted in increased serum 3,3′,3′-triiodothyronine (reverse T_3) concomitant with decreased serum T_3 in both hypothyroid and hyperthyroid patients (22). However, a small decline in T_4 secretion may also partially account for the glucocorticoid induced reduction in serum T_3.

Our study indicates that short-term administration of high dose glucocorticoids blunts both the PRL and TSH responses to TRH in normal men. The decreased T_3 and T_4 response following TRH is most likely the result of the inhibitory effect of glucocorticoids on TSH secretion by the pituitary but a direct inhibitory effect on thyroid release of T_3 and T_4 cannot be eliminated. The finding of a blunted TSH response to TRH in normal man confirms the results of previous studies (11,13). In the previous studies where no blunting of the basal TSH or the TSH response to TRH were observed, the subjects received small doses of glucocorticoids (60 mg of cortisol or less per day) (9) or high doses of glucocorticoids for 2 days or less (9,10). These results suggest that both the dose and duration of glucocorticoid administration are important factors in the suppression of basal and TSH response to TRH. Our finding of a blunted PRL response to TRH and metoclopramide has not previously been reported. Dussault (13) reported that administration of 2 mg of dexamethasone per day for 3 days suppressed baseline serum PRL but not the PRL response to TRH. Our observation that administration of 8 mg of dexamethasone for 5 days suppresses both the basal and PRL response to TRH suggests that the dose and duration of glucocorticoid administration are also important factors in the blunting of the PRL response to TRH.

TRH acts directly on the anterior pituitary to stimulate PRL release (23) and metoclopramide induces PRL release probably by antagonizing the dopamine-dependent hypothalamic inhibition of PRL secretion (15). The present observations suggest that pharmacological doses of glucocorticoids probably suppress both basal secretion and stimulated release of PRL at the pituitary level.

Acknowledgments

The authors are grateful to Jung Park, Nancy Meyer, and Allan Reed for their skillful technical assistance and to Becci Kinnamon and Carolyn Schaefer for their excellent secretarial service in preparation of the manuscript.

References

1. Copinschi, G., M. l'Hermite, R. LeClercq, J. Golstein, L. Vanhaelst, E. Virasoro, and C. Robyn, Effects of glucocorticoids on pituitary hormonal response to hypoglycemia. Inhibition of prolactin release, J Clin Endocrinol Metab 40: 442, 1975.
2. Nakagawa, K., Y. Horiuchi, and K. Mashimo, Further studies on the relation between growth hormone and corticotrophin secretion in insulin-induced hypoglycemia, J Clin Endocrinol Metab 32: 188, 1971.
3. Harnes, P. G., P. Langlier, and S. M. McCann, Modification of stress-induced prolactin release by dexamethasone or adrenalectomy, Endocrinology 96: 475, 1975.
4. Kreiger, D. T., P. J. Howanitz, and A. G. Frantz, Absence of nocturnal elevation of plasma prolactin concentration in Cushing's disease, J Clin Endocrinol Metab 42: 260, 1976.
5. Wilber, J. F., and R. D. Utiger, The effects of glucocorticoids on thyrotropin secretion, J Clin Invest 48: 2096, 1969.
6. Nicoloff, J. T., D. A. Fisher, and M. D. Appleman, The role of glucocorticoids in the regulation of thyroid function in man, J Clin Invest 49: 1922, 1970.
7. Hershman, J. M., and J. A. Pittman, Response to synthetic thyrotropin-releasing hormone in man, J Clin Endocrinol Metab 31: 457, 1970.
8. Saito, S., K. Abe, H. Yoshida, T. Kaneko, E. Kaneko, N. Nakamura, N. Shinizu, and N. Yanaihara, Effects of synthetic thyrotropin-releasing hormone

on plasma thyrotropin, growth hormone and insulin levels in man, *Endocrinol Jap* 18: 101, 1971.
9. Woolf, P. D., D. Gonzalez-Barcena, D. S. Schalch, L. A. Lee, J. P. Arzac, A. V. Schally, and A. J. Kastin, Lack of effect of steroids on thyrotropin-releasing hormone (TRH) mediated thyrotropin (TSH) release in man, *Neuroendocrinology* 13: 56, 1974.
10. Haigler, E. D., J. A. Pittman, J. M. Hershman, and C. M. Baugh, Direct evaluation of pituitary thyrotropin reserve utilizing synthetic thyrotropin releasing hormone, *J Clin Endocrinol Metab* 33: 573, 1971.
11. Otsuki, M., M. Dakoda, and S. Baba, Influence of glucocorticoids on TRF-induced TSH response in man, *J Clin Endocrinol Metab* 36: 95, 1973.
12. Dannies, P. S., and A. H. Tashjian, Effects of thyrotropin-releasing hormone and hydrocortisone on synthesis and degradation of prolactin in a rat pituitary cell strain, *J Biol Chem* 248: 6174, 1973.
13. Dussault, J. H., The effect of dexamethasone on TSH and prolactin secretion after TRH stimulation, *Can Med Assoc J* 111: 1195, 1974.
14. Delitala, G., A. Masala, S. Alagna, and L. Devilla, Metoclopramide and prolactin secretion in man: Effects of pretreatment with L-dopa and 2-Bromo-α-Ergocryptine (CB-154), *IRCS Med Sci (Endocrinol Syst)* 3: 274, 1975.
15. McCallum, R. W., J. R. Sowers, J. M. Hershman, and R. A. L. Sturdevant, Metoclopramide stimulates prolactin secretion in man, *J Clin Endocrinol Metab* 42: 1148, 1976.
16. Sinha, Y. N., F. W. Selby, U. J. Lewis, and W. P. Vanderlaan, A homologous radioimmunoassay for human prolactin, *J Clin Endocrinol Metab* 36: 509, 1973.
17. Pekary, A. E., J. M. Hershman, and A. F. Parlow, A sensitive and precise radioimmunoassay for human thyroid stimulating hormone, *J Clin Endocrinol Metab* 41: 676, 1975.
18. Chopra, I. J., R. S. Ho, and R. Lum, An improved radioimmunoassay of triiodothyronine in serum: Its application to clinical and physiological studies, *J Lab Clin Med* 80: 729, 1972.
19. Chopra, I. J., A radioimmunoassay for measurement of thyroxine in unextracted serum, *J Clin Endocrinol Metab* 34: 938, 1972.
20. Duick, D. S., D. W. Warren, J. T. Nicoloff, C. L. Otis and M. S. Croxson, Effect of single dose dexamethasone on the concentration of serum triiodothyronine in man, *J Clin Endocrinol Metab* 39: 1151, 1974.
21. Chopra, I. J., U. Chopra, and J. Orgiazzi, Abnormalities of hypothalamo-hypophyseal-thyroid axis in patients with Graves' opthalmopathy, *J Clin Endocrinol Metab* 37: 955, 1973.
22. Chopra, I. J., D. E. Williams, J. Orgiazzi, and D. H. Solomon, Opposite effects of dexamethasone on serum concentrations of $3,3',5'$-triiodothyronine (reverse T_3) and $3,3',5$-triiodothyronine (T_3), *J Clin Endocrinol Metab* 41: 911, 1975.
23. Bowers, C. Y., H. G. Friesen, P. Hwang, H. J. Guyda, and K. Folkers, Prolactin and thyrotropin release in man by synthetic pyroglutamylhistidyl-prolinamide, *Biochem Biophys Res Commun* 45: 1033, 1971.

53

Copyright © 1977 by J. B. Lippincott Company
Reprinted from *Endocrinology* 100:238-241 (1977)

STIMULATION IN VIVO OF THE SECRETION OF PROLACTIN AND

GROWTH HORMONE BY β-ENDORPHIN

C. Rivier, W. Vale, N. Ling, M. Brown and R. Guillemin

Laboratories for Neuroendocrinology

The Salk Institute, La Jolla, California 92037

Several laboratories have recently reported the isolation and characterization of morphinomimetic brain oligopeptides. Hughes et al. (1) isolated Leu^5-enkephalin and Met^5-enkephalin from porcine brain; Met^5-enkephalin is identical to the sequence (61-65) of β-lipotropin, while Leu^5-enkephalin shows the sequence (61-64). Guillemin and co-workers (2,3) isolated two opiate-like peptides, termed endorphins, from porcine posterior pituitary and hypothalamic extracts; α-endorphin and γ-endorphin are respectively identical to the sequence β-LPH-(61-76) and β-LPH-(61-77). The entire C-terminal fragment of β-lipotropin, β-LPH-(61-91), identified by Bradbury et al. (4) and Li and Chung (5) from whole pituitary extracts, also has morphinomimetic properties.

This laboratory has engaged in the isolation of the endogenous ligand of the opiate receptors on the hypothesis (2,9) that the endogenous opiate-like peptides might be involved in the mechanisms of release of pituitary hormones, since the opiate alkaloids are well known to stimulate secretion of prolactin and growth hormone (6-9). We report here on the effects of three opioid peptides on the secretion of prolactin and growth hormone.

MATERIALS AND METHODS

Cell Culture Assay: Enzymatically dispersed normal rat pituitary cells were maintained in culture for 4 days, then exposed to the peptides for 4 hours (10).

Rat Bioassay: Male Sprague-Dawley rats, 44-46 days old, were treated with estrogen (50 μg) and progesterone (25 mg) for 3 days, then anesthetized with urethane (150 mg/100 g body weight)(11). The test materials were injected into the jugular vein (iv) in a volume of 1 ml or into the cisterna magna (ic) in a volume of 25 μl. Blood samples were taken immediately prior to the injection, and 10 min later.

Hormone Determinations: PRL and GH levels were measured by double antibody methods as previously described (6,11).

Drugs and Peptides: Morphine sulfate was purchased from Merck Sharpe and

---

Submitted September 27, 1976

Stimulation of Prolactin and Growth Hormone Release

Dohme. Naloxone hydrochloride (N-allyl-nor-oxymorphone) was a gift from Endo Labs., Garden City, New York. Met[5]-enkephalin, β-LPH-(61-65), α-endorphin (β-LPH-(61-76)) and β-endorphin (β-LPH-(61-91)) were synthesized using solid phase methodology (12).

Statistical Analysis: All experiments were carried out in a randomized block design. Following analysis of variance, differences between treatments were determined by the multiple range tests of Dunnett and Duncan.

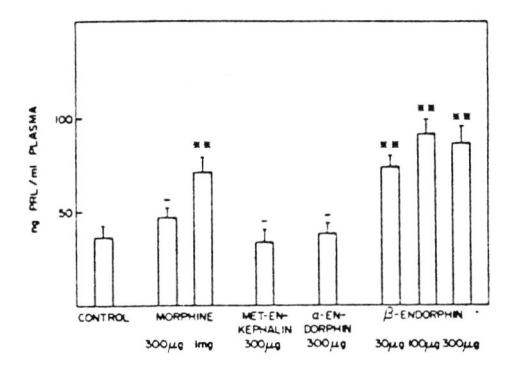

Figure 1: Effect of several doses of iv administered morphine sulfate (MS) and opioid peptides on PRL secretion in steroid-primed rats. Each bar represents the mean and standard error of the mean for groups of 5 rats. -, $p > 0.05$; **, $p < 0.01$.

RESULTS AND DISCUSSION

Figure 1 illustrates the effect of several doses of iv administered morphine sulfate (MS) and opioid peptides on PRL secretion. Met[5]-enkephalin and α-endorphin do not elevate plasma PRL levels. On a molar basis, β-endorphin is at least 20 times more potent than MS, Met[5]-enkephalin or α-endorphin. These results were obtained in steroid-primed rats; similar observations have been made in non-treated animals. In the myenteric plexus bioassay (3) as well as in studies of

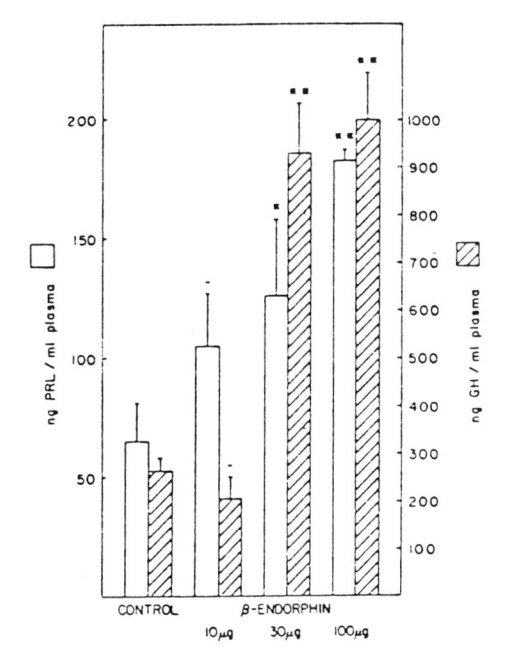

Figure 2: Effect of ic administered β-endorphin on PRL and GH secretion in steroid-primed rats. Details as in Fig. 1. *, $p < 0.05$.

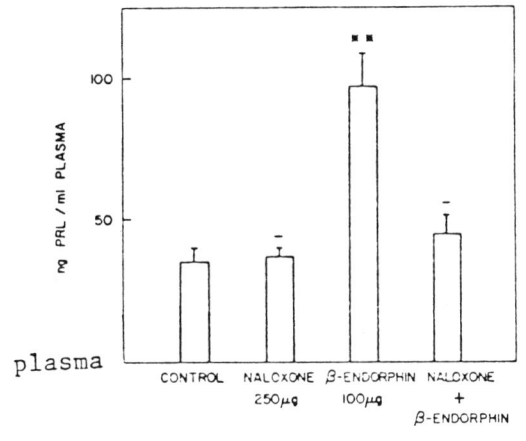

Figure 3: Effect of naloxone on β-endorphin induced secretion of PRL in steroid-primed rats. Details as in Figure 1.

TABLE 1: Effect of β-endorphin, Met[5]-enkephalin and α-endorphin on PRL and GH secretion by cultured rat pituitary cells

Treatment		ng PRL dish.hr	SEM	P	ng GH dish.hr	SEM	P
Experiment 1:							
Control		109	2		792	107	
β-endorphin	0.01 µg/ml	120	4	-(a)	827	159	-
"	0.1 µg/ml	118	4	-	767	90	-
"	1.0 µg/ml	132	5	-	940	63	-
"	10. µg/ml	125	4	-	860	84	-
Met[5]-enkephalin	0.01 µg/ml	107	3	-	808	60	-
"	0.1 µg/ml	121	3	-	770	107	-
"	1.0 µg/ml	126	4	-	797	128	-
"	10. µg/ml	117	2	-	797	196	-
Experiment 2:							
Control		143	4		417	13	
α-endorphin	0.01 µg/ml	141	3	-	474	23	-
"	1.0 µg/ml	139	6	-	474	27	-

(a) $p > 0.05$

competition for the opiate receptor in synaptosomal preparations (3,13-15) β-endorphin is at least 5 times as potent as normorphine or levorphanol, whereas Met[5]-enkephalin and Leu[5]-enkephalin have relative affinities of ca. 0.3 (3,13,14). β-endorphin is also a potent stimulator of PRL and GH secretion when injected ic (Fig. 2). Pharmacological effects of MS on several receptors are reversed or prevented by the opiate antagonist naloxone (9,15,16); similarly naloxone, at doses which do not affect PRL secretion, inhibits the stimulatory effect of β-endorphin on the secretion of PRL (Fig.3). Most effects of the opioid peptides, but not all, have been found to be prevented or reversed by naloxone (17). As is the case for MS (9), all three morphinomimetic peptides are devoid of in vitro activity (Table 1), suggesting a central nervous system site of action of these substances in their releasing GH and PRL in vivo. These results are at variance with the recent findings of Lien et al. (18) who reported that as little as 5 ng/ml Met[5]-enkephalin and Leu[5]-enkephalin significantly increases PRL secretion by cultured pituitary cells. Since we have repeatedly failed to observe any stimulatory effect of these two peptides in vitro, the reason for this discrepancy is unknown.

We have previously found that a variety of pharmacological stimuli of PRL secretion, including TRF, neurotensin, substance P, histamine and α-adrenergic agonists, are not affected by concomitant naloxone administration (9). These results would indicate that the stimulatory activity of these latter substances does not involve an opiate-receptor dependent step. Although the significance of opiate-like peptides in the physiological control of PRL and GH secretion remains to be determined, these results indicate one more biological activity shared by MS and the neurotropic brain peptides related to β-lipotropin.

ACKNOWLEDGEMENT

The authors thank E. Tucker, C. Douglas, A. Wolfe, M. Mercado, L.

Koski, R. Kaiser, and S. Minick for excellent technical assistance, and Jean Rivier for his contribution in assembling the protected β-endorphin onto the chloromethylated resin. We are indebted to the National Institute of Arthritis, Metabolism and Digestive Diseases, Rat Pituitary Hormone programs, for supplying the rat PRL and GH radioimmunoassay kits, and Endo Labs for the gift of naloxone. Research supported by NIH grants Nos. AM-18811, AM-16707, National Foundation 1-411, and the William Randolph Hearst Foundation.

REFERENCES

1. Hughes, J., T.W. Smith, H.W. Kosterlitz, L.A. Fothergill, B.A. Morgan, and H.R. Morris, Nature 258: 577, 1975.

2. Guillemin, R., N. Ling, and R. Burgus, C R Acad Sci, Series [D] (Paris) 282:1821, 1976.

3. Lazarus, L.H., N. Ling, and R. Guillemin, Proc Natl Acad Sci USA 73:2156, 1976.

4. Bradbury, A.F., D.G. Smyth, C.R. Shepp, N,J.M. Birdsall, and E.C. Hulme, Nature 206:793, 1976

5. Li, C.H., and D. Chung, Proc Natl Acad Sci USA 73:1145, 1976.

6. Brown, M., and W. Vale, Endocrinology 97:1151, 1975.

7. McCann, S.M., S.R. Ojeda, C. Libertun, P.G. Harms, and L. Krulich. In Zimmerman, E., and H. Hecht (eds.), Narcotics and the Hypothalamus, Raven Press, New York, 1974, p. 121.

8. Martin, J., Neuroendocrinology 13: 339, 1974.

9. Rivier, C., M. Brown and W. Vale, Program 58th Endocrine Society Meeting, San Francisco, 1976, p. 119 (Abstract).

10. Vale, W., G. Grant, M. Amoss, R. Blackwell, and R. Guillemin, Endocrinology 91:562, 1972.

11. Rivier, C., and W. Vale, Endocrinology 95:978, 1974.

12. Ling, N., and W. Vale, Biochem. Biophys Res Commun 63:801, 1975.

13. Cox, B.M., A. Goldstein, and C.H. Li, Proc Natl Acad Sci USA 73: 1821, 1976.

14. Terenius, L., A. Wahlstrom, G. Lindesbert, S. Karlsson, and U. Ragnasson, Biochem Biophys Res Commun 71:175, 1976.

15. Packman, P.M., J.A. Rothchild, Endocrinology 99:7, 1976.

16. Vale, W., C. Rivier, and M. Brown, Ann Review Physiol (in press).

17. Bloom, F., D. Segal, N. Ling, and R. Guillemin, Science 194, 1976 (in press).

18. Lien, E.L., R.L. Fenichet, V. Garsky, D. Sarantakis, and N.H. Grant, Life Sci 19:837, 1976.

Part VII
MORPHOLOGY AND NEUROENDOCRINE ROLE OF HYPOTHALAMIC CATECHOLAMINE NEURONS

Editor's Comments
on Papers 54 and 55

54   CARLSSON, FALCK, and HILLARP
Excerpt from *Cellular Localization of Brain Monoamines*

55   FUXE and HÖKFELT
Further Evidence for the Existence of Tubero-infundibular Dopamine Neurons

Carlsson et al. (Paper 54) developed a histochemical technique permitting visualization of neurohumoral amines within cells of the central nervous system. Studies with this staining technique demonstrated that 5-hydroxytryptamine (5-HT), norepinephrine (NE), and dopamine (DA) are found primarily in nerve cells and not in glia cells, as had been previously speculated. Fuxe and Hökfelt (Paper 55) used this technique to identify large numbers of DA-containing nerve terminals in close apposition to the portal vessels in the median eminence of the hypothalamus. Thus, the best early evidence that DA is a synaptic neurotransmitter was the demonstration by Carlsson et al. (Paper 54) and Fuxe and Hökfelt (Paper 55) that DA is present in terminal buttons of hypothalamic neurons. They also demonstrated high levels of NE in preoptic, supraoptic, paraventricular, arcuate, retrochiasmatic nuclei, and the internal layer of the median eminence. Fuxe and Hökfelt (Paper 55) showed that, in the arcuate nucleus of the medial basal hypothalamus, there are clusters of dopaminergic neurons with fiber projections into the median eminence. They showed that other axonal terminals from NE and possibly serotonergic fibers arriving from mesencephalic structures were also found in the median eminence.

As summarized by Hökfelt and Fuxe (1971), there is a cluster of neurons in the medial basal hypothalamus that contain DA and project into the median eminence and are associated with hormonal control. These tubero-infundibular dopaminergic (TIDA) neurons have been found to undergo changes in DA content, as well as turnover rates under different reproductive stages. Extrahypothalamic, as well as hypothalamic monoaminergic, neurons modulate the release of hypothalamic releasing and inhibitory hormones. There is a nor-adrenergic system originating outside the hypothalamus and passing into the basal hypothalamus via the medial forebrain bundle and innervating various nuclei concerned with releasing hormone formation. Fuxe and Hökfelt have demonstrated that many of the tubero-infundibular neurons from the medial basal hypothalamus with nuclei located mostly in the arcuate nucleus and, to a lesser extent, in the ventromedial nuclei with projections to the median eminence, elaborate the release of TRF, CRF and LH-RH.

REFERENCE

Hökfelt, T., and K. Fuxe. 1971. *Brain Endocrine Interaction, Median Eminence: Structure and Function.* International Symposium, Munich, 1971, p. 181.

54

Copyright © 1962 by Acta Physiological Scandinavica

Reprinted from pages 23-27 of *Acta Physiol. Scand.* 56(suppl. 196), 1962, 28pp.

CELLULAR LOCALIZATION OF BRAIN MONOAMINES

By

ARVID CARLSSON, BENGT FALCK and NILS-ÅKE HILLARP

[*Editor's Note:* In the original, material precedes this excerpt.]

Discussion

The dominating structure which develops fluorescence in the hypothalamus is the fine varicose fibres assumed to be the terminal parts of axons forming synaptic contacts. There is almost conclusive evidence that these fibres contain NA but it cannot be excluded that they contain also DA or that some of them have DA exclusively. The most significant facts are summarized below.

1. The fluorescence method shows a high specificity for certain catecholamines and tryptamines (see the introduction to Results). All the characteristics of the reaction and the properties of the fluorescent product indicate that a compound is demonstrated which belongs to one or the other of these groups. The colour of the emitted light suggests a catecholamine rather than a tryptamine. If the fluorescence is due to a catecholamine, the characteristics of the reaction strongly implicate a primary amine and almost exclude a secondary amine such as A. The fact that A exists in only very low concentrations in the hypothalamus (BERTLER and ROSENGREN 1959) strengthens the view that this amine can be excluded. — The fluorescence method is discussed further in another paper (FALCK 1962).

2. Of the known monoamines which yield intensely fluorescent condensation products with formaldehyde only A, NA, DA and 5-HT have been found in significant amounts in the hypothalamus of normal animals. The corresponding amino acid precursors may develop fluorescence but are normally present — if at all — in too small amounts to interfere.

3. After administration of reserpine the disappearance and recovery of the fluorescence as function of dose and time agree very well with those of the catecholamines (CARLSSON et al. 1957, BRODIE 1958, BRODIE, MAICKEL and WESTERMAN 1961, and unpublished data).

4. When the hypothalamic catecholamines — but not 5-HT — are depleted through the administration of m-tyrosine and α-methyl-m-tyrosine the fluorescence also disappears. This finding in itself almost conclusively proves that a catecholamine and not 5-HT is accumulated in the varicose fibres. Since α-methyl-m-tyrosine under the conditions employed affects DA but slightly, the data indicate that the catecholamine in question is predominantly NA.

5. When a reaccumulation of 5-HT — but not catecholamines — is brought about through administration of nialamide to reserpinized animals no fluorescence reappears in the fibres.

6. Finally, the distribution of NA — but not 5-HT and DA — in the different parts of the hypothalamus (BERTLER 1961) is similar to that of the fluorescent varicose fibres which, furthermore, have been found to be scarce in all brain parts with a low NA content (e.g. cerebellum and cerebral cortex). Table 1 gives the content of this amine in some parts of the rat brain. It is seen that the preoptic region, which has abundant varicose fibres, also shows a high concentration of NA. The somewhat unexpectedly high content in the posterior hypothalamus may be due to the presence of NA in the big fluorescent nerve cells (see below).

von EULER and his co-workers (cf. von EULER 1956, 1961) have presented strong evidence for the view that the adrenergic transmitter is NA and that

[*Editor's Note:* Table 1 is not reproduced here.]

this amine — although present in the whole neuron — is accumulated and stored in very high concentrations in the "terminals" of the adrenergic nerves. This accumulation has recently been directly demonstrated (FALCK and TORP 1962). The fluorescent varicose fibres in the hypothalamus have the same charateristic appearance and must — as judged from the fluorescence intensity — accumulate and store similar very high concentrations of NA as the "terminals" in peripheral tissues. Besides the morphological evidence (section I) there is thus also biochemical evidence for the view that the fluorescent fibres represent the terminal parts of axons. The very high accumulation of NA in these terminal parts is just what would be expected if they are "terminals" belonging to adrenergic neurons in the brain.

There are thus reasons to believe that adrenergic neurons exist in the central nervous system. From this point of view it is highly interesting that some nerve cells in the hypothalamus and also other regions develop a fluorescence in the cell bodies and larger processes which suggest the presence of a catecholamine in low concentrations. The findings that this fluorescence may be caused to disappear through administration of reserpine, m-tyrosine and α-methyl-m-tyrosine strongly support this view. These nerve cells may thus represent the cell bodies of adrenergic neurons.

The fluorescent zone in the median eminence is puzzling. The results obtained so far indicate that a catecholamine is accumulated here but its cellular localization has not been revealed. However, the intimate relation of the zone to the hypophysial portal system suggests a rôle in the humoral regulation of the pituitary functions. Preliminary examinations (J. HÄGGENDAL, unpublished data) of the monoamines in the median eminence suggest a high DA content. The finding that much of the fluorescence still persisted after α-methyl-m-tyrosine — in contrast to m-tyrosine — also might suggest the presence of this amine (cf. CARLSSON and LINDQVIST 1962).

Like NA, 5-HT easily gives an intensely fluorescent condensation product with formaldehyde under the conditions used and the fluorescence method readily demonstrates the 5-HT present in the mast cells of some species (FALCK 1962). However, it has proved difficult to visualize the brain stores of this amine. This might be due to a localization to submicroscopic structures which are not closely packed or to a so widespread distribution that the concentration does not reach the limit of detection. The very fine smooth fibres with a more yellowish fluorescence may well contain 5-HT, however. The colour of the emitted light and the findings that the fluorescence disappears after administration of reserpine — but not m-tyrosine or α-methyl-m-tyrosine — favour this view.

The diffuse fluorescence of the circumscribed and more or less continuous areas, including the amygdala, surrounding the anterior hypothalamus and preoptic region seems to be due to the presence of a catecholamine, possibly both NA and DA. The characteristics of the fluorescence reaction, the properties of the fluorescent material, and the results obtained in the experiments with drugs strongly support this view. The cellular localization is unknown but it does not seem probable that a monoamine is present diffusely throughout the tissue. A more attractive hypothesis is that the amine is stored in the terminal parts of submicroscopic nerve fibres which lie fairly close together.

The caudate nucleus has a very high DA, much lower 5-HT and very low NA content (BERTLER and ROSENGREN 1959, BERTLER 1961). This nucleus as a whole has a fairly high fluorescence which is quite diffuse. All data hitherto obtained — histochemical as well as pharmacological — strongly indicate that this fluorescence — mainly at least — is due to the DA present. The pharmacological data are summarized in Table 2. The fact that m-tyrosine did not cause the fluorescence to disappear completely may probably be explained on the basis that both m-tyrosine and its decarboxylation product, m-tyramine, 2 hours after the last injection are present in concentrations high enough to produce a significant fluorescence on formaldehyde condensation.

It is quite improble that the DA present in the caudate nucleus has a diffuse distribution in the tissue, and it does not seem very likely that it is accumulated in the glia cells throughout the nucleus. The amine is thus probably localized to submicroscopic structures belonging, for instance, to the neuropil.

This work has been supported by grants from the Swedish Medical Research Council, the Directorate of Life Sciences, AFOSR, Office of Aerospace Research, United States Air Force, monitored by the European Office of Aerospace Research under Grant No. AF-EOAR-61-64, and by a grant (B-2854) from the United States Public Health Service.

[*Editor's Note:* Table 2 is not reproduced here.]

SUMMARY

The cellular localization of brain monoamines has been studied with the use of a fluorescence method for histochemical demonstration of certain catecholamines and tryptamines in combination with a pharmacological approach. Mainly the hypothalamus and caudate nucleus of mouse and rat were examined. The following are the most important results.

1. Noradrenaline in the hypothalamus shows a high accumulation in fine varicose fibres which are present almost everywhere, but highly concentrated to some areas (especially a large area in the preoptic region, the supraoptic and paraventricular nuclei, and the periventricular nuclei in the anterior hypothalamus). There is good evidence that these fibres represent the terminal parts of axons forming synaptic contacts. Consequently, adrenergic neurons may exist and noradrenaline may serve as a synaptic transmitter in the central nervous system.

2. Similar fibres are present also in other parts of the central nervous system, including the spinal cord. More dense accumulations have so far been found only in some areas in the pons and medulla oblongata.

3. There is good evidence that the perikarya and processes of some nerve cells in the hypothalamus (and also other brain regions) contain a catecholamine (probably noradrenaline) in low concentrations. These nerve cells may represent the cell bodies of adrenergic neurons.

4. There is good evidence that a catecholamine is accumulated in high concentration in the superficial zone of the median eminence. Its cellular localization has not been revealed. Dopamine may be the main amine present. The intimate relation of this zone to the hypophysial portal system suggest a rôle in the humoral regulation of the pituitary functions.

5. Some circumscribed and more or less continuous areas, including the amygdala, surrounding the anterior hypothalamus and preoptic region develop a fluorescence which seems to be due the presence of a catecholamine, possibly both noradrenaline and dopamine. The cellular localization is unknown but it may well be that the amines are stored in the terminal parts of submicroscopic nerve fibres which lie fairly close together.

6. The caudate nucleus as a whole develops a fairly high fluorescence. All histochemical as well as pharmacological data strongly indicate thas this fluorescence — mainly at least — is due to the dopamine present. The amine is probably localized to submicroscopic structures belonging, for instance, to the neuropil.

REFERENCES

Bertler, Å. 1961. Occurrence and Localization of Catechol Amines in the Human Brain. *Acta Physiol. Scand.* **51**:97-107.

Bertler, Å., and E. Rosengren. 1959. Occurrence and Distribution of Catechol Amines in Brain. *Acta Physiol. Scand.* **47**:350-361.

Brodie, B. B. 1958. Storage and Release of 5-hydroxytryptamine. In *5-hydroxytryptamine*, G. P. Lewis, ed. London: Pergamon Press, pp. 64-83.

Brodie, B. B., R. P. Maickel, and E. O. Westerman. 1961. Action of Reserpine on Pituitary-Adrenocortical System Through Possible Action on Hypothalamus. In *Regional Neurochemistry*, S. S. Kety and J. Elkes, eds. Oxford: Pergamon Press, pp. 351-361.

Carlsson, A, and M. Lindqvist. 1962. In Vivo Decarboxylation of α-methyl Dopa and α Methyl Metatyrosine. *Acta Physiol. Scand.* **54**:87-94.

Carlsson, A., E. Rosengren, Å. Bertler, and J. Nilsson. 1957. Effect of Reserpine on the Metabolism of Catechol Amines. In *Psychotropic Drugs*, S. Garattini and V. Ghetti, eds. Amsterdam: Elsevier, pp. 363-372.

Falck, B. 1962. Observations on the Possibilities for the Cellular Localization of Monoamines with a Fluorescence Method. *Acta Physiol. Scand. Suppl. 197.*

Falck, B., and A. Torp. 1962. New Evidence for the Localization of Noradrenaline in the Adrenergic Nerve Terminals. *Med. Exp.* **6**:169-172.

von Euler, U. S. 1956. *Noradrenaline*, Springfield, Ill.: C. C Thomas.

von Euler, U. S. 1961. Neurotransmission in the Adrenergic Nervous System. *The Harvey Lectures*, Series 55 (N.Y.), pp. 43-63.

55

Copyright © 1966 by Acta Physiologica Scandinavica

Reprinted from *Acta Physiol. Scand.* **66**:245-246 (1966)

Further Evidence for the Existence of Tubero-infundibular Dopamine Neurons

By

KJELL FUXE and TOMAS HÖKFELT

Previous studies (Fuxe 1964) have given strong support for the existence of a tubero-infundibular dopamine (DA) neuron system. Further evidence for this view is given in the present paper, using the histochemical fluorescence method for the cellular demonstration of catecholamines (CA) and 5-hydroxytryptamine (Falck *et al.*) in combination with an experimental pharmacological approach.

About 25 adult Sprague-Dawley rats were used. Two types of experiments were made: (1) Hypophysectomy was performed on 15 rats via the parapharyngeal or transauricular approach in order to damage the median eminence. The animals were sacrificed 1, 2 and 3 days after the operation. (2) 10 rats were treated with reserpine (10 mg/kg i.p., 24 hrs before killing) — nialamide (100 mg/kg—300 mg/kg i.p., 5 hrs before killing) — 3,4-dihydroxy-phenylalanine (l-dopa) (50 mg/kg—100 mg/kg s.c., 30 min before killing) in order to increase the amine contents of the central CA neurons. — All the animals were killed by decapitation after light chloroform anesthesia. The hypothalamus with the infundibular stalk was dissected out, freeze-dried, treated with formaldehyde gas, embedded, sectioned and mounted as previously described in detail (Dahlström and Fuxe 1964).

The operated animals that had an intact median eminence showed a normal fluorescence microscopical picture with only a small number of weakly green-fluorescent CA nerve cells in the anterior part of the nucleus arcuatus (Fig. 1) and the ventral part of the anterior, periventricular nucleus (group A12, see Dahlström and Fuxe 1964). The DA terminals in the external layer of the median eminence of these animals formed a strongly fluorescent zone of a dotted appearance. In the operated animals that had a damaged median eminence, however, a marked increase was observed in the number and intensity of the CA nerve cells of group A12 (Fig. 2). The increase was related to the size of the lesion, *i.e.* an extensive damage caused a strong increase in intensity and number of cellbodies. The most pronounced changes were observed one day after operation. These changes in the amine contents of the CA cell bodies in all probability represent retrograde cell body changes (*cf.* Dahlström and Fuxe 1965).

In those animals that had been treated with reserpine-nialamide-l-dopa, it was possible in some cases to trace weakly green fluorescent axons from the cell-bodies of

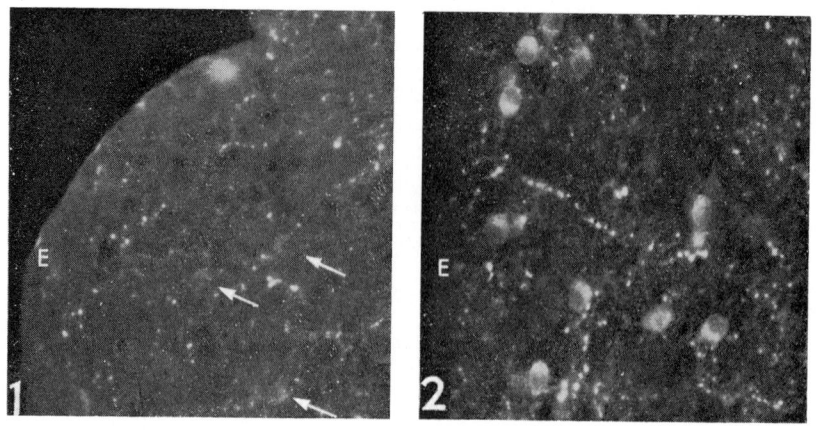

Fig. 1. Nuc. arcuatus of normal rat. A small number of weakly green-fluorescent CA nerve cells (→) are observed. E = ependyma of the third ventricle. × 270.

Fig. 2. Nuc. arcuatus of a rat with a damaged median eminence. The operation was made 1 day before killing. A large number of CA nerve cells with an increased fluorescence intensity are present. E = ependyma of the third ventricle. × 270.

the nuc. arcuatus to the DA terminals of the median eminence (see also Fuxe 1965). The A12 nerve cells showed a very marked increase in number and fluorescence intensity as did the DA terminals of the median eminence. These findings are supported by other workers (Lichtensteiger and Langemann 1965).

The present study together with previous studies (Fuxe 1964) give final evidence for the existence of tubero-infundibular DA neurons. Their function is at present under study.

The skilful technical assistance of miss Vivian Bring is gratefully acknowledged.
This work has been supported by the Swedish Medical Research Council (Project No 12× — 715-01) and by a Public Health Service Research Grant (NB 05236-01).

References

DAHLSTRÖM, A. and K. FUXE, Evidence for the existence of monoamine containing neurons in the central nervous system. I. Demonstration of monoamines in the cell bodies of brain stem neurons. *Acta physiol. scand.* 1964a. *62.* Suppl. 1—55.

DAHLSTÖM, A. and K. FUXE, Evidence for the existence of monoamine neurons in the central nervous system. II. Experimentally induced changes in the intraneuronal amine levels of bulbospinal neuron systems. *Acta physiol. scand.* 1965. *64.* Suppl. 247.

FALCK, B., N.-Å. HILLARP, G. THIEME and A. TORP, Fluorescence of catecholamines and related compounds condensed with formaldehyde. *J. Histochem. Cytochem.* 1962. *10.* 348—354.

FUXE, K., Cellular localization of monoamines in the median eminence and the infundibular stem of some mammals. *Z. Zellforsch.* 1964. *61.* 710—724.

FUXE, K., The distribution of monoamine nerve terminals in the central nervous system. *Acta physiol. scand. 64.* Suppl. 247.

LICHTENSTEIGER, W. and H. LANGEMANN, Aufnahme exogener Katecholamine in monoaminhaltige Neurone des ZNS. *Helv. physiol. pharmacol. Acta* 1965. *23.* c 31—c33.

Part VIII
ENDOGENOUS OPIATE AGONISTS IN THE BRAIN

Editor's Comments
on Papers 56 and 57

56 LAZARUS, LING, and GUILLEMIN
  β-Lipotropin as a Prohormone for the Morphinomimetic Peptides Endorphins and Enkephalins

57 GUILLEMIN et al.
  β-Endorphin and Adrenocorticotropin Are Secreted Concomitantly by the Pituitary Gland

Hughes and his colleagues (Hughes, 1975; Hughes et al., 1975a,b) described the existence of an endogenous substance in the brain that acts as an agonist of (synaptosomal) opiate receptor sites and characterized the substance, termed *enkephalin,* as a low molecular weight peptide. They isolated enkephalin from extracts of whole porcine brain and determined that it is composed of two pentapeptides, which they were able to characterize and synthesize. The C-terminal amino acids of these two pentapeptides were methionine and leucine, respectively; thus, they were called *methionine-enkephalin* and *leucine-enkephalin*. Both enkephalins were shown to have potent agonist activity at opiate receptor sites, the potency of natural enkephalin in the vas deferens assay system being fifteen times greater than that of normorphine. The enkephalins were shown to produce a dose-related inhibition of electrically evoked contractions of mouse vas deferens and guinea pig ileum; these inhibitory effects could be completely antagonized by naloxone. There was close agreement between the pharmacologic activities of the natural and synthetic peptides. The methionine-enkephalin sequence was noted to be present as amino acid residues 61 to 65 in β-lipotropin. Hughes and co-workers speculated that β-lipotropin is a common precursor for the enkephalins and for the peptides residing in the hypophysis with opiate activity. The discovery of the presence in brain of these two endogenous pentapeptides with opiate agonist activity set the stage for testing the hypothesis set forth by these investigators that these peptides act as neurotransmitters or neuromodulators at synaptic junctions. The generic name *endorphin* was set forth to denote the morphinomimetic activity of these peptides endogenous to the brain (Pasternak et al., 1975; Teschemacher et al., 1975).

Lazarus et al. (Paper 56) demonstrated that β-lipotropin (β-LPH), a 91 amino acid polypeptide isolated from the hypophysis of a number of species, displayed no morphinomimetic activity in bioassays. However, incubating β-LPH with aqueous brain extracts at neutral pH was found to generate peptides, including methionine-enkephalin, with morphinomimetic biological and opiate receptor binding activity. This study showed conclusively that β-LPH is a prohormone, endorphins and enkephalins being fragments of the β-lipotropin molecule. β-lipotropin, however, is the first prohormone found to be the parent of several breakdown products with different physiological functions. Subsequent evidence has shown that enkephalins may be derived from a different precursor, larger than β-LPH, that happens to share with β-LPH the same sequence of 5 amino acid residues making up the enkephalins. Guillemin has proposed that the evanescent action of the enkephalins and their wide distribution in the nervous system suggest that they may act as neurotransmitters. Furthermore, he suggests that the endorphins and enkephalins play an important role in brain functions involving mood, emotion, behavior, and pain perception.

Guillemin et al. (Paper 57) reasoned that since adrenocorticotropin hormone (ACTH) and β-endorphin were both fragments of the precursor β-lipotropin and all are stored and released in the same secretory granules, it was likely that ACTH and β-endorphin are secreted concomitantly. In rats exposed to stress, plasma and hypophysial levels of ACTH and β-endorphin rose concomitantly. In hypophysectomized rats, neither ACTH nor β-endorphin was detectable in the plasma, and there was no response to stress, indicating that both of the peptides were of hypophysial origin. Addition of purified corticotropin-releasing factor to cultures of adenohypophysial cells stimulated concomitant secretion of ACTH and β-endorphin, indicating that the regulatory mechanisms governing secretion and synthesis of the peptides are identical. Adrenalectomy resulted in increased secretion of both β-endorphin and ACTH, and administration of dexamethasone suppressed secretion of both peptides, indicating that β-endorphin secretion is regulated by the same adrenal steroid feedback mechanisms as ACTH. Secretion of ACTH closely paralleled that of β-endorphin from fragments of hypophysis of a patient with Nelson's syndrome. Also, extracts from an ACTH-secreting adenoma of the pancreas were shown to contain ACTH, β-endorphin and β-lipotropin. The authors concluded that the hypophysis secretes ACTH and β-endorphin as part of a holistic response of the organism to stress. The knowledge of the existence of the endorphins and enkephalins and further understanding of their functions and physiology will quite likely revolutionize our understanding of neuroendocrinology.

REFERENCES

Hughes, J. 1975. Isolation of an Endogeneous Compound from the Brain with Pharmacological Properties Similar to Morphine. *Brain Res.* **88**:295.

Hughes, J., T. W. Smith, H. W. Kosterlitz, L. Fothergill, B. A. Morgan, and H. R. Morris. 1975a. Identification of Two Related Pentapeptides from the Brain with Potent Opiate Agonist Activity. *Nature* **259**:577.

Hughes, J., T. Smith, B. A. Morgan, and L. Fothergill. 1975b. Purification and Properties of Enkephalin—the Possible Endogenous Ligand for the Morphine Receptor. *Life Sci.* **16**:1753.

Pasternak, G. W., R. Goodman, and S. H. Snyder. 1975. An Endogenous Morphine-like Factor in Mammalian Brain. *Life Sci.* **16**:1753.

Teschemacher, H., K. E. Opheim, B. M. Cox, and A. Goldstein. 1975. Peptide-like Substance from Pituitary That Acts Like Morphine. *Life Sci.* **16**:1777.

56

Reprinted from *Natl. Acad. Sci. Proc.* 73:2156–2159 (1976)

β-Lipotropin as a prohormone for the morphinomimetic peptides endorphins and enkephalins

LARRY H. LAZARUS, NICHOLAS LING, AND ROGER GUILLEMIN

The Salk Institute, La Jolla, California 92037

ABSTRACT   The hypophysial homomeric peptide β-lipotropin (β-LPH-[1-91]) has no morphinomimetic activity in a bioassay (myenteric plexus-longitudinal muscle of the guinea pig's ileum) or binding assays with stereospecific opiate-receptors of rat brain synaptosome preparations. Incubating β-LPH-[1-91] at neutral pH with the supernatant aqueous extracts of rat brain generates (fragments of β-LPH with) morphinomimetic activity in the same assay systems. These results are related to the recently recognized structural relationships between β-LPH, the newly isolated peptides met-enkephalin (β-LPH-[61-65]) and α-endorphin (β-LPH-[61-76]) and also to the biologically active fragments or analogs: β-LPH-[61-64], β-LPH-[61-65]-NH$_2$, (Met(O)[65])-β-LPH-[61-65], β-LPH-[61-69], and β-LPH-[61-91]. Enzymatic biogenesis of these morphinomimetic peptides would preclude localizing them as such in cellular or subcellular elements with currently available methodology.

Two laboratories have recently reported the isolation and primary structure of novel oligopeptides of whole brain or hypothalamus-neurohypophysis origin, endowed with biological characteristics similar to those of the alkaloids of opium in bioassays *in vitro* and stereospecific binding assays on synaptosomal opiate-receptors: Hughes *et al.* (1) characterized *enkephalin*, extracted from whole (pig) brain, to be in fact a mixture in the ratio 4/1 of the two pentapeptides H-Tyr-Gly-Gly-Phe-Met-OH (met-enkephalin) and H-Tyr-Gly-Gly-Phe-Leu-OH (leu-enkephalin). Guillemin *et al.* (2) isolated several *endorphins* from an extract of (pig) hypothalamus-neurohypophysis and characterized one of them, α-endorphin, as the hexadecapeptide H-Tyr-Gly-Gly-Phe-Met-Thr-Ser-Glu-Lys-Ser-Gln-Thr-Pro-Leu-Val-Thr-OH. Hughes *et al.* recognized that met-enkephalin is identical to the sequence which extends from Tyr[61] to Met[65] of the various β-lipotropins, and Guillemin *et al.* observed that the primary structure of α-endorphin is identical to that of the sequence from Tyr[61] to Thr[76] of the β-lipotropins, met-enkephalin thus being the NH$_2$-terminal pentapeptide of α-endorphin. Moreover, in their original report (2) Guillemin, Ling, and Burgus stated that the (synthetic) nonapeptide H-Tyr-Gly-Gly-Phe-Met-Thr-Ser-Glu-Lys-OH, i.e., β-LPH-[61-69] also had considerable morphinomimetic activity. It was then obvious that the relationship between β-lipotropins (β-LPHs) and the opioid peptides was more than accidental. In fact, after the statement of Hughes *et al.* appeared (1), and before the structure of α-endorphin was completed, both our group and Goldstein's (see 3) observed that while β-LPH had no morphinomimetic activity even at high doses, the COOH-terminal fragment β-LPH-[61-91], available from previous isolation studies (4, 5), had considerable activity in the morphine-bioassay and opiate receptor binding assays (in ref. 4, the proposal is made to name β-LPH-[61-91] as β-endorphin).

Isolated in 1964 from sheep pituitary glands (6), β-LPH was

Abbreviation: β-LPH, β-lipotropin; β-MSH, β-melanocyte stimulating hormone.

subsequently isolated and characterized from the pituitary of a variety of species; in all cases it is a homomeric 91-residue polypeptide with minor species variances in its amino acid sequence (see ref. 7 and references therein). The physiological significance of β-LPH has remained obscure to this day. It has lipolytic activity in several systems and minimal melanophoretic and adrenocorticotropic activity (7). It has been reported in blood (8) and has been located in discrete cells of the anterior and intermediate lobes of the pituitary by immunofluorescence (9). Long recognized (6) to be a possible source of β-melanocyte stimulating hormone β-MSH (β-LPH-[41-58]) and perhaps its only artefactual source (10), β-LPH was investigated here as a possible prohormone for the morphinomimetic peptides in view of the relationships of primary structures recalled above. There is ample evidence that *brain* extracts contain endopeptidases with the ability to produce the expected or suspected fragments (11, 12).

The morphinomimetic activity of several synthesized fragments of β-LPH and analogs are also reported here.

MATERIALS AND METHODS

(*a*) For bioassays (myenteric plexus-longitudinal muscle of the guinea pig's ileum) (13), ovine β-LPH (25 μg/25 μl of H$_2$O) was incubated, in several experiments, up to 2 hr at 37° with 25 μl of the supernatant of a sucrose (0.32 M) extract of whole rat brain centrifuged at 100,000 × g for 1 hr. At chosen times, aliquots of the total incubation mixture (see Fig. 1) were added to the incubation fluid (5 ml chamber) of the bioassay.

(*b*) For studies of binding to synaptosomal opiate-receptors, ovine β-LPH (2 μg/2 μl of H$_2$O) was incubated for up to 2 hr at 37° with 10 μl of the same rat brain extract as above. At chosen times, aliquots of the mixture were removed and boiled for 5 min. Rat brain synaptosomal fractions were prepared by discontinuous gradients (14). Aliquots of these fractions (513 μg or 189 μg of protein for P$_2$ or F fraction respectively) were incubated with 0.025 μCi of [^{3}H]etorphine (41 Ci/mol, Amersham-Searle), 10 mM Tris·HCl at pH 7.4, 1 mg of bovine serum albumin (BSA) and β-LPH (0.5 μg), or the same weight of β-LPH after incubation with the aqueous brain extract, in a total volume of 0.1 ml, for 20 min at 37° or 60 min at 0° in a dimly lit room (15). For measurement of specific binding, 10 μg of normorphine or 10 μg of levorphanol was added to the reaction mixtures. Two ml of ice-cold isotonic buffer containing 0.2% BSA was added to the above mixture at the end of incubation, the solution was filtered on Whatman glass fiber discs (GF/C), and rinsed once. The entire operation took less than 10 sec. The filters were dried and the radioactivity was determined with a standard toluene based scintillation fluid. Specific binding was determined by the difference between [^{3}H]etorphine displaced by either the normorphine or levorphanol and the total [^{3}H]etorphine bound. Nonspecifically bound [^{3}H]-

317

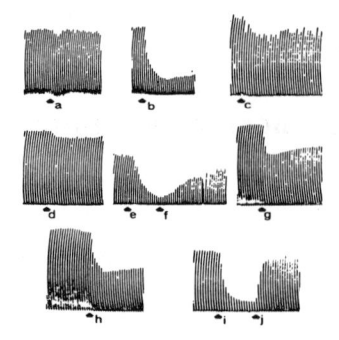

FIG. 1. Electrically evoked contractions of the myenteric plexus-longitudinal muscle of guinea pig ileum. a, β-LPH-[1-91], 1 μM; b, normorphine, 30 nM; c, 0.5 μM β-LPH-[1-91] incubated with brain extract for 30 min; d, as in c, but incubated for 2 hr—the small decrease in amplitude is identical to that produced by brain extract alone; e, β-LPH-[61-91], 0.6 μM; f, naloxone, 1 μM; g, β-LPH-[61-69], 1 μM; h, met-enkephalin, (β-LPH-[61-65]), 0.1 μM; i, α-endorphin, (β-LPH-[61-76]), 50 nM; j, naloxone, 1 μM.

etorphine amounted to 55–70% of the total bound. In other experiments, solutions (10 μg/ml) of synthetic peptides were diluted in aqueous BSA (1 mg/ml) and incubated as above with [^{3}H]etorphine.

(c) Synthetic peptides were prepared by solid phase methodology, purified, and their homogeneity ascertained by the methods routinely used in this laboratory (16). The peptides so prepared were: H-Tyr-Gly-Gly-OH, i.e., β-LPH-[61-63]; H-Tyr-Gly-Gly-Phe-OH, i.e., β-LPH-[61-64]; H-Tyr-Gly-Gly-Phe-Met-OH, i.e., β-LPH-[61-65] also known as met-enkephalin (1); H-Tyr-Gly-Gly-Phe-Met-NH$_2$, i.e., (met)-enkephalin-amide; (Met(O)^{65})-β-LPH-[61-65]; H-Tyr-Gly-Gly-Phe-Met-Thr-Ser-Glu-Lys-OH, i.e., β-LPH-[61-69]; and α-endorphin, i.e., β-LPH-[61-76].

RESULTS

Even at the high doses tested (up to 10 μg/ml), β-LPH has no morphinomimetic activity (Fig. 1a), in a bioassay sensitive to 10 ng of normorphine per ml (Fig. 1b). Incubation of β-LPH with the aqueous extract of rat brain generates opioid activity (Fig. 1c) which disappears after a 2 hr incubation (Fig. 1d). The morphine-like activity of the mixture in the bioassay is increased rather than reversed by naloxone, indicating an unusual involvement of the opiate-receptors of the myenteric plexus tissue; such unmasking of agonist activity of naloxone has been seen occasionally by us when dealing with mixtures of peptides or with some peptides related to sequences of ACTH. In the opiate receptor binding assay, competing activity displacing [^{3}H]-etorphine is observed after incubation of β-LPH with aqueous brain extract, while intact β-LPH has no statistically significant activity (Table 1); as in the bioassay, prolonged incubation with the brain extract (2 hr) leads to disappearance of the opiate-receptor binding activity. As shown in Fig. 2, the peptides compete with [^{3}H]etorphine in the synaptosomal binding assay in a manner that parallels the effects of levorphanol or normorphine. The minor activity of the highest dose of β-LPH, occasionally observed, is best explained by the ample possibility for peptide cleavage during the incubation with the synaptosomal fraction known to carry proteases.

Fig. 1e and g–i show the morphine-like activity of some fragments of β-LPH of known structure, and its reversal by naloxone (Fig. 1f and j). The tripeptide H-Tyr-Gly-Gly-OH, i.e., β-LPH-[61-63] has no opioid activity in the bioassay at doses as high as 10 μg/ml (0.1 mM). The tetrapeptide H-Tyr-Gly-Gly-Phe-OH has definite activity at the same doses, its specific activity being thus ca. 1/100 that of met-enkephalin. H-Tyr-Gly-Gly-Phe-Met-NH$_2$ has considerable activity in the bioassay, its specific activity being ca. 5 times that of the free acid form of the pentapeptide, while the methionine sulfoxide analog has ca. ½ the specific activity of the free acid of the pentapeptide. The duration of activity of met-enkephalin-amide is considerably increased over that of the free acid form.

DISCUSSION

Though far from exhaustive, these experiments show that incubation of β-LPH with aqueous brain extracts at neutral pH generates (peptides with) morphinomimetic activity. It will be of interest to determine the primary structure of the fragments produced to relate them to those of characterized peptides with opioid activity (no attempt was made here even to assess the cleavage points of β-LPH). The opioid activity of many syn-

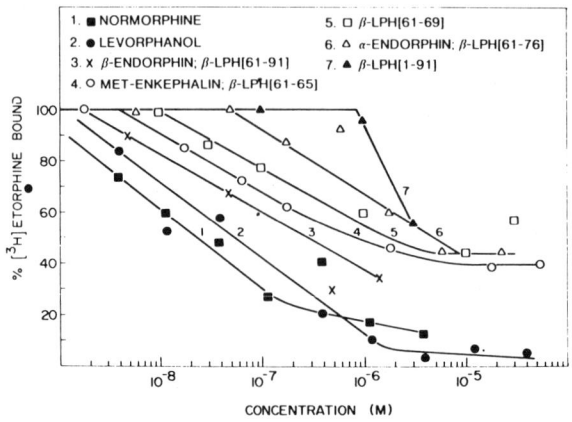

FIG. 2. Competition of the binding of [^{3}H]etorphine by opiates and morphinomimetic peptides. Stock solutions of all compounds were diluted in water containing 1 mg of bovine serum albumin/ml. Each point represents the average value of assays carried out in triplicate as given in Materials and Methods (0° for 60 min with a synaptosomal membrane preparation P_2).

Table 1. Stereospecific binding of [^{3}H]etorphine in the presence of various competitors

Condition	Addition	Radioisotope bound (cpm) No. 1	No. 2	No. 3	P*
(I)					
	Control	2655	2676	2913	
	3×10^{-5} M normorphine	1623	1687	1791	0.01
	1×10^{-6} M β-LPH	2497	2339	2729	—
(II)					
	Control	3801	3773	4061	
	3×10^{-5} M normorphine	2606	2601	2431	0.01
	3×10^{-5} M levorphanol	2445	2442	2514	0.01
	5×10^{-7} M β-LPH preincubated with brain extract for 30 min	3166	3366	2613	0.01
	5×10^{-7} M β-LPH	3986	3986	3374	—

Condition	Addition	No. of replicates	Radioisotope bound (cpm)†	
(III)				
	Control	5	9897 ± 295	
	3×10^{-5} M normorphine	5	3488 ± 89	0.01
	5×10^{-7} M β-LPH preincubated with brain extract for 30 min	3	8222 ± 295	0.05
	5×10^{-7} M β-LPH preincubated with boiled brain extract for 5 min	3	10,433 ± 895	—
	5×10^{-7} M β-LPH	5	10,828 ± 315	—

Conditions I and III were a 20 min incubation at 37° with synaptosomes. Condition II was a 60 min incubation at 0° with synaptosomes.
* Values of P were calculated by multiple comparison tests of Dunnett or Duncan after analysis of variance on original data.
† Values are the mean ± SEM.

thesized fragments of the COOH-terminal [61-91]-portion of β-LPH, as reported here, is in keeping with these observations.

Thus, β-LPH, containing the sequences of met-enkephalin (β-LPH-[61-65]), of α-endorphin (β-LPH-[61-76]), of β-endorphin (β-LPH-[61-91]), of β-MSH (β-LPH-[41-58]), and also of the fragment Met[4] to Gly[10] of adrenocorticotropin (β-LPH-[47-53]) may well be involved in those circumstances, physiological and experimental in which enkephalin, α-endorphin, β-MSH and ACTH-[4-10] have been reported to have profound and diverse neurotropic or behavioral activities (review in ref. 17). The various opioid peptides so far characterized from whole brain, hypothalamus or pituitary all have primary structures related to fragments of β-LPH; so far the only recognized source of β-LPH is the pituitary gland. These results are, thus, in agreement with and probably explain the earlier work of Goldstein et al. (18) who originally reported the presence of substances possibly of peptide nature with opioid activity in extracts of the pituitary. The results reported here, along with knowledge of the primary structure of enkephalins and endorphins raise a remarkable possibility: while the biogenesis of the hypothalamic hypophysiotropic peptides thyrotropin- releasing factor (TRF), luteinizing hormone-releasing factor (LRF), and somatostatin is probably by protein synthesis of the oligopeptides or more likely of proto-forms from ribosomal templates, the likely biogenesis of the neurotropic peptides discussed here is reminiscent of that of the angiotensins (19). With β-lipotropin as clearly the circulating and available substrate, it will be of major physiological importance to characterize, locate, and study the regulation of the several enzymes involved in the multiple cleavages of β-lipotropin that yield the neurotropic peptides. The resemblance with the biogenesis of angiotensins is even more striking considering the demonstration of angiotensin-converting enzyme in discrete locations of the brain (caudate nucleus) (ref. 20 and references therein). There is also renin-like activity in aqueous extracts of the brain of several species (21, 22), though a purely lysosomal origin of such brain-renin, as recently proposed (23), would raise doubts about its physiological availability. Should the various neurotropic peptides be generated by enzymatic cleavages of β-LPH as a substrate available in extracellular spaces, attempts to localize them by the currently available methods of immuno-histochemistry would be futile. The search will have to be for the converting enzymes after they have been characterized. By that time, the physiological significance, if any, of these peptide-ligands of the opiate receptors should have been critically evaluated.

Note Added in Proof. The primary structure of γ-endorphin isolated from hypothalamus-neurohypophysis extracts (2) has now been established as being identical to that of β-LPH-[61-77]; also β-LPH-[61-91] has been isolated from the same extracts on the basis of the bioassay described here for opiate-like activity.

Dr. C. H. Li, Hormone Research Laboratories, University of California, San Francisco, kindly provided on December 16, 1975 samples of ovine β-LPH and β-LPH-[61-91] used in these studies. We are happy to acknowledge the technical assistance of M. Mercado, L. Koski and S. Minnick. Research supported in part by Grant HD-09690-01 from NICHD and by the William Randolph Hearst Foundation.

1. Hughes, J., Smith, T. W., Kosterlitz, H. W., et al. (1975) Nature 258, 577–579.
2. Guillemin, R., Ling, N. & Burgus, R. (1976) C.R. Acad. Sci., Paris, Ser D. 282, 783–785.
3. Cox, B. M., Goldstein, A. & Li, C. H. (1976) Proc. Natl. Acad. Sci. USA 73, 1821–1823.
4. Li, C. H., & Chung, D. (1976) Proc. Natl. Acad. Sci. USA 73, 1145–1148.
5. Bradbury, A. F., Smyth, D. G., & Snell, C. R. (1975) in Peptides, Chemistry, Structure and Biology, Proc. 4th Amer. Pept. Symp., eds. Walter, R. & Meienhofer, J. J. (Ann Arbor Science Publ., Ann Arbor, Mich.), pp. 609–615.
6. Li, C. H. (1964) Nature 201, 924–925.
7. Yamashiro, D. & Li, C. H. (1974) Proc. Natl. Acad. Sci. USA 71, 4945–4949.

8. Lohmar, P. & Li, C. H. (1968) *Endocrinology* **82**, 898–904.
9. Moon, H. D., Li, C. H. & Jennings, B. M. (1973) *Anat. Rec.* **175**, 529–538.
10. Scott, A. P. & Lowry, P. J. (1974) *Biochem. J.* **139**, 593–605.
11. Marks, N. & Stern, F. (1975) *FEBS Lett.* **55**, 220–224.
12. Long, J. M., Krivoy, W. A. & Guillemin, R. (1961) *Endocrinology* **69**, 176–181.
13. Paton, D. M. & Zar, M. A. (1968) *J. Physiol.* **194**, 13–33.
14. Whittaker, V. P., Michaelson, I. A. & Kirland, R. J. A. (1964) *Biochem. J.* **90**, 293–303.
15. Klee, W. A. & Streaty, R. A. (1974) *Nature* **248**, 61–63.
16. Ling, N. & Vale, W. (1975) *Biochem. Biophys. Res. Commun.* **63**, 801–806.
17. DeWied, D. (1975) *Biochem. Pharmacol.* **24**, 1463–1477.
18. Cox, B. M., Opheim, K. E., Teschemacher, H. & Goldstein, A. (1975) *Life Sci.* **16**, 1777–1782.
19. Peart, W. S. (1965) *Pharmacol. Rev.* **17**, 143–169.
20. Poth, M. M., Heath, R. G. & Ward, M. (1975) *J. Neurochem.* **25**, 83–85.
21. Ganten, D., Minnich, J. L., & Granger, P., et al. (1971) *Science* **173**, 64–65.
22. Daul, C. B., Heath, R. G. & Gasey, R. E. (1975) *Neuropharmacology* **14**, 75–80.
23. Day, R. P. & Reid, I. A. (1976) *Endocrinology* **99**, 93–100.

β-ENDORPHIN AND ADRENOCORTICOTROPIN ARE SECRETED CONCOMITANTLY BY THE PITUITARY GLAND

Roger Guillemin, Therese Vargo, Jean Rossier, Scott Minick, Nicholas Ling, Catherine Rivier, Wylie Vale, and Floyd Bloom

Salk Institute for Biological Studies, La Jolla, Calif.

The two biologically active polypeptides adrenocorticotropin (ACTH) and β-endorphin have been shown by Mains, Eipper, and Ling (1) originally to be part of a much larger precursor glycoprotein (31,000 daltons, referred to as 31K-precursor), as synthesized by the cloned pituitary cells of the (mouse) cell line AtT-20/D-16v. The common precursor concept is supported by earlier data on immunocytochemistry of normal pituitary tissue: ACTH [1–39] (residues 1 to 39); β-lipotropin (β-LPH [1–91]) the immediate endorphin-precursor, and the biologically active peptides β-endorphin (that is, β-LPH [61–91]) and α-endorphin (that is, β-LPH [61–76]) are all present in the same cells in the anterior and intermediate lobes of the pituitary gland (2). These observations raise the possibility that the biologically active forms of ACTH and β-endorphin might be normally secreted concomitantly. While work over the last 30 years has elucidated the physiological mechanisms involved in the secretion of ACTH, particularly as it relates to the response to stress, the recently discovered endorphins could not be studied in similar circumstances until specific methods to measure their concentration in blood or tissue extracts became available. We have recently devised, described, and validated such methodology (3). We now show that, in all conditions studied so far, ACTH and β-endorphin are secreted simultaneously by the pituitary gland.

Thirty-three male rats (Holtzman, 200 ± 15 g of body weight) were kept for 3 weeks, six animals per cage, with lights on at 0700 hours and off at 2000 hours. For studies on acute response to stress, each animal had the right tibia-fibula broken instantaneously, trunk blood being collected by decapitation in tubes containing EDTA (sodium salt) at intervals ranging from 60 seconds to 30 minutes. To study a possible adrenal steroid feedback mechanism on the secretion of endorphin, rats received dexamethasone acetate, a total of 12 mg over 12 days, in two daily subcutaneous injections; other animals were bilaterally adrenalectomized and maintained for 16 weeks on 1 percent NaCl as drinking fluid. Finally three rats from a larger pool of hypophysectomized animals were stressed and processed as above 10 months after total hypophysectomy.

As is shown in Fig. 1 and Table 1, plasma and pituitary concentrations of ACTH and β-endorphin vary concomitantly and in remarkable parallelism in all experimental situations described here, indicating that ACTH and endorphins are secreted simultaneously.

Hypophysectomy abolishes the response to stress, indicating that the peptides (β-endorphin and ACTH) measured in these studies are of hypophysial origin. Addition of purified corticotropin-releasing factor and of other secretagogues to monolayer cultures of adenohypophysial cells also stimulates concomitant secretion of immunoactive ACTH and β-endorphin (4). Thus it would appear that the regulatory mechanisms (hypothalamic releasing factor, feedback by glucocorticoids) involved in the secretion and biosynthesis of both ACTH and β-endorphin are common and identical (5).

The antiserum used here (RB100-10/76) to measure plasma and tissue levels of β-endorphin is directed to the region Asn[20]-His[27] (Asn, asparagine; His, histidine) of the primary sequence of β-endorphin (3). Because of the commonality of that sequence in β-endorphin and its precursor β-LPH, the antiserum recognizes the two peptides as well as 31K-precursor on an equimolar basis (1, 3). Estimation of the molecular size by well-calibrated filtration columns (P-60 Biogel in 4M guanidine hydrochloride) has shown that the major component (about 90 percent) in the rat pituitary extracts recognized by the antiserum used here corresponds to β-endorphin (3200 daltons) with a minor (about 10 percent), larger component corresponding to β-LPH (10,000 daltons) and a still smaller amount (< 1 percent) corresponding to 31K-precursor; moreover, gel filtration on Sephadex G75 of the plasma of stressed rats shows also a large peak of immunoreactive endorphin with a retention coefficient identical to that of synthetic β-endorphin.

In other studies, we have observed that the elevated spontaneous secretion of ACTH by fragments incubated in vitro of the hyperplastic pituitary of a patient with the Nelson syndrome was also accompanied by correspondingly elevated secretion of β-endorphin (6); also extracts of an ectopic ACTH-secreting adenoma of the pancreas were shown to contain ACTH, β-LPH, and β-endorphin (7). In normal rats, electric shocks to the footpad, a type of acute stress other than that described above, also led to elevated levels of plasma β-endorphin.

Thus, the conclusion appears inescapable that, in all conditions studied here in which the pituitary secretes ACTH, it also secretes β-endorphin.

Since the early studies of Selye (8), ACTH has been recognized as the primary pituitary hormone secreted in response to acute stress in all species studied. The teleological proposal has been to relate the acute secretion of ACTH to the corresponding immediate activation of the adrenal cortex for the secretion of glucocorticoids necessary for immediate increase of neoglucogenesis and the ensuing availability of energy rich carbohydrates. In many, although not all, species, prolactin and growth hormone may also be released in similar conditions (9). Growth hormone, ACTH, and prolactin are pituitary responses to stress, all affecting metabolism. Our results show that β-endorphin is also released in response to acute stress.

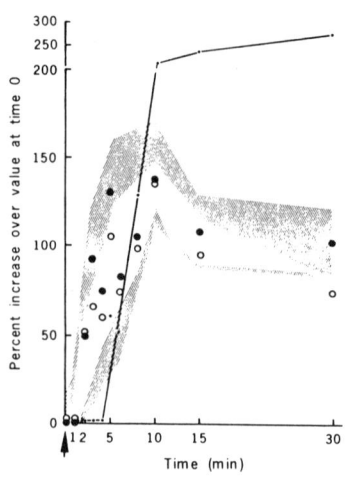

Fig. 1. Plasma levels of ACTH (closed circles) and β-endorphin (open circles) measured by radioimmunoassays (3, 15) in trunk blood obtained from rats killed at times shown on the abscissa; acute stress occurred at time zero. Solid line shows plasma levels of adrenal corticosterone measured by fluorometry (16). Shaded areas show confidence limits of the measurements. The correlation coefficient, ρ, between the two populations of ACTH and β-endorphin concentrations is 0.9708 for values of means (d.f. = 20) and 0.7785 for all individual values (d.f. = 64).

Evidence has been presented (10) that peripheral injection of β-endorphin in mice produces analgesia; this result was obtained with doses of the peptide leading to plasma concentrations four to five orders of magnitude greater than those observed in response to stress. We have failed to observe in rats such central effects of similarly large doses of β-endorphin (up to 20 mg per kilogram of body weight) injected in a peripheral vein. This is in contradistinction to the profound effects (analgesia, catatonia) exerted by small amounts (≥ 0.5 μg) of β-endorphin when injected directly in the brain and unanimously observed (11). It may be that our current criteria for assessing possible central effects of the circulating endorphins are naive and of small power. Should such effects of the peripherally released β-endorphin eventually be detectable, our results demonstrate that the system necessary for its immediate secretion and availability in response to stress is highly functional and coupled with activation of the ACTH-adrenal cortex axis.

Thus, a holistic response of the organism to stress would involve the immediate secretion of pituitary hormones, some (such as ACTH and growth hormone) involved in somatotropic (metabolic) adaptive reactions, whereas others (such as β-endorphin, β-melanocyte stimulating hormone, or γ-lipotropin) are endowed with neurotropic (12), comportmental, or psychotropic adaptive reactions. Suggestive of a vascular pathway from pituitary to brain, recent observations (13) have shown high

Table 1. Plasma and pituitary concentrations of adrenocorticotropin (ACTH) and β-endorphin as modified by adrenalectomy, administration of dexamethasone, and for plasma levels, as modified by hypophysectomy. Plasma and pituitary samples were obtained in nonstress conditions, after decapitation in all groups, except in the case of hypophysectomy. The hypophysectomized animals were first bled through the jugular vein within 2 minutes of initiating ether anesthesia. This provided baseline sample. The right tibia and fibula were then broken as in the stress procedures (Fig. 1); blood was obtained again 10 minutes later by decapitation. In these hypophysectomized animals, either before stress or after stress, neither ACTH nor β-endorphin were measurable. For the radioimmunoassay, plasma samples were processed with no concentration procedure; whole pituitary glands or adenohypophyses were frozen on Dry Ice within 1 minute of the animals' decapitation; later (1 to 2 hours) they were extracted in 1N acetic acid at 100°C for 10 minutes.

Treatment	Plasma (ng/ml) ACTH	Plasma (ng/ml) β-Endorphin	Whole pituitary (μg/gland) ACTH	Whole pituitary (μg/gland) β-Endorphin	Adenohypophysis (μg/gland) ACTH	Adenohypophysis (μg/gland) β-Endorphin
None (controls)	0.8 ± 0.2 (3)*	1.5 ± 0.2 (9)	4.8 ± 0.3 (3)	2.6 ± 0.2 (11)	2.7 ± 0.5 (3)	1.1 ± 0.2 (3)
Adrenalectomy	8.8 ± 1.6 (3)	8.8 ± 1.0 (6)†	9.9 ± 1.1 (3)†	10.8 ± 1.5 (3)†	8.3 ± 1.1 (3)†	5.4 ± 0.7 (3)†
Dexamethasone	< 0.2 (6)‡	< 1 (7)‡	2.1 ± 0.1 (6)§	1.2 ± 0.1 (7)†		
Hypophysectomy	< 0.2 (3)‡	< 1 (3)‡				

*Numbers in parentheses represent the number of replicates for that treatment; a total of 40 rats was used in three separate experiments, the results of which were pooled after demonstration of homogeneity of their variance (χ² test); results were studied by analysis of variance in a randomized (no block) design. †$P < .01$. ‡Indicates that the content of each (plasma) sample was at or below the lower limits of sensitivity of the assay. §$P = .05$ between experimental group and control group.

concentrations of pituitary hormones from all three lobes of the pituitary, in the long portal vessels. Functional significance of these observations remains to be proved; there is as yet no evidence that blood flows retrograde from pituitary into brain in a functional mechanism able to deliver pituitary peptides. On the contrary, we have evidence that profound variations in the pituitary secretion of β-endorphin are not reflected in concomitant variations of brain levels of β-endorphin (14). Thus, with all this conflicting evidence, we have to search for one or several peripheral targets for the β-endorphin secreted in response to stress in the dynamic fashion and large amounts that we have demonstrated here.

References and Notes

1. R. Mains, E. Eipper, N. Ling, *Proc. Natl. Acad. Sci. U.S.A.* **74**, 3014 (1977).
2. F. Bloom, E. Battenberg, J. Rossier, N. Ling, J. Leppaluoto, T. M. Vargo, R. Guillemin, *Life Sci.* **20**, 43 (1977); see also the following reports demonstrating β-LPH and ACTH in the same cells: H. D. Moon, C. H. Li, B. M. Jennings, *Anat. Rec.* **175**, 529 (1973); G. Pelletier, R. Leclerc, F. Labrie, J. Cote, M. Chrétien, M. Lis, *Endocrinology* **100**, 770 (1977); M. P. Dubois, *Lille Med.* **17**, 1391 (1972).
3. R. Guillemin, N. Ling, T. M. Vargo, *Biochem. Biophys. Res. Commun.* **76**, 361 (1977).
4. W. Vale *et al.*, in preparation.
5. Thus the still uncharacterized hypothalamic corticotropin releasing factor (CRF) would also be the endorphin releasing factor. This is reminiscent of what happened with the hypothalamic "luteinizing hormone releasing factor" (LRF), later shown to release both luteinizing hormone and follicle stimulating hormone [A. V. Schally *et al.*, *Biochem. Biophys. Res. Commun.* **43**, 393 (1971); M. Amoss *et al.*, *ibid.* **44**, 205 (1971)].
6. In collaboration with X. Bertagna and F. Girard, Paris.
7. In collaboration with D. Orth, Nashville, Tenn.
8. H. Selye, *Stress* (Acta, Montreal, Canada, 1950).
9. S. M. Glick, *Ann. N.Y. Acad. Sci.* **148**, 471 (1968); G. D. Bryant, J. L. Linzell, F. C. Greenwood, *Hormones* **1**, 26 (1970).
10. L. F. Tseng, H. H. Loh, C. H. Li, *Nature (London)* **263**, 239 (1976).
11. F. Bloom, D. Segal, N. Ling, R. Guillemin, *Science* **194**, 630 (1976); Y. F. Jacquet and N. Marks, *ibid.*, p. 632; E. Wei and H. Loh, *ibid.* **193**, 1262 (1976); A. F. Bradbury, D. G. Smyth, C. R. Snell, N. J. Birdsall, E. C. Hulme, *Nature (London)* **260**, 793 (1976).
12. W. Krivoy and R. Guillemin, *Endocrinology* **69**, 170 (1961).
13. C. Oliver, R. S. Mical, J. C. Porter, *ibid.* **101**, 598 (1977); R. B. Page, B. L. Munger, R. M. Bergland, *Am. J. Anat.* **146**, 273 (1976).
14. J. Rossier, T. M. Vargo, S. Minick, N. Ling, F. E. Bloom, R. Guillemin, *Proc. Natl. Acad. Sci. U.S.A.*, in press.
15. W. Vale and C. Rivier, *Fed. Proc. Fed. Am. Soc. Exp. Biol.*, in press; when the WHO 3rd International Reference Standard for adrenocorticotropin is used, the antiserum (D. Orth) reads the NH_2-terminal [1–24] region of ACTH [1–39].
16. R. Guillemin, G. W. Clayton, H. S. Lipscomb, J. D. Smyth, *J. Lab. Clin. Med.* **53**, 830 (1959).
17. Supported by NIH grants AM-18811 and HD-09690, and by grants from the William Randolph Hearst Foundation. We thank J. Tabin and E. Guillemin for technical assistance.

AUTHOR CITATION INDEX

Abe, K., 109, 247, 296
Abel, J. J., 32
Abrams, R. L., 224
Abrams, R. M., 172, 270
Abramson, E. A., 224
Aceto, T., Jr., 231
Adamsons, K., 153
Ahlquist, R. P., 128
Ajador, L., 200
Akbar, A. M., 200
Alagna, S., 297
Allsop, L. B., 109
Amarger, J., 133
Amenomori, Y., 166, 228, 270, 288, 292
Amoss, M., 101, 190, 242, 247, 253, 301, 323
Anand, B. K., 61
Anden, N. E., 292
Andersen, R. N., 91
Anderson, E., 56, 61
Anderson, M. S., 109, 247, 280
Antanehak, N., 133
Antunes-Rodrigues, J., 190, 239
Aono, T., 208
Appleman, M. D., 296
Arfania, J., 208
Arimura, A., 97, 101, 109, 180, 185, 190, 195, 196, 199, 200, 204, 224, 239, 242, 247, 253
Arky, R. A., 224
Armentrout, R. W., 185
Arzac, J. P., 297
Aschner, B., 75
Asdell, S. A., 122, 146
Ashheim, P., 162, 190
Assenmacher, I., 44, 61
Astwood, E. B., 70
Attramadal, A., 204
Audibert, A., 133
Averill, R. L. W., 106, 234
Axelrod, J., 109, 204, 253

Baba, S., 297

Baba, Y., 180, 185, 190, 195, 196, 204, 242
Bachman, C., 146
Baddeley, R. M., 270
Bahn, R. C., 217
Bailey, J. D., 224
Bailey, P., 122
Bakke, J. L., 234
Ball, J., 146, 224
Bard, P., 146
Bárdos, V., 141, 172
Bargmann, W., 32, 36
Barnett, J. A., 224
Barowsky, N. J., 280
Barraclough, C. A., 133, 141, 146, 171, 172
Barrett, J. F., 97, 101, 185, 190, 247
Barrnett, R. J., 70, 71
Barry, J., 204
Bartosik, D., 162
Bassiri, R. M., 109, 253
Bates, R. W., 231
Batson, H. C., 270
Battenberg, E., 323
Baugh, C. M., 297
Becht, F. C., 122
Beck-Peccoz, P., 208
Beecham, A. F., 101
Behnsen, G., 15
Benfey, B. G., 153
Benoit, J., 44, 61
Benson, G. K., 166, 270
Bergland, R. M., 323
Bergman, A. J., 264
Bernardis, L. L., 106, 224, 228, 231, 234, 253
Bernstein, R. I., 247
Berson, S. A., 200, 220, 224
Berthold, A. A., 2, 39
Bertler, Å., 310
Biasotti, A., 25, 109
Biegelman, P. M., 277
Birdsall, N. J. M., 301, 323
Birge, C. A., 292
Birk, S. A., 208

325

Author Citation Index

Bishop, P. M., 146
Bishop, W., 292
Bissell, A., 70
Bissonnette, T. H., 122
Bittner, J. J., 141
Bloom, F. E., 323
Bogdanove, E. M., 61, 75, 85, 172, 217, 227
Bogdanski, D. F., 153
Bogdonoff, M. D., 224
Bøler, J., 106, 109, 242
Bollinger, J., 106, 247, 253
Bongiovanni, A., 239
Boop, W. C., 106
Boryzcka, A., 247
Boshans, R. L., 106
Bourgery, J. M., 22
Bowers, C. Y., 97, 101, 106, 109, 162, 180, 185, 190, 195, 239, 242, 247, 280, 297
Box, B. M., 228
Blackwell, R., 190, 242, 247, 253, 301
Blair, C. B., 75
Blanco, S., 224
Bliss, C. L., 239, 277
Bloom, F., 301
Blount, R. F., 61
Bradbury, A. F., 301, 319, 323
Bradbury, J. T., 146
Brazeau, P., 247, 253
Breese, G. R., 109, 247
Bremer, F., 122
Brewer, H. B., 190
Brobeck, J. R., 39, 56, 61, 70, 75, 86
Brodie, B. B., 153, 310
Brolin, S. E., 71
Bronzert, R. J., 190
Brooks, C. M., 22, 122, 128, 146
Brown, G. M., 208
Brown, J. G., 217
Brown, M., 301
Brown-Grant, K., 85
Brownstein, M., 109, 204, 253
Bryant, G. D., 280
Bucy, P. C., 128
Buffett, R. F., 217
Buhi, W. C., 208
Burgess, J. A., 224
Burgus, R., 2, 97, 101, 106, 109, 190, 242, 247, 253, 280, 301, 319
Burrows, G. N., 208
Buse, M. G., 234
Butcher, M., 190, 242, 247, 253
Butler, A. W., 153

Cacicedo, G. L., 247
Cahane, M., 109
Cahane, T., 109

Cajal, S. R. y., 22, 122
Campbell, H. J., 91, 106, 162, 166, 190
Camus, J., 122
Canales, E. S., 208
Canales, F. S., 208
Cantalamessa, L., 208
Cantarow, A., 75
Carlson, H. E., 208, 247, 283
Carlsson, A., 224, 310
Casa, L. D., 224
Catania, A., 208
Cerasi, E., 224
Chaffee, E. L., 52
Chambon, Y., 133
Chang, Y. H., 242
Cheek, W. R., 153
Chen, C. L., 288, 292
Chen, R. F., 190
Cheng, C. P., 39, 56, 75
Chenoweth, M. B., 224
Chess, D., 128
Chickedel, E., 247
Chieffo, V., 247, 280
Chocobski, J., 122
Chopra, I. J., 297
Chopra, U., 297
Chowers, S., 162, 172
Chretien, M., 323
Chung, D., 301, 319
Claesson, L., 128
Clamen, M., 86
Clark, J., 292
Clayton, G. W., 323
Clemens, J. A., 292
Cobb, S., 122
Cochrane, R. L., 44
Cohn, C., 217
Coleman, D., 101
Colfer, H. F., 52, 85
Collin, R., 122
Connors, M., 247
Copinschi, G., 296
Coppola, J. A., 224, 288
Cote, J., 321
Courrier, R., 162, 190
Cowell, S. J., 224
Cox, B. M., 301, 316, 319, 320
Coy, D. H., 200, 253
Coy, E. J., 200
Crighton, D. B., 204
Critchlow, V., 141, 146, 171, 172
Croll, M. M., 22
Croxson, M. S., 297
Cuatrecasas, P., 223
Cushing, H., 122
Cutting, W. C., 61

326

Author Citation Index

Cyon, A. von, 122

Dahlström, A., 292, 312
Daily, W. J. R., 217
Dakoda, M., 297
Dandy, W. E., 122
D'Angelo, S. A., 85, 97, 106, 109, 172, 234
Dannies, P. S., 297
Danon, A., 270, 277
Dasgupta, S. R., 133
Dattatreyamurty, B., 208
Daughaday, W. H., 224, 292
Daul, C. B., 320
Davidson, J. M., 172, 204
Davis, J. O., 217
Day, R. P., 320
Debeljuk, L., 180, 185, 190, 196, 200, 204
DeFeo, V. J., 133
de Groot, J., 52, 56, 75, 85, 106, 141
De Jongh, S. E., 264
Del Conte, E., 86
Delitala, G., 297
Del Vecchio, A., 217
Dempsey, E. W., 22
Derbyshire, A. J., Jr., 22, 86
Desclin, L., 109, 133, 172, 204, 264, 277
Desiderio, D., 2, 106, 109, 190, 242
Deuben, R., 228, 239
DeVane, G., 247
Devilla, L., 297
DeWied, D., 320
Dey, F. L., 22
Dhariwal, A. P. S., 190, 204, 224, 239, 242, 247, 253
Diaz-Infante, A., Jr., 195
Dickerman, E., 292
Dickerman, S., 292
Dikstein, S., 270, 277
Dodds, E. C., 122
Donoso, A. O., 292
Doolittle, R. F., 185
Doughady, W., 109
Dougherty, T. F., 52
Drager, G. A., 32
Dua, S., 61
Dubois, M. P., 204, 323
Dubreuil, R., 86
Ducommun, P., 234
Duick, D. S., 297
Dunn, J. D., 200, 204
Dunn, T. F., 2, 101, 106, 109, 190, 242, 247, 280
Dury, A., 146
Dussault, J. H., 297
Du Vigneaud, V., 36
Duyek, C., 277

Eayrs, J. T., 270
Ebbighausen, W., 190
Eberlein, W., 239
Echertova, A., 97, 228
Edelmann, A., 39
Edman, P., 190
Efendic, S., 253
Ehrensing, R. H., 109
Eipper, E., 323
Elftman, H., 44
Ellis, S., 288
Endröczi, E., 253
Engel, S. L., 153
Ensinck, J., 247
Enzmann, F., 106, 109, 199, 242
Erwin, H. L., 86
Escobar del Ray, F., 247
Eskin, I. A., 128
Estes, E. H., Jr., 224
Evans, H. M., 228, 239, 264
Everett, J. W., 44, 52, 91, 133, 141, 146, 162, 172, 199, 264, 271, 277
Eversole, W. J., 39
Ezdinli, E. Z., 224

Faglia, G., 208
Faiman, C., 208
Falck, B., 310, 312
Falconi, G., 239
Fales, H., 190
Farr, A. L., 109, 239, 253
Fawcett, C. P., 204, 247, 253, 292
Fayez, J., 283
Fee, A. R., 22, 128, 146
Fellows, R., 190, 242
Fenichet, R. L., 301
Ferin, M., 204
Ferrel, A. L., 204
Feuer, G., 91, 162, 166, 190
Fevold, H. L., 141
Fielding, U., 22, 25
Fineberg, S. E., 208
Finesinger, J. E., 122
Fink, G., 199
Fiorindo, R. P., 280
Fisher, A. E., 146
Fisher, C., 22, 52
Fisher, D. A., 296
Flament-Durand, J., 109, 171, 172, 204
Fleischer, N., 190, 280
Flerkó, B., 91, 109, 133, 141, 146, 172, 204
Fochi, M., 162
Folkers, K., 106, 109, 242, 297
Folley, S. J., 166, 270
Fontham, E. H., 292
Forsham, H. P., 247

Author Citation Index

Fortier, C., 56, 61
Fothergill, L. A., 301, 316
Franc, M., 228
Frantz, A. G., 296
Franz, J., 97, 228
Fraschini, F., 204
Fredrickson, D. S., 75, 86
Friedberg, S. J., 224
Friedgood, H. B., 122
Friedman, H. M., 91, 153, 162, 166, 204, 270
Friedman, M. H., 146
Friesen, H. G., 109, 280, 297
Frohman, L. A., 106, 224, 231, 234, 253
Fry, E. G., 39, 56, 75
Frykman, H. M., 22
Fujimoto, Y., 180
Fulmer, J. D., 234
Fuxe, K., 288, 292, 305, 312

Gaarenstroom, J. H., 264
Gage, C., 133
Gagliardino, J. J., 224
Gaillard, P. J., 61
Gala, R. R., 277
Gale, C. C., 247
Ganong, W. F., 61, 75, 86, 91, 217
Ganten, D., 320
Garcia, J., 91, 162, 166, 190, 239
Gard, D. A., 97, 247
Gardner, W. J., 86
Gardner, W. U., 39
Garsky, V., 301
Gasey, R. E., 320
Gaunt, R., 39, 133
Gay, V. L., 288
Geiger, R., 199
Geiling, E. M. K., 22
Geisen, K., 199
Gemelli, A., 22
Genovese, E., 217
George, R., 106
Gepts, W., 172
German, W. I., 75
Gersh, I., 22, 36, 128
Gershon, R., 133
Gerstenfeld, S., 224
Geschwind, I. I., 228, 239
Gibson, J. G., 85
Gilliland, I. C., 86
Gilman, M., 133
Gilon, C., 247, 253
Glick, S. M., 220, 223, 224, 323
Glowinski, J., 253
Goldberg, R. C., 91
Goldman, B. D., 234
Goldstein, A., 301, 316, 319, 320
Goldstein, J., 296

Gomez-Perez, F., 195
Gomori, G., 32, 36
Gonzales-Barcena, D., 109, 200, 297
Goodman, L. S., 39, 56, 75, 128
Goodman, R., 316
Goodner, C. J., 247
Gordon, J., 36
Gordon, R. S., 239
Gorski, R. A., 171, 172
Gott, C., 224
Granger, P., 320
Grant, G., 242, 247, 253, 301
Grant, K. J., 234
Grant, N. H., 301
Gray, W. R., 180, 190
Green, J. D., 25, 52, 109, 128, 156, 166
Greenspan, F. S., 228, 239
Greenwood, F. C., 280
Greep, R. O., 39, 44, 70, 71, 91, 146, 264
Greer, M. A., 67, 70, 75, 86, 109, 277
Gregorova, I., 228
Greulich, W. W., 146
Greving, R., 122
Griffiths, J. Q., 39
Grodin, J. M., 106, 109, 234
Gross, C., 180, 185
Grosvenor, C. E., 277
Grumbach, M. M., 247
Gual, C., 195, 196, 280
Guiliani, G., 162
Guillemin, R., 2, 61, 91, 97, 101, 106, 109, 153, 162, 190, 228, 234, 242, 247, 253, 280, 301, 319, 320, 323
Guyda, H. J., 109, 280, 297

Haar, F. v. d., 190
Haberland, P., 153, 239
Hagenmaier, H., 190
Haigh, C. P., 86
Haigler, E. D., 297
Hair, G. W., 22
Halász, B., 91, 109, 162, 171, 204
Halmi, N. S., 61, 75, 85, 217, 227
Halsted, W. S., 39
Hammer, C. T., 292
Hammond, J., 122, 146
Hanström, B., 32
Harada, G., 200
Hare, K., 32
Hare, R. S., 32
Harlan, W. R., 224
Harms, P. G., 301
Harnes, P. G., 296
Harris, G. W., 2, 22, 25, 32, 39, 44, 52, 56, 61, 67, 75, 85, 86, 91, 97, 106, 109, 122, 141, 146, 153, 156, 162, 166, 190, 195, 228
Harrison, F., 86

Author Citation Index

Hartley, B. S., 180
Hartman, F. A., 217
Haselbach, C. H., 228
Haterius, H. O., 22, 86, 122, 146
Haun, C. K., 270
Hawley, W. D., 97, 101
Haworth, C., 185
Haymaker, W., 61
Heape, W., 146, 156
Hearn, W. R., 61, 153
Heath, B. G., 320
Heathcote, J. G., 185
Heatherington, A., 86
Hechst, B., 32
Hedlum, M. T., 200
Hershman, J. M., 208, 283, 296, 297
Hertz, R., 91, 217
Hickey, R. C., 32
Higgins, G. M., 39
Hild, W., 32, 36, 61
Hill, R. L., 190
Hill, R. T., 39
Hillarp, N.-Å., 32, 128, 172, 312
Hilliard, J., 196, 292
Hines, F. M., 234
Hinsey, J. C., 22, 122, 166
Hirs, C. H. W., 180
Hisaw, F. L., 146
Hinton, G. G., 217, 253
Ho, R. S., 297
Hohlweg, W., 172
Hökfelt, T., 253, 288, 292, 305
Hollander, C. S., 223
Hollenberg, C. H., 220
Hollevsovsky, V., 190
Hollinshead, W. H., 22, 52, 86, 114, 128, 156
Holmgren, B., 87, 156, 247
Holsinger, J., 172
Hopkins, T. F., 228, 270
Horino, M., 239
Horiuchi, Y., 296
Hoskins, R. G., 247
Houssay, B., 25, 109
Householder, D. E., 153
Howanitz, P. J., 296
Howard, H., 242
Hsu, K. C., 204
Huggins, R. A., 128
Hughes, J., 301, 316, 319
Hulme, E. C., 301, 323
Hume, D. M., 56, 61, 75, 86, 91
Hutchens, T. T., 52
Hwang, P., 109, 280, 297

Ichikawa, Y., 200
Igarashi, M., 166, 193, 228
Iino, S., 106

Illner, P., 247, 253
Imai, S., 101
Ingle, D. J., 39
Ingram, W. R., 22, 52, 227
Innes, I. R., 288
Irie, M., 106, 109
Ishida, Y., 239
Ishii, J., 106
Iverson, L. L., 253

Jackson, I. M. D., 109
Jacobs, L. S., 109, 292
Jacobsohn, D., 39, 44, 52, 56, 75, 91, 141, 153, 172, 264, 292
Jacobson, C., 122
Jacquet, Y. F., 323
Jaffe, R. B., 200, 208
Javid, R., 224
Jennings, B. M., 320, 323
Jensen, D. K., 280
Jeppson, S., 208
Jirgl, V., 228
Johansson, O., 253
Johnson, D. C., 141
Jolly, W. A., 39
Jones, I. C., 146, 264
Joseph, D., 217
Jubiz, W., 200
Junkmann, K., 172
Jutisz, M., 97, 109, 162, 190, 247

Kahlson, G., 153
Kahn, R. H., 270
Kameko, T., 101
Kamberi, I. A., 288, 292
Kaneko, E., 296
Kaneko, T., 247, 296
Kanematsu, S., 172, 270, 292
Kansal, P. C., 234
Kant, K. J., 106, 253
Kaplan, S. L., 247
Karisson, S., 301
Kastin, A. J., 97, 101, 109, 180, 185, 190, 195, 196, 200, 280, 297
Katayama, K., 208
Katsoyannis, P. G., 36
Katz, S. H., 224, 239
Kawaguchi, K., 208
Kawai, T., 109
Kawakami, M., 133, 141, 146, 162
Kayashima, F., 208
Keeler, R., 217
Keeton, R. W., 122
Kegawa, T., 228
Kehl, R., 133
Kelch, R. P., 200
Kellaway, C. H., 224

Author Citation Index

Keller, A. D., 75
Kendal, J. W., 277
Kennedy, G. C., 217, 253
Kennedy, T. H., 106
Kent, G. C., 133, 146
Keye, W. R., Jr., 200
Kigawa, T., 166, 270
Kimentova, V., 97
King, L. S., 15, 22, 25
Kipnis, D. M., 224, 239
Kirland, R. J. A., 320
Kirshner, N., 224
Klee, W. A., 320
Klein, M., 146
Klein, R. F., 224
Klein, S. P., 75
Kliman, B., 217
Kmentova, V., 228
Knobil, E., 91, 224, 239, 247
Kobayashi, H., 180
Kobayashi, R. M., 109, 253
Kobayashi, T., 166, 228, 270
Koch, Y., 288
Koei, J., 97
Koelle, G. B., 288
Koerker, D. J., 247
Kohler, P. O., 224
König, W., 199
Kontoz, J. A., 253
Kopech, G., 61
Korenman, S. G., 280
Kosterlitz, H. W., 301, 316, 319
Kovács, S., 106, 253
Kozlowski, G. P., 204
Kratzsch, E., 32
Kravatz, A. A., 172
Kreiger, D. T., 296
Krieg, W. J. S., 68
Krivoy, W. A., 320, 323
Krulich, L., 204, 224, 239, 242, 247, 253, 292, 301
Krylow, L., 15
Kulcsar, S., 133
Kullander, S., 208
Kumasaka, T., 200, 204
Kuroshima, A., 162, 239

LaBella, F. S., 280
Labouesse, B., 180, 185
Labrie, F., 253, 323
Langlier, P., 296
Lachtensteiger, W., 312
Lackey, R. W., 239
Lameyer, L. D. F., 86
Landgrebe, F. W., 32
Langermann, H., 312

Laqueur, G. L., 36, 56
Lara, P. P., 109
Laszlo, J., 224
Lawler, H. C., 36
Lawrence, N. L., 234
Lawrence, W. E., 75
Lazarus, L. H., 301
Leach, R. B., 75
Leclerc, R., 296, 323
Lee, K. L., 97, 247
Lee, L. A., 109, 297
Lehmeyer, J. E., 292
Leininger, C. R., 22
Leonardello, J., 204
Leonardi, R., 224
Leppaluoto, J., 323
Levin, S. E., 247
Lewis, M. R., 61
Lewis, P. R., 224
Lewis, U. J., 297
l'Hermite, M., 296
Li, C. H., 228, 239, 301, 319, 320, 323
Liberman, M. J., 133, 146
Libert, O., 228
Libertun, C., 301
Lien, E. L., 301
Light, R. U., 52
Lindesbert, G., 301
Lindqvist, M., 310
Ling, N., 190, 242, 247, 253, 301, 319, 320, 323
Lipner, H. L., 217
Lippmann, W., 224
Lipscomb, H. S., 91, 228, 323
Lipsett, M. B., 224
Lipton, M. A., 109
Lis, M., 323
Lisk, R. D., 172
Lissák, K., 253
Liu, T. Y., 242
Locke, W., 196
Loeb, L., 39, 122
Löfgren, F., 91
Loh, H. H., 323
Lohmar, P., 320
Long, C. N. H., 39, 56, 75
Long, J. M., 91, 320
Lovinger, R., 247
Lowry, O. H., 109, 204, 239, 253
Lowry, P. J., 320
Lu, K. H., 288, 292
Luft, R., 224, 253
Lum, R., 297
Lyons, W. R., 264, 277

McCallum, R. W., 283, 297
McCann, S. M., 56, 61, 75, 91, 153, 162, 166,

330

172, 190, 193, 195, 204, 217, 224, 228,
   234, 239, 242, 247, 253, 270, 277, 292,
   296, 301
McCleery, D. P., 22
McCullagh, E. P., 86
McDermott, W. V., 39, 56, 75
MacGillivray, M. H., 231
Machlin, L. J., 239
McKennee, C. T., 280
McKeown, T., 122
Macklin, C. C., 15
Macklin, M. T., 15
MacLeod, R. M., 292
Maddock, W. O., 75
Madison, L. L., 224
Magoun, H. W., 22, 32, 86
Maickel, R. P., 310
Mains, R., 323
Makepeace, A. W., 146
Malacara, J. M., 199, 247, 253
Mandell, A. J., 247
Mandelstamm, M., 15
Mann, E. B., 75
Maran, J. W., 253
Marine, D., 39
Mariz, I., 247
Markee, J. E., 22, 52, 86, 114, 122, 128, 146,
   156, 162, 172, 264, 292
Marks, N., 320, 323
Marshall, F. H. A., 22, 39, 122
Martin, J., 106, 109, 208, 224, 242, 247, 253,
   301
Martinez, C., 141
Martini, L., 86, 153, 162, 166, 204, 217, 239
Martinovitch, P. N., 61
Martin-Zurro, A., 247
Masala, A., 297
Mashimo, K., 296
Matsubara, H., 180, 190
Matsuda, K., 206, 277
Matsukura, S., 200
Matsuo, H., 180, 185, 190, 196, 199, 204, 242
Matsuzaki, F., 106
May, R. M., 39
Mayer, G., 146, 264
Mead, P., 253
Meites, J., 97, 101, 133, 166, 196, 208, 228,
   239, 264, 270, 277, 288, 292
Melville, E. V., 32
Mercier-Parot, L., 133
Merckel, C., 146
Merimee, T. J., 208, 224
Mesrob, B., 190
Mess, B., 91, 109, 204
Meyer, R. K., 44
Meyer, V., 224, 247

Mical, R. S., 288, 292, 323
Michael, R. P., 133, 146, 270
Michaelson, I. A., 320
Midgley, A. R., Jr., 195, 196, 208, 288
Mikkelsen, W. P., 52
Miller, G. T., 133
Miller, R., 61
Milne, G. W. A., 190
Mindlin, R. L., 153
Minick, S., 323
Minnich, J. I., 320
Mira, L., 153, 166
Mirsky, A., 61
Mishell, D. R., 208
Mittler, J. C., 196
Miyake, A., 208
Mizuno, M., 166, 228, 270, 288
Mochizuki, M., 208
Mohindra, S., 61
Monahan, M., 190, 242
Moon, H. D., 320, 323
Moon, R. C., 277
Moore, C. R., 39
Moore, E. A., 162, 277
Morato, M. J. X., 25
Morgan, B. A., 301, 316
Morgenstern, L. L., 280
Morikawa, H., 208
Morris, H. R., 301, 316
Moss, R. L., 247
Mota, M., 204
Müller, E., 239, 242
Müller, E. E., 97, 224
Munger, B. L., 323
Murray, M. R., 61
Myers, G. B., 75

Naftolin, F., 195, 200
Nagai, Y., 190
Nagasawa, H., 288
Nagata, Y., 208
Nagataki, S., 106
Nair, R. M. G., 180, 185, 190, 196, 199, 204,
   242
Nakagawa, K., 296
Nakamura, N., 247, 296
Nakano, R., 208
Nallar, R., 162, 199, 277
Naocco, C., 247
Narita, K., 180
Nedde, N. R., 162
Nelson, M. M., 228
Nelson, W. O., 146, 264
Nett, T. M., 200
Neuhoff, V., 190
Newlon, M., 172

Author Citation Index

Nicholson, G., 180
Nickerson, M., 128, 288
Nicoll, C. S., 228, 270, 277, 280
Nicoloff, J. T., 296, 297
Nikitovitch-Winer, M., 44, 91, 133, 162, 166, 277
Nilson, H. W., 39
Nilsson, J., 310
Nishi, K., 109
Niswender, G. D., 200, 288
Noble, R. L., 122
Nowakowski, H., 91
Nussey, A., 247, 253

O'Connor, W. J., 32
Odell, W. D., 200, 224
Ojeda, S. R., 301
Okinaka, S., 106
Oldham, F. K., 22
O'Leary, J. L., 22, 52, 128
Oliver, C., 323
O'Malley, B. W., 224
Opheim, K. E., 316, 320
Orden, L. S. van, 224
Orgiazzi, J., 297
Ortmann, R., 32
Otis, C. L., 297
Otsuki, M., 297

Packman, P. M., 301
Page, E., 277
Page, R. B., 323
Palay, S. L., 32
Palka, Y. S., 172
Palkovits, M., 109, 204, 253
Palmer, J., 247
Parker, M. L., 224
Parkes, A. S., 22, 128, 146
Parlow, A. F., 153, 162, 166, 171, 297
Parsons, J. A., 280
Paschkis, K. E., 75
Pasteels, J. L., 270, 277
Pasternak, G. W., 316
Paton, D. M., 320
Peart, W. S., 320
Pecile, A., 153, 162, 166, 239, 242
Pekary, A. E., 172, 208, 297
Pelletier, G., 253, 323
Pencharz, R. I., 146
Penfield, W., 122
Perez Pasten, E., 280
Peter, R. E., 247
Peters, J. P., 75
Peterson, R. E., 217
Pfeiffer, C. A., 141

Phillips, S. L., 239
Pichette, J. W., 264
Pickford, M., 22
Pierce, J. G., 106
Pincus, G., 122, 146
Pines, J. L., 22, 122
Pisano, J. J., 190
Pittman, J. A., 296, 297
Pizzolato, P., 97
Plotnikoff, N. P., 109, 247
Pohley, F., 196
Polishuk, W. Z., 133
Popa, G. T., 22, 25
Popenhoe, E. A., 36
Porte, D., Jr., 224
Porter, J. C., 109, 204, 234, 288, 292, 323
Porter, R. W., 56, 86
Poth, M. M., 320
Poulain, P., 204
Prange, A. J., 109, 247
Prasad, M. R. N., 44
Pugsley, L. I., 228
Pupp, L., 91, 109, 171
Purandare, T. V., 208
Purves, H. D., 86
Putnam, T. J., 15

Querido, A., 86
Quijada, M., 204, 247, 253

Raben, M. S., 220
Rabinowitz, D., 208, 224
Rachmanow, A., 15
Radford, H. M., 172
Raghunath, P., 61
Ragnasson, U., 301
Ramirez, V. D., 162, 166, 172, 195, 247, 270
Randall, R. J., 109, 204, 239, 253
Rannevik, G., 208
Ranson, S. W., 22, 32, 52, 86
Rasmussen, A. T., 22
Ratner, A., 166, 208, 228, 270, 277
Ravello, J. J., 86
Rayford, P. L., 200, 224
Redding, T. W., 97, 101, 162, 180, 185, 190, 195, 196, 200, 234, 247
Redgate, E. S., 44
Reece, R. P., 264, 270, 277
Reeves, J. J., 195
Reichert, L. E., 208
Reichlin, S., 85, 86, 97, 106, 109, 199, 208, 217, 224, 227, 231, 234, 247, 253
Reid, I. A., 320
Reineke, E. P., 87
Reiss, J. M., 86

Reiss, M., 86
Rennels, E. G., 44
Renzi, A. A., 133
Repass, R. L., 234
Reschini, I., 208
Ressler, C., 36
Reyes, F. I., 208
Reynolds, G. A., 97, 101
Reynolds, S. R. M., 133
Richter, C. P., 122
Riggs, L., 224
Rioch, D. McK., 22, 52, 56, 128
Rivier, C., 247, 253, 301, 323
Rivier, J., 190, 242, 247, 253
Roberts, C. W., 36
Roberts, S., 277
Robyn, C., 296
Roovete, A., 224
Rosebrough, N. J., 109, 204, 239, 253
Rosemberg, E., 56
Rosen, S. H., 39
Rosenberg, B., 61, 91
Rosengren, E., 310
Ross, G. T., 200, 208
Rossier, J., 323
Roth, J., 220, 223, 224
Rothballer, A. R., 224
Rothchild, I., 133
Rothchild, J. A., 301
Roush, M. E., 292
Roussy, G., 122
Royce, P. C., 44, 91, 153
Rubin, A. L., 247
Ruch, W., 247
Rybak, M., 97, 228

Saavedra, J. M., 109, 204, 253
Saffran, M., 97, 153
Saifer, A., 224
Saito, S., 109, 153, 166, 247, 296
Saito, T., 97, 239
Sakiz, E., 97, 109, 162, 190, 234, 247
Salaman, P. F., 106, 234
Sammartino, R., 25
Sanchez-Franco, F., 247
Sandberg, D. K., 204
Sanders, A., 44
Sanford, J. P., 224
San Martino, R., 109
Sarantakis, D., 301
Sasaki, R. M., 180, 190
Sato, G., 32
Sato, H., 200, 204, 253
Saul, G. D., 146
Sawano, S., 97, 101, 180, 190, 195, 224

Sawyer, B. D., 292
Sawyer, C. H., 22, 52, 86, 114, 128, 133, 141, 146, 156, 162, 172, 196, 204, 264, 270, 292
Sayers, G., 39, 44, 56, 61, 75, 91, 153
Schalch, D. S., 106, 109, 200, 224, 234, 280, 297
Schally, A. V., 91, 97, 101, 106, 109, 153, 162, 180, 185, 190, 195, 196, 199, 200, 204, 224, 228, 234, 239, 242, 247, 253, 280, 297, 323
Scharrer, B., 32, 36
Scharrer, E., 32, 36
Schiebler, T. H., 32, 36
Schlimme, E., 190
Schneider, H. P. G., 204, 288
Schreiber, V., 97, 109, 228
Schreiner, L. H., 56
Schulemann, W., 15
Schwartz, N. B., 162
Scott, A. P., 320
Scott, P. P., 146
Segal, D., 247, 301, 323
Segal, S. J., 141
Selby, F. W., 297
Selye, H., 122, 323
Seyler, L. E., Jr., 199
Sheehan, H. C., 75
Shepp, C. R., 301
Sheps, M. C., 162, 277
Sheth, A. R., 208
Shiba, T., 101
Shibusawa, K., 109
Shimizu, N., 247
Shina, D., 97
Shinizu, N., 296
Shirota, K., 109
Shizume, K., 106
Shore, P. A., 153
Shrago, E., 217
Shute, C. C. D., 224
Siler, T. M., 247, 280
Simpson, M. E., 228, 239, 264
Sinha, Y. N., 297
Skelton, F. R., 232
Sklow, J., 146
Slater, G. G., 277
Slusher, M. A., 277
Smalstig, E. B., 292
Smelik, P. G., 292
Smith, A. J. K., 234
Smith, G., 239
Smith, K. R., 234
Smith, M. G., 122
Smith, P. E., 75, 91, 122

Author Citation Index

Smith, S. W., 32
Smith, T. W., 301, 316, 319
Smyth, D. G., 301, 319, 323
Smyth, J. D., 321
Snell, C. R., 319, 323
Snyder, J., 106, 109, 234
Snyder, P. J., 109, 280
Snyder, S. H., 316
Solomon, D. H., 297
Soria, J., 208
Soskin, S., 22, 128
Sowers, J. R., 208, 283, 297
Spatz, H., 91
Spellacy, W. N., 208
Spirtos, B. N., 85, 217, 227
Srebnik, H. H., 228
Stachura, M. E., 253
Statt, W. H., 224
Steelman, S. L., 196, 239
Stein, M., 61
Stern, F., 320
Stevens, H. M., 22
Stevenson, J. A. F., 217, 228, 253
Stewart, J. M., 185
Stikeleather, R. A., 109
Story, J., 106
Streaty, R. A., 320
Strudwick, J. L., 86
Stumpf, W. E., 204
Sturdevant, R. A. L., 283, 297
Stux, M., 86
Sullivan, J., 70
Sulman, F. G., 133, 270, 277
Summer, V. K., 75
Sutin, J., 224
Swan, J. M., 36, 39, 56, 75
Sydnor, K. L., 61
Szentágothai, J., 91, 109, 133, 141, 146, 162, 172, 204

Talas, M., 208
Taleisnik, S., 91, 153, 162, 166, 190, 204
Talwalker, P. K., 166, 228, 270, 277, 288
Tanezawa, O., 208
Tashjian, A. H., Jr., 280, 297
Tatsuno, T., 180
Taubenhaus, M., 22, 128
Taymor, M. I., 208
Theobald, G. W., 122
Thieme, G., 312
Thompson, I. E., 208
Thorn, G. W., 217
Thorneycraft, I. H., 208
Tima, L., 171
Timiras, P. S., 86
Tobin, C. E., 264

Tomie, S., 109
Tomizawa, K., 109
Tommie, W., 162
Torp, A., 310, 312
Townsend, B. F., 52, 146, 292
Tello, J. F., 22
Terenius, L., 301
Teschemacher, H., 316, 320
Traum, R. E., 85
Travaglini, P., 208
Trendelenburg, P., 32
Trout, D. L., 224
Truscott, B. L., 22, 128
Tsai, C. C., 200
Tseng, L. F., 321
Tshida, Y., 162
Tsushima, T., 109
Tuchmann-Duplessis, H., 133
Turkington, R. W., 292
Turner, C. W., 264, 270, 277
Turpeinen, K., 264
Tyler, F. H., 200
Tyrrell, J. B., 247
Tyslowitz, R., 70

Udenfriend, S., 153
Uhlarik, S., 91, 109, 171
Uotila, U. U., 75
Utiger, R. D., 109, 234, 253, 280, 296

Vale, W., 2, 101, 106, 190, 242, 247, 253, 280, 301, 320, 323
Valverde-R, C., 247, 253, 280
Vandenberg, G., 200, 247
VanderLaan, J. W., 68
Vanderlaan, W. P., 297
Van Dyke, H. B., 153, 208
Vanhaelst, L., 296
VanMaanen, J. H., 292
Vargo, T. M., 323
Varterkaitus, J. L., 208
Velardo, J. T., 133
Verney, E. B., 122
Vernikos-Dannellis, J., 270
Vertes, M., 106
Vertes, Z., 106
Virasoro, E., 296
Vivian, S. R., 280
Vogt, M., 22, 36, 122
von Euler, C., 86, 87, 156, 247
Von Euler, U. S., 224, 310
Voss, B. J., 22
Vötsch, W., 190

Wahlstrom, A., 301
Wallach, D. P., 87

Walton, A., 146
Wang, K. T., 180, 190
Ward, D. N., 2, 97, 101, 190
Ward, M., 320
Waring, H., 32
Warren, D. W., 297
Watanabe, S., 190
Weaver, T. A., Jr., 128
Webster, B., 280
Wedig, J., 288
Weed, L. H., 122
Wei, E., 323
Weil-Malherbe, H., 224
Weinstein, G. L., 146
Weise, M., 190
Weiss, P., 32
Weissback, H., 153
Welt, L. G., 75
West, C. D., 200
Westerman, E. O., 310
Westman, A., 39, 52, 172, 264
White, A., 52
White, W. F., 180, 185, 190, 195, 196, 200
Whitelaw, J. M., 133
Whittaker, V. P., 320
Wilber, J. F., 234, 280, 296
Wilder, J., 231
Williams, D. E., 297
Williams, P. C., 146
Wilson, I. C., 109, 247
Winnik, H. Z., 133
Winokur, A., 109
Winter, J. S. D., 208
Wise, A. J., 280
Wislocki, G. B., 15, 22, 25, 52, 128

Wissman, H., 199
Wittenstein, G. J., 56, 86
Woeber, K. A., 224
Wolthuis, O. L., 270
Wood, K. R., 180, 190
Woodbury, D. M., 86
Woodbury, R. A., 128
Woods, J. W., 86, 106
Woolf, P. D., 297
Worcester, J., 234
Worobec, R. B., 200, 204
Worthington, W. C., Jr., 199, 217, 234
Wuttke, W., 288
Wyman, L. C., 217

Yalow, R. S., 200, 220, 224
Yamamoto, T., 109
Yamashiro, D., 319
Yamazaki, E., 97, 109, 247
Yanaihara, N., 247, 296
Yankopoulos, N. A., 217
Yardley, J., 247, 253
Yen, S. S. C., 200, 247
Yonkman, F. F., 128
Yoshida, H., 247, 296
Young, J. D., 185
Young, M. W., 22

Zar, M. A., 320
Zarato, A., 208
Zellforsch, Z., 292
Zelter, G., 32, 36
Zimmerman, F. A., 204
Zonder, B., 146
Zuckerman, S., 36

SUBJECT INDEX

Acetylcholine
  adrenocorticotropic hormone secretion and, 47
  prolactin secretion and, 257
  releasing factors and, 47
  and tuberoinfundibular neurones, 257
Acromegaly
  growth hormone responses to hyperglycemia in, 218, 219
  LH-RH testing in, 205, 207–208
ACTH. See Adrenocorticotropic hormone
Adenohypophysis
  anatomical diagram, 8
  blood supply, 7–8
  parts of, 6–8, 17
Adrenergic pathways
  α-adrenergic blocking drugs, 113, 123–128, 142–144, 211, 300
  β-adrenergic blocking drugs, 113, 211
  influence on gonadotropin secretion, 113
  influence on growth hormone secretion, 212
  influence on ovulation, 113, 123–128
  influence on prolactin secretion, 257, 292
Adrenocorticotropic hormone (ACTH)
  adrenal ascorbic acid depletion as an indicator of release of, 46, 54
  β-endorphin and, 321
  corticotropin secretion (CRF), 47
  electrical stimulation and, 45, 50–52
  feedback regulation of, 322
  hypothalamus and, 47
  lymphopenic response and, 46–52
  neurotransmitter regulation of, 315
  pituitary-adrenal regulation of, 322
  stress and, 46–52, 322
  tissue culture studies of secretion, 57–60
Amenorrhea galactorrhea syndrome
  associated with adenomas, 193
  drug-induced, 129–132, 257
  LH-RH stimulating test in, 193
  prolactin in, 129–132, 257
Androgens
  effects on gonadotropin secretion, 134–140
  mechanism of action on the brain, 134–135
Angiotensin
  brain, 319
  -like immunoreactivity in CNS, 319
Antidiuretic hormone
  gonadotropin secretion and, 147
  paraventricular nucleus and, 26–35
  secretion of
    factors affecting, 31–35
    pars nervosa and, 32
    supraoptic nucleus and, 26–35
  supraoptic nucleus and, 26–35
Apomorphine, prolactin release and, 289, 292
Arcuate nucleus
  gonadotropin secretion and, 114, 134
  growth hormone secretion and, 210–214
  LH-RH synthesis in, 192
  thyrotropin secretion and, 91
Arginine vasopressin. See Antidiuretic hormone
Atropine, pseudopregnancy and, 142–144

Catecholamines. See Dopamine; Epinephrine; Norepinephrine
Chlorpromazine
  gonadotropin secretion and, 129–132
  prolactin secretion and, 129–132, 291
  pseudopregnancy and, 129–132
Corticotropin releasing factor (CRF)
  assay of, 57–60
  β-endorphin release by, 315
  hypothalamic nuclei and, 46, 50–52
  release of corticotropin and, 47
  stalls median eminence and, 46–52
  stress and, 46–48

Deoxyglucose, and GH secretion, 220–222

Subject Index

Dexamethasone
  effect on gonadotropin secretion, 206
  growth hormone secretion and, 293
  prolactin secretion and, 281–283, 293–295
Diabetes insipidis, supraopticohypophysial tract and, 31
Dibenamine, and gonadotropin secretion, 113, 123–128, 142–144
Dopamine
  hypothalamic distribution, 304–310
  prolactin secretion and, 257, 281–284, 289–292

Endorphins
  assay for, 314, 322
  β-endorphin, 313, 321, 323
  behavioral effects, 315
  breakdown of, 315
  conversion into enkephalin, 315
  corticotropin releasing factor and, 321
  ectopic production, 322
  growth hormone release by, 283, 298–300
  as pituitary opiate peptides, 298–300, 321
  pituitary secretion, 323
  prolactin release by, 281, 298–300
  tuberoinfundibular dopamine systems and, 312
Enkephalins
  analgesic effects of, 315
  bioassay for, 314–318
  behavior effects of, 315
  biotransformation of, 315
  brain opiate peptides, 314–319
  β-endorphin, conversion into, 315
  growth hormone release and, 298–300
  interaction of, with opiate receptor, 314
  prolactin release by, 298–300
  tuberoinfundibular dopamine pathways and, 311–314
Epinephrine, 306
  gonadotropin secretion and, 147
  prolactin secretion and, 275
Estradiol
  effect on gonadotropin secretion, 142–145, 205–209
  effect on prolactin secretion, 257, 265–269

Follicle stimulating hormone (FSH), secretion of, 134, 163–165
  feedback regulation of, 164
  neural pathways of control of, 134, 163–165

Glucocorticoids, modulatory role of
  adrenocorticotropin secretion and, 322
  β-endorphin secretion and, 322
  gonadotropin secretion and, 206
  growth hormone secretion and, 293–295
  prolactin secretion and, 281, 282, 293–295
  thyrotropin secretion and, 65, 282, 293–295
Glucose, effects on growth hormone secretion, 210–221
Gonadotropins, secretion of, 114–156
  androgens and, 132–138
  biogenic amines and, 113, 123–128, 142–144
  cyclic secretion, 114, 134, 159, 171
  estrogen effects on, 145
  neural pathways of control of, 114
  sites of estradiol feedback in, 114, 167, 206
  tonic secretion, 114, 134, 138, 171
Growth hormone (GH)
  acromegaly and, 219, 220
  secretion of
    adrenergic control of, 211, 221
    β-endorphin and, 298–300
    enkephalins and, 298–300
    exercise and, 211–221
    noradrenergic control of, 210–211, 221–223
    radioimmunoassay of, 210, 230, 298–300
    somatostatin and, 235, 248
    stress and, 211, 221, 248
    tibial epiphysial cartilage with assay for, 225–227, 237
    TRH-induced release of, 687
Growth hormone release inhibiting hormone (GHR-IH). See Somatostatin

Haloperidol, prolactin release and, 289, 291–292
Histamine
  gonadotropin secretion and, 147, 150
  prolactin release by, 300
  tuberoinfundibular neuron and, 304
5-Hydroxytryptamine (5-HT, serotonin)
  ACTH secretion and, 47
  gonadotropin secretion and, 147
  hypothalamic neurons, effects on, 304–312
  luteinizing hormone-releasing hormone, 151, 152
  prolactin release and, 300
Hypoglycemia, release of growth hormone during, 211–223
Hypophysial portal circulation, 4–24, 154–156, 323
  retrograde flow and, 323

Subject Index

Hypothalamo-hypophysial tract
  oxytocin release and, 26–35
  vasopressin release and, 26–35
Hypothalamus
  adrenocorticotropic hormone secretion and, 47
  afferent connections of, 147
  catecholamines and, 304–310
  control of anterior pituitary secretion, 35–44, 112
  electrical stimulation of, and thyrotropin release, 76–82, 232–234
  factors of
    CRF, 305
    GH-RF, 211–223, 225–227, 235
    PIF, 257–289
    PRF, 257
  gonadotropin secretion and, 111–199
  growth hormone secretion and, 113, 209–234
  hormones
    distribution of, 305
    LH-RH, 150–199, 305
    somatostatin, 235–236, 248–253
    TRH, 305
  hypophysiotropic area, 65, 88, 167
    arcuate nucleus and, 90, 167, 305
    thyrotropin secretion and, 88–91, 103
    TRH localization in, 103, 107–109
  infundibular stalk, growth hormone secretion and, 232–234
  median eminence of, 36–44
  neurosecretion of, 26–35, 304–310
  nuclei of, and TRH concentration, 107–109, 305
  peptides of, 300–310
  prolactin secretion and, 113
  thyrotropin secretion and, 63–109, 113
  tuberoinfundibular system of, 304–312
  vital dye staining of, 10–13

Lactogenic hormone. *See* Prolactin
Lesions, hypothalamic
  adrenocorticotropic hormone secretion and, 74, 75
  gonadotropin secretion and, 74, 75
  growth hormone secretion and, 74, 75
  thyrotropin secretion and, 64–75
Leucine enkephalin, 298–300, 315
LH. *See* Luteinizing hormone
LH-RH. *See* Luteinizing hormone-releasing hormone
β-Lipotropin (β-LPH), 315–317
  ACTH secretion and, 315
  growth hormone secretion and, 283, 298–300

  morphinomimetic activity, 298–300, 317
  MSH secretion and, 319
  as prohormone, 315, 317
  prolactin secretion and, 282–283, 298–300
Luteinizing hormone, secretion of, 134
  biogenic amines and, 113
  feedback control, 134–162, 191, 206
  glucocorticoid effects on, 282–283
  neural pathways of control of, 134
  radioimmunoassay for, 205–206
Luteinizing hormone-releasing hormone
  antidiuretic hormone and, 153, 154
  bioassay of, 148
  chemical identification of, 173–190
  distribution of, 147–171, 319
  gonadotropin secretion and, 113, 147–171
  hypothalamic nuclei and, 148–155, 167–171, 192
  isolation of, 173
  norepinephrine and, 113
  prolactin secretion and, 193
  radioimmunoassay of, 192, 205
  synthesis of, 173–190
  tuberoinfundibular system and, 192

Medial basal hypothalamus, 305
  gonadotropin hormone secretion, 147–149
  neural afferents to, 147–149, 167–171
Median eminence (SME), 17, 36–44
  adrenocorticotropic hormone secretion and, 82–85
  dopaminergic neurons in, 309
  follicle stimulating hormone secretion and, 165
  lesions of, and anterior pituitary hormone secretion, 64–85
  LH-RH in, 147–165
  noradrenergic neurons in, 309
  somatostatinergic neurons in, 249–252
  thyrotropin secretion and, 73–85
  TRH in, 102
Melanocyte stimulating hormone (MSH)
  characterization of, 319
  secretion
    control of, 322
    neurotransmitters and, 319
    relation to ACTH secretion, 319, 322
Methionine-enkephalin, 298–300, 315. *See also* Enkephalin
  tuberoinfundibular dopamine systems and, 312
Metoclopramide, prolactin secretion and, 281, 293–296
MIF. *See* Melanocyte stimulating hormone
Morphine
  ACTH and, 317–322

339

Subject Index

growth hormone and, 282–283
prolactin secretion and, 282–283, 300
MSH. *See* Melanocyte stimulating hormone

Naloxone
opiate receptors and, 298–300, 318
prolactin secretion and, 282, 300
Neurohypophysis, 16–21
hormones of, 21–32
nerve tracts from hypothalamus, 16–35
neurosecretory material from hypothalamus, 26–35
Neurons
adrenergic, 113, 306
catecholaminergic, 303, 304
dopaminergic, 304
neurosecretory, 26–35
peptidergic, 26, 113, 253
tuberoinfundibular, 304, 311, 312
Neuropeptides. *See also* Peptides; *specific peptides*
β-endorphin, 314–322
enkephalins, 315–318
LH-RH, 319
lipotropins, 314–318
opioid peptides, 314–322
somatostatin, 248–253
TRH, 319
Neurosecretory granules, 26–35
Norepinephrine, pathways containing, 304–310
ACTH secretion, 47
growth hormone secretion, 221
LH-RH secretion, 113
TRH secretion, 113

Opiate receptor, enkephalin interactions with, 313–318
Opiate-receptor peptides, endogenous, 313
analgesia, 315, 322
assay for, 318
endorphins, 314
enkephalins, 314–318
Ovulation
estrogen effects on, 138, 142–144
gonadotropin secretion and, 112, 115–128, 138
inhibition, 113, 129
progesterone, effects on, 136
Oxytocin
cells producing, 21–34
distribution, 21–35
in hypothalamus, 21–35
release of, 32

transport of, 26–35

Paraventricular nucleus (PVN), 26–35
Pars distalis, nomenclature, 17
Peptides. *See also* Hypothalamus; Neuropeptides
CNS, biotransformation of. *See* Neuropeptides
morphinomimetic, 298–300, 317
as neurotransmitters, 304
oligopeptides, 317
tuberoinfundibular system and, 312
Perphenazine, and prolactin release, 289, 290–292
Phenobarbital, hormone release, 142–144
Phenothiazines
gonadotropin secretion and, 129
prolactin secretion and, 257, 290–292
Phentolamine
growth hormone secretion and, 211, 221
prolactin secretion and, 289
PIF. *See* Prolactin-inhibitory factor
Pimozide, prolactin secretion and, 291
Pituitary
anterior
action of PIF on, 257–292
blood supply to, 4–24
hormomes of, 40–44
hypothalamic control of secretions of, 4–24, 36–46
parts of, 6–8, 17
secretory cell types of, 71
chromophobe adenomas of, 192–193, 205
control of secretion
ACTH secretion, 36–44, 46–60
gonadotropin secretion, 36–44, 112–171
growth hormone secretion, 36–44, 210–253
intermediate lobe, 17
opiate peptides of, 315, 322
prolactin secretion, 256–296
thyrotropin secretion, 36–44, 63–109
Pregnancy, LH-RH stimulation tests in, 205–208
Preoptic area-anterior hypothalamic area (POA-AHA)
gonadotropin release and, 112, 114, 134, 138, 148
nerve tracts of, 30
TRH localization, 102–109
Prolactin (PRL)
amphetamines and, 284–288
catecholamines and, 289–292
dopamine and, 257, 281–282, 284, 289–292
β-endorphin secretion and, 281, 288–300

Subject Index

enkephalins, 298–300
ergot alkaloids and, 289, 292
5-HT and, 300
lactogenic hormone, 130–132
luteotropic hormone, 130–132, 256–264
methylodopa and, 284–286
monoamine oxidose inhibitors, 281, 284, 285
norepinephrine and, 292
opiate peptides and, 281, 298–300
phenothiazines and, 129–132, 257, 281–282
radioimmunoassay of, 278–280, 286
reserpine and, 129–132, 257
secretion of
  abnormalities of, 193
  enhanced after stalk section, 131, 256
  estradiol effects on, 256–269
  hypothalamic control of, 256–296
  lactation and, 257, 269
  pregnancy and, 193
  pseudopregnancy and, 130–132
  stress and, 257
  suckling stimulus and, 256, 257
  TRH stimulation, 278–280
Prolactin-inhibitory factor (PIF)
  characterization of. 288–289
  estradiol effects, 256–269
  hypothalamic location, 257–269
  regulation of prolactin secretion, 257
  stress and, 271–275
  suckling effects, 256–275
Prolactin releasing factor (PRF)
  evidence for, 257
  regulation of prolactin secretion, 257
Prolactin secretory reserve, tests of, 278–280, 293–296
Propranolol
  growth hormone secretion and, 211, 221
  prolactin secretion and, 289
Propylthiouracil, effect on thyrotropin secretion, 64–67, 70, 72
Pseudopregnancy
  corpus lutea and, 129–132, 259–269
  dopamine antagonists and, 129, 142–144
  prolactin in, 130–132, 257–269
PVN. See Paraventricular nucleus

Radioimmunoassays
  adrenocorticotropic hormone, 322
  β-endorphin, 322
  follicle stimulating hormone, 205–206
  growth hormone, 300
  luteinizing hormone, 205–206
  luteinizing hormone-releasing hormone, 192, 198–199

prolactin, 278–280, 300
thyrotropin, 104
TRH, 107–109
Reserpine
  gonadotropin secretion and, 113, 129, 142–144
  growth hormone secretion and, 113
  ovulation and, 113
  prolactin secretion and, 113, 129
  pseudopregnancy and, 129

Serotonin. See 5-Hydroxytryptamine
SME. See Median eminence
Somatostatin
  acromegaly and, 246
  actions of, 235–248
  biochemical characterization of, 240–242
  cyclic form, 235
  distribution of, 235, 236, 248–253
  effects of
    on growth hormone secretion, 235
    on prolactin secretion, 243–246
    on thyrotropin secretion, 235, 236, 243–246
  hypothalamic nuclei and, 249–252
  isolation of, 236–240
  neurotransmitter role, evidence for, 236, 253
  radioimmunoassay, 249–250
Stalk section, effects on
  ACTH secretion, 54, 55
  gonadotropin secretion, 54, 55
  growth hormone secretion, 54, 55
  prolactin secretion, 131, 256
Sterotaxic instrument, 67, 102, 229
Stress
  adrenocorticotropin secretion and, 46, 315, 322
  β-endorphin secretion and, 315, 322
  growth hormone secretion and, 211, 221, 322
  melanocyte stimulating hormone, 322
  prolactin secretion and, 256, 293, 322
Substance P, 300
  effects on LH-RH, 147
Suckling, prolactin release and, 256, 257
Suprachiasmatic hypothalamic nucleus
  gonadotropin secretion and, 112, 138
  lesions of, and thyrotropin secretion, 69–71, 79–83
Supraoptic nucleus (SON)
  diabetes insipidus and, 31
  neurosecretory neurons, 28–32
  oxytocinergic neurons in, 32
  vasopressinergic neurons in, 32
Supraoptico-hypophysial system

Subject Index

growth hormone secretion and, 215–216
thyrotropin secretion and, 65, 79–85

Thiouracil, effect on thyrotropin secretion, 70–71
Thyroid-stimulating hormone. See Thyrotropin
Thyrotropin (TSH), secretion of, 64–109
  glucocorticoids and, 65, 293–295
  hypothalamic control of, 76–85
  pituitary-thyroid feedback and, 96–100
  radioimmunoassay of, 104
  tests of, 92–97
Thyrotropin-releasing hormone (TRH)
  antisera, 102
  biochemical characterization, 92–94, 98–100
  distribution of, 102–103, 107–109, 253
  identification, 98–100
  isolation, 92
  prolactin secretion and, 256, 278–281
  radioimmunoassay, 107–109

regulation of effects
  by glucocorticoids, 293–295
  somatostatin, 235–248
  thyroid hormones, 95–105
  secretion, and neurotransmitters, 300
Thyroxine, 98–100
Triiodothyronine, 96–100
Tuberoinfundibular dopaminergic (TIDA) system, 290
  definition of, 304, 311–312
  5-HT and, 311
  medial preoptic-anterior hypothalamic area, 311–312
  monoamines and, 311–312
  prolactin secretion and, 290

Ventromedial hypothalamic nucleus (VHN), 305
  growth hormone secretion and, 210–234
  thyrotropin secretion and, 69, 102
Vital dyes, use in studing anatomy of hypothalamus-pituitary system, 10–13, 26

About the Editor

JAMES RUSSELL SOWERS, M.D., is an associate professor of medicine at the University of Missouri, Kansas City. He obtained his medical degree from the University of Missouri in Columbia. He took a residency in internal medicine and then completed a fellowship in endocrinology at Wadsworth Veterans Administration Medical Center/UCLA. Dr. Sowers is a fellow of the American College of Physicians and the Endocrine Society and he has his boards in internal medicine and in endocrinology. He has published approximately 40 papers dealing with the general field of neuroendocrinology since completing his fellowship. His research interests include the field of controlled prolactin secretion and neuroendocrine releasing hormones, as well as the role of central control mechanisms in the etiology of essential hypertension.